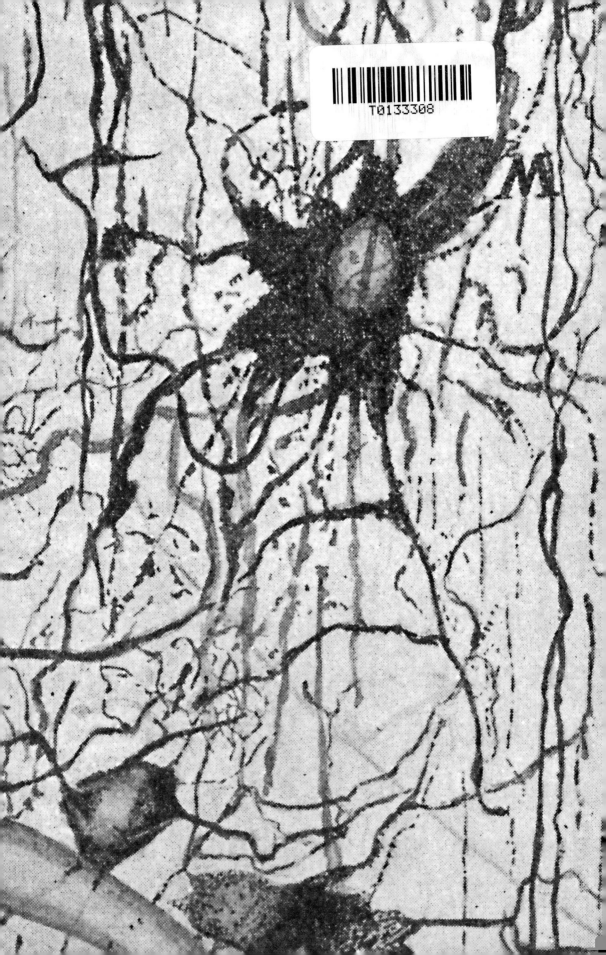

Radical Treatment

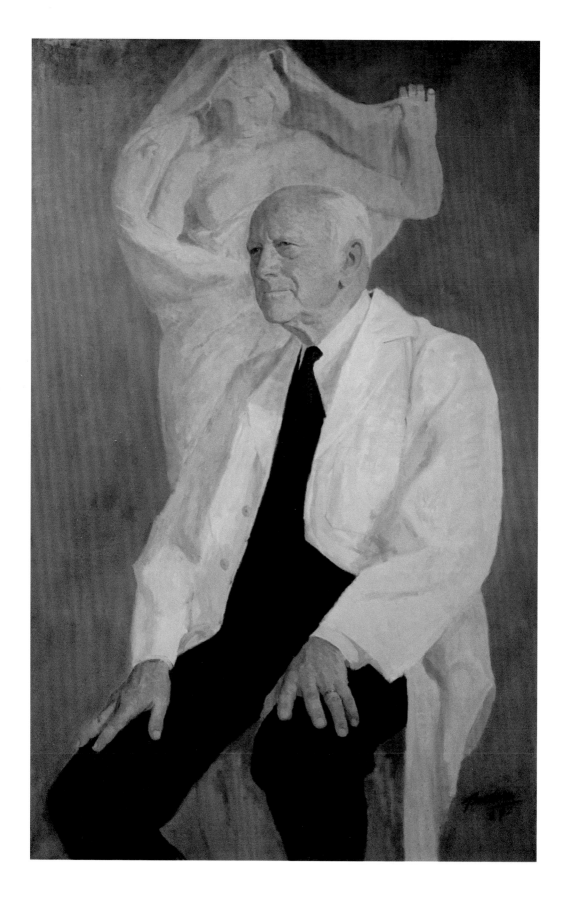

Radical Treatment

Wilder Penfield's Life in Neuroscience

RICHARD LEBLANC

McGill-Queen's University Press

Montreal & Kingston • London • Chicago

ISBN 978-0-7735-5928-8 (cloth)
ISBN 978-0-2280-0019-8 (ePDF)
ISBN 978-0-2280-0020-4 (ePUB)

Legal deposit first quarter 2020
Bibliothèque nationale du Québec

Printed in Canada on acid-free paper

This book has been published with the help of a grant from the Montreal Neurological Institute.

  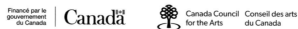

We acknowledge the support of the Canada Council for the Arts.

Nous remercions le Conseil des arts du Canada de son soutien.

Library and Archives Canada Cataloguing in Publication

Title: Radical treatment : Wilder Penfield's life in neuroscience / Richard Leblanc.
Other titles: Wilder Penfield's life in neuroscience
Names: Leblanc, Richard (Neurosurgeon), author.
Description: Includes bibliographical references and index.
Identifiers: Canadiana (print) 20190191015 | Canadiana (ebook) 20190191058 | ISBN 9780773559288 (cloth) | ISBN 9780228000198 (ePDF) | ISBN 9780228000204 (ePUB)
Subjects: LCSH: Penfield, Wilder, 1891–1976. | LCSH: Neuroscientists—Canada—Biography. | LCSH: Neurosurgeons—Canada—Biography. | LCSH: Neurosciences. | LCSH: Nervous system—Surgery. | LCSH: Neuro-sciences—Philosophy. | LCGFT: Biographies.
Classification: LCC R464.P46 L43 2019 | DDC 610.92—dc23

Frontispiece: Portrait of Wilder Penfield in front of *Nature Unveiling Herself before Science*. Lynn Buckham. Montreal Neurological Institute and McGill University.

Drawing is the honesty of art – Dalí

Contents

Acknowledgments

I am very grateful to all who have supported the Thomas Willis and the Neuro History Funds of the Montreal Neurological Institute. This book would not have been published without their generosity. I also owe a great debt of gratitude to Helmut Bernhard who photographed the brain maps that illustrate this book and to Ann Watson for so many things. This book is dedicated to Kathleen and Katherine, who will always be in the front row with me.

Radical Treatment

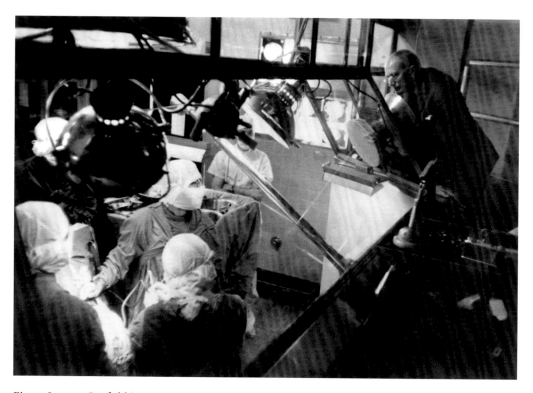

Figure Intro.1. Penfield is seen giving advice to William Feindel from the gallery of the Montreal Neurological Institute's Theatre One. Feindel later became the third director of the Montreal Neurological Institute, succeeding Theodore Rasmussen. Montreal Neurological Institute and McGill University.

Introduction

This book addresses Penfield's thinking as it evolved from his description of brain scars at the beginning of his career, to his last thoughts on the human condition. It is based on a review of Penfield's clinical charts, my reading of his writings over the course of my career as a neurosurgeon and physician-scientist at the Montreal Neurological Institute (MNI), and my encounters with his pupils, who were also my teachers in the care of epileptic patients.

Penfield's clinical charts are the foundations that support his scientific edifice. Each chart contains a patient's history, physical examination, and radiological findings. The charts of patients admitted to the MNI after 1938 also contain Herbert Jasper's EEG reports and the minutes of the Clinical EEG Conference, where every patient's case was discussed before a decision was made to operate. The heart of each patient's chart is Penfield's detailed operative report and the meticulously detailed recording of the effects of electrocortical stimulation. Penfield or his assistant initially wrote these down on the side or on the back of each patient's brain map, and, after the MNI opened its doors, they were dictated to a secretary in the gallery of the operating room. Each map illustrates Penfield's operative findings and the cortical and subcortical pathology that he encountered at craniotomy. They localize the points where electrical stimulation of the cortex produced somatosensory, visual, verbal, or motor responses. The brain maps also illustrate the sites from which epileptic activity was recorded and from which epileptic seizures were generated by cortical stimulation. Intraoperative photographs were also taken to complement the sketches, but the sketches were Penfield's principal tools. The photographs are accurate but they have limitations. The exposed brain is a half-sphere and the early cameras had limited depth of field. The brain pulsates when it is exposed, and the early photographs are sometimes blurred. The camera captures every detail without discernment, but it can't capture what is not exposed to the lens – the medial aspect of the frontal lobe where the supplementary motor area resides, the undersurface of the temporal lobe, the hippocampus at the depth of the surgical exposure, the insula in shadow, the subcortical infiltration of a brain tumour. All of these were recorded in the sketches.

Sketches eliminate the superfluous. They are selective in what they highlight – a constricted artery, a reddish draining vein, the feel of a sclerosed hippocampus. Photographs don't speak to us the way that sketches do: the sketches were annotated as insight arose from observation, and the notes found their way into Penfield's lectures and texts.

Readers will be surprised at Penfield's informal training in neurosurgery. Although he met Harvey Cushing early in his career, he was one of the few North American neurosurgeons of his generation who did not train with him. Penfield's formal training in neurosurgery, such as it was, was with Percy Sargent, the senior neurosurgeon at the National Hospital for the Paralyzed and Epileptic at Queen Square, London. Penfield assisted Sargent in the operating room and cared for his postoperative patients on the wards. His first published paper on a neurosurgical topic was a review of Sargent's cases of osseous brain tumours. But Sargent taught Penfield more than how to turn a bone flap or remove a brain tumour. Penfield would also have observed Sargent resect cortical scars from epileptic patients, and from Sargent he would have learned of the vascular hypothesis of epileptogenesis, to which he devoted the first decade of his career. This is an aspect of Sargent's influence on Penfield that has not previously been addressed. It was however Otfrid Foerster, a German neurosurgeon of international repute, who had the most profound influence on Penfield, as he adopted Foerster's method of investigating and treating posttraumatic epilepsy. Penfield's career took flight after his stay with Foerster.

Penfield's first academic interest in Montreal was the investigation of the vascular hypothesis of epileptogenesis. This held that posttraumatic seizures arise as a result of transient ischemia of the cortex surrounding a cortical scar. Penfield was the first to describe the components of cortical scars, their gradual contraction, and the resultant pull on cortical arteries that he thought triggered reflex vasoconstriction and posttraumatic seizures. This led Penfield to discover intracranial vasoactive nerves, which supported the vascular hypothesis, and to study cortical blood flow, which disproved it.

Penfield's reputation rests largely on his contributions to the structure–function relationship of the brain as idealized by the sensory-motor homunculus and on the treatment of temporal lobe epilepsy. The homunculus is the result of cortical stimulations performed during operations for the treatment of extratemporal epilepsy and of brain tumours within the frontal and parietal lobes. Penfield performed these operations early in his career in Montreal. It was only two decades after his arrival in Montreal, with his discovery of mesial temporal sclerosis, that temporal epilepsy became the focus of his attention.

Most of Penfield's discoveries were based on intraoperative observations – he famously remarked that the operating room was his laboratory. Although the functions of the pre- and postcentral convolutions were known before Penfield took up the stimulating electrode, he discovered the role of the motor strip in vocalization, the language function of the supplementary motor area, and the second sensory area in man.

Penfield's greatest contribution to clinical neurology was undoubtedly his discovery of what is now referred to as mesial temporal sclerosis, which led him to devise the most successful operation for the treatment of medically refractory epilepsy. It also led to the discovery, with Brenda Milner and Herbert Jasper, of the role of the hippocampi in immediate recall, which established the duality of memory before Milner encountered patient H.M.

Penfield's thoughts on memory, and on its interaction with what he described as the centrencephalic integrating system, heretofore a neglected topic, are discussed in these pages. Penfield's idea was that memory sensation, motility, cognition, and emotions are integrated into a whole, to which he referred as an experiential phenomenon, whose function was greater than the sum of its parts. Penfield referred to the integration of experiential phenomena through mutual interconnections between the cortex and the diencephalon as the "physiology of mind." Penfield was prescient in his largely forgotten concept of the centrencephalic integrating system, as modern neurobiology has turned from the structure–function relationship of the brain to the study of neural circuits and how they interact to create the human experience. Penfield's concept of the centrencephalic system and of its role in the stream of consciousness is discussed in the following pages for the first time.

Similarly, Ivan Pavlov's influence on Penfield has not previously been discussed, but Penfield was fully conversant with Pavlov's work, onto the details of specific experiments that Pavlov and his students had performed. And, as I show, it is Pavlov and the conditioned reflex to which Penfield turned to formulate his concept of the biological mechanism by which chronic epileptic seizures arise.

A note on "radical treatment" is warranted. The word *radical* was used in the early part of the twentieth century to distinguish surgical intervention from the "conservative," nonsurgical, treatment of illness and disease. Thus, "radical" appears in the title of Penfield's first papers on the surgical treatment of epilepsy, and he refers to it in many of his publications.[1] Penfield used the term "radical" to mean the "complete" resection of a localized cortical scar. He defined his use of the term in these words: "Radical operation depends, for its rationale, upon the conception … that every epileptic seizure begins with ganglionic discharge in some area of grey matter. The aim of surgical excision is to remove the focal area in which epileptogenic discharges originate and thus put an end to the seizures."[2] In the context of the time, Penfield's low surgical complication rate is a testament to his meticulous surgical technique and to superlative postoperative nursing care.

Penfield's contributions to neurobiology and to epileptology came at a time when descriptive neurology was ebbing and being surpassed by experimentation. Thus, his work can be considered as marking the end of nineteenth-century neurology. The new paradigm would be pursued within the walls of his creation, the Montreal Neurological Institute.

A Note on Anatomy

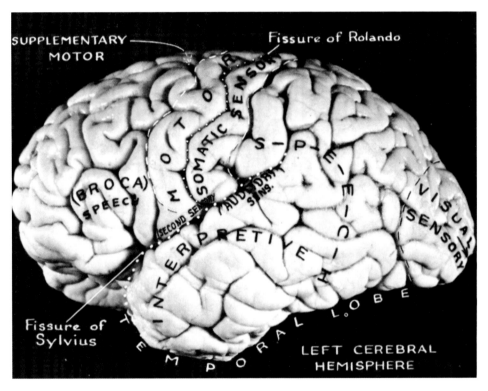

Figure Ana.1. The left hemisphere of the human brain labelled by Penfield. The pre- and post-central gyri, which are respectively labelled "motor" and "somatic sensory," are on either side of the fissure of Rolando. The supplementary motor area is on the medial aspect of the superior, or first, frontal convolution, immediately in front of the foot area of the motor strip. It is not visible as the brain is viewed from its lateral aspect, but its medial location is indicated by the curve at the end of the arrow. Broca's area is indicated in the posterior aspect of the third frontal convolution. Wernicke's area is indicated by the label "speech." This includes the posterior aspects of the first and second temporal convolutions and the inferior parietal lobule. The "interpretive" area occupies the first temporal convolution, exclusive of Wernicke's area. A more extensive interpretive area is present in the right temporal lobe. Montreal Neurological Institute and McGill University.

THE COVERINGS OF THE BRAIN

A thick but flexible membrane called the dura mater covers the brain. Its consistency is not unlike kid leather. The dura separates the epidural space from the subdural space. The epidural space is between the dura and the inner aspect of the skull and the subdural space is between the dura and the arachnoid membrane. The thin, transparent, gossamer-like arachnoid membrane is so named because it reminded early anatomists of a spider's web. The arachnoid membrane overlies a third membrane, the pia mater, which envelops the undulating convolutions of the brain. This space between the arachnoidal and pial membranes is referred to as the subarachnoid space, which contains the cerebrospinal fluid, or CSF. The arachnoid and pia constitute the meninges. Infection of the meninges is referred to as meningitis. The inflammatory process can also irritate the cortex and cause epileptic seizures. Blood can accumulate in any of the spaces delineated by these membranes but only the slow accumulation of blood in the subdural space, which causes pressure to be applied to the underlying cortex, is associated with epilepsy.

FISSURES AND CONVOLUTIONS

The external anatomy of the brain is defined by the great fissures that separate each hemisphere into lobes and by the secondary fissures that separate the lobes into convolutions. The Rolandic, or central, fissure separates the frontal and parietal lobes from one another, and the Sylvian fissure separates the frontal and parietal lobes above from the temporal lobe below. The insular lobe, also referred to as the island of Reil, or the insula, lies deep within the Sylvian fissure. The inferior borders of the frontal and parietal lobes and the superior border of the temporal lobe cover the insula, which is not visible unless the Sylvian fissure is opened widely. The superior and inferior borders of the Sylvian fissure are referred to as the opercula. Thus, there is a frontal, a parietal, and a temporal operculum. The second sensory area is located within the frontal and parietal opercula. The occipital lobe is the fifth lobe of the brain. It is poorly delineated on the lateral surface of the cerebral hemisphere, but it is clearly separated from the medial aspect of the parietal lobe by the parieto-occipital fissure.

Each frontal lobe is divided into four convolutions or gyri. The first three convolutions run parallel to each other as they course horizontally from the frontal pole to the fourth frontal convolution, which stretches vertically upward across the hemisphere along the Rolandic fissure. The three horizontal convolutions are referred to as the superior (first), the middle (second), and the inferior (third) frontal convolutions. The fourth frontal convolution is referred to as the precentral gyrus or as the motor strip. It constitutes the anterior bank of the Rolandic fissure. The supplementary motor area is found in the medial aspect of the superior frontal gyrus, immediately in front of the motor region of the foot. Broca's area resides within the posterior aspect of the third frontal convolution. It is separated from the precentral gyrus by a small, unnamed convolution. It is composed of the *pars opercularis*, which is nearest to the precentral gyrus, and the larger *pars triangularis*, which is immediately in front of the *pars opercularis*. The orbito-frontal region of the frontal lobe lies above the roof of the orbit.

The parietal lobe includes the postcentral gyrus, which constitutes the posterior bank of the Rolandic fissure. The postcentral gyrus runs parallel to the motor strip and it is the site where sensations originating from sensory receptors of the skin, muscles, and tendons terminate. The bulk of the parietal lobe lies behind the postcentral gyrus. It extends inferiorly to the Sylvian fissure and posteriorly to its junction with the occipital lobe. The parietal lobe is divided into the superior and inferior parietal lobules by the intraparietal sulcus. The inferior parietal lobule is composed of the supramarginal and angular gyri, which are part of Wernicke's area.

The occipital lobe occupies the posterior aspect of the hemisphere. The primary visual area, the area that receives light perception and the images projected upon the retina, is referred to as the calcarine cortex. It is situated in the medial aspect of the occipital lobe as horizontal, parallel bands on both sides of the calcarine fissure. Visual associative areas, which extend into the parietal lobe, surround the primary visual area.

The temporal lobe resides within the part of the skull called the middle fossa. It is composed of five convolutions. The superior, or first, temporal convolution is bordered superiorly by the Sylvian fissure, and it extends from the temporal pole to the supramarginal gyrus. The opercular aspect of the first temporal convolution contains the smaller Heschl's gyri, which constitute the primary auditory area. The area behind Heschl's gyri is referred to as the *planum temporale*, which is larger on the left, language-dominant temporal lobe than on the right. The second temporal convolution parallels the first. It extends from the temporal pole to the angular gyrus. The posterior aspects of the first and second temporal convolutions are also part of Wernicke's area. Thus, Wernicke's area is composed of the posterior aspects of the first and second temporal gyri and the supramarginal and angular gyri. The third temporal convolution lies between the second temporal convolution and the fusiform gyrus, which is on the inferior surface of the temporal lobe. The most medial temporal convolution is referred to as the hippocampal or, more commonly, as the parahippocampal gyrus. Its anterior-most aspect ends in a knuckle-like projection referred to as the uncus, which contains the amygdala and the anterior part of the hippocampus called the *pes hippocampi*. The *pes hippocampi* continues posteriorly for six centimetres or so as the hippocampus proper, before it curves upwards to join the other components of the limbic system.

THE CORTICAL MANTLE AND
FUNCTIONAL INTEGRATION

The cortex of the lateral aspect of the temporal lobe, like the cortex of the other lobes of the brain, is referred to as *neocortex*, to reflect its late arrival in the evolutionary development of the brain. The neocortex is composed of six intercalated layers of neurons and white matter fibres. The cortex of the medial temporal lobe – the parahippocampal gyrus and the hippocampus – is composed of only three layers. It is the phylogenetically oldest cortex of the brain, and it is thus referred to as the *archicortex*. These distinctions were important in the shift of focus from the lateral neocortex to the medial archicortex in the surgery of temporal lobe epilepsy.

The neocortex of each convolution communicates with its neighbour through small, U-shaped white matter fibres. Through these short, interconnecting fibres the pre- and postcentral gyri communicate with each other, assuring coordination – or integration – of sensorimotor function. Groups of convolutions with similar function communicate with each other through longer, thicker white matter fibres joined into fascicles. Thus, Wernicke's area is joined to Broca's area through the arcuate fasciculus. These two systems, the U fibres and the fasciculi, assure the integration of *intra*-hemispheric functions. Similarly, *inter*-hemispheric functional integration is assured by interconnecting fibre bundles that join homologous area of both hemispheres to each other through the corpus callosum and the anterior and posterior commissures.

Penfield was fully aware of the existence of these interconnecting pathways, but he felt that they were of lesser importance in the integrative function of the brain. Rather, he ascribed this function to bidirectional connections between the cortex and diencephalon – a way station between the cerebral hemispheres and the lower brain stem and spinal cord. The integration of brain function through the cortex and diencephalon would preoccupy Penfield throughout his career. The integration of higher cognitive functions, such as memory, speech, and perception by the cortical-diencephalic circuit, to which Penfield referred as the *centrencephalic integrating system*, for Penfield, constituted the mind.

EPILEPTIC SEIZURES

Traumatic scars, brain tumours, haemorrhagic cysts, and other pathologies cause epilepsy only when they encroach upon the cerebral cortex. A traumatic cortical scar, or cicatrix, results from the loss of neurons due to the initial injury and from the infiltration of astrocytes and their projections, collagen fibres, and reactive blood vessels into the traumatized cortex. The scar can also contain retained skull fragments if it

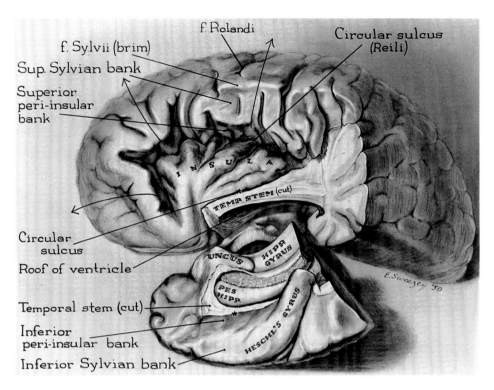

Figure Ana.2. Drawing by Eleanor Sweezey to illustrate the external aspect of the insula and the inner structure of the temporal lobe. The insula is exposed by retracting the superior bank of the Sylvian fissure, as indicated by the arrows. The anterior temporal lobe has been amputated by cutting through the white matter that constitutes the temporal stem and the temporal lobe has been reflected inferiorly to expose its inner structure. The uncus is illustrated at the anterior aspect of the hippocampal gyrus. Current nomenclature refers to this convolution as the *para*-hippocampal gyrus. The amygdala is not illustrated, but it is located within the white matter of the uncus, just anterior to the *pes hippocampi*. The *pes hippocampi* continues posteriorly as the body of the hippocampus. Heschl's gyrus is seen within the first temporal convolution. It is composed of three or four smaller gyri rather than the single one illustrated here. Heschl's gyri constitute the primary auditory area. The *planum temporale* is immediately behind Heschl's gyrus. It is larger in the left, language-dominant hemisphere than it is in the right, nondominant hemisphere. The planum temporale is part of Wernicke's area that is related to the interpretation of spoken language. Montreal Neurological Institute and McGill University.

was caused by penetrating head trauma. Penfield referred to such a scar as a meningo-cerebral cicatrix, to distinguish it from the simpler cortical scar.

The major manifestations of a seizure are referred to as the ictus. The site that triggers an epileptic seizure can often be localized by the manifestations that it produces at its onset. Thus, head and eye turning often indicate that the epileptogenic area lies within the frontal lobe in front of the motor strip, opposite to the side to which the head and eyes are turned. The seizure is then referred to as aversive, and the patient is said to be looking away from his lesion. Focal lesions involving the motor strip often produce a Jacksonian march, named after John Hughlings Jackson who first drew attention to this phenomenon. In a Jacksonian march, the seizure begins with movement of a particular part of the body, for example the face, and spreads progressively along the motor strip in a somatotopic fashion, in which the hand, the arm, and finally the leg participate. A Jacksonian seizure often leads to loss of consciousness and generalized convulsions. As the patient recovers from the attack he or she might experience a temporary, focal paralysis that can also indicate the site of origin of the seizure. A seizure that involves motor and sensory phenomena, whether in isolation or as part of a Jacksonian march, is said to be of central origin because the motor and sensory strips are within the pre-and postcentral convolutions that line the central fissure. Penfield discovered that head turning is also associated with seizures arising in the occipital lobe. If this is the case, the seizure is often preceded by the appearance of coloured lights in the patient's visual field, or by other visual phenomena.

Temporal lobe, or psychomotor, seizures are often manifested by a blank stare and stereotypic behaviour of which the patient is unaware and of which he or she has no memory. These episodes are referred to as automatisms. Automatisms can be simple, such as smacking of the lips or fidgeting with the buttons of a shirt, or they can be complex, such as when a patient performs his usual activities as if in a trance and has no recollection of them. Such complex automatisms may, unusually, last for hours or days, during which the patient can travel long distances and have no memory of how she got to where she is when she comes out of the spell. This is called a fugue state, and is often used as a dramatic device in motion pictures.

THE SURGEON'S VIEWPOINT

What has not been drawn has not been seen[1]

Penfield first recorded his operative observations with a sterilized pencil on a blank piece of sterile paper onto which he drew the surgical exposure, his operative findings, and the effects of electrico-cortical stimulation. His sketches can be disorienting at first glance because Penfield drew them from the surgeon's viewpoint, as he stood at the head of the operating table. From this vantage point, the brain appears to be upside down when compared to the usual anatomical view, as is seen when the patient is upright. The accompanying sketch that Penfield drew of a patient with a left frontal brain tumour is typical of his technique. The patient was lying on his right side with the left cerebral hemisphere exposed to the surgeon's view. Penfield

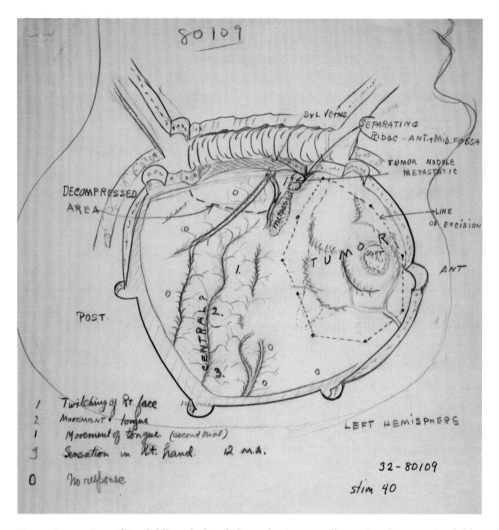

Figure Ana.3. One of Penfield's early, hand-drawn brain maps illustrating the operative field from the surgeon's viewpoint. The patient was lying on her right side, and the left hemisphere has been exposed. The surgeon stood at the head of the table, where the patient's head rested. A left frontal lobe tumour is indicated within the dotted lines. The results of cortical stimulation are indicated and prominent vessels are illustrated. Montreal Neurological Hospital, case I.H., 1932.

sometimes drew a faint outline of the head around the operative field, as he did in this case, to help with orientation. Some details of the sketch are common to all of Penfield's sketches. The semicircular openings in the skull represent the sites where burr holes were placed, and the parallel lines that join them indicate the edges of the craniotomy. The reflected bone flap is seen at the top of the drawing, where the curved, parallel lines represent the temporalis muscle, which remained attached to the bone flap. Penfield identified the postcentral gyrus and the motor strip from the responses elicited by electrocortical stimulation. This also identified the Rolandic fissure and the limits of the frontal and parietal lobes, respectively. Penfield could then follow the Rolandic fissure as it coursed downward to its junction with the Sylvian fissure, thus identifying the temporal lobe. Following the Sylvian fissure posteriorly led Penfield to the supramarginal gyrus, which curves around the end of the Sylvian fissure. Similarly, following the sulcus between the first and second temporal gyri led him to the angular gyrus.

Prominent arteries and veins were frequently illustrated in Penfield's operative sketches. The Y-shaped vessel in the illustration represents a prominent vein draining blood away from the central region to the superior sagittal sinus, the major draining channel of the cerebral hemispheres. The pathology found at surgery, in this case a brain tumour, is sketched in, and the resected area is indicated by dotted lines. The Sylvian fissure is not indicated in the sketch reproduced here because it was not necessary to expose the temporal lobe since the tumour was in the frontal lobe. Nonetheless, Penfield performed a temporal decompression by removing the inferior aspect of the temporal bone in order to accommodate the brain swelling that often followed the removal of a large brain tumour. The decompressed area is also delineated and labelled in the drawing.

CHAPTER I

1954 – Outside Looking In

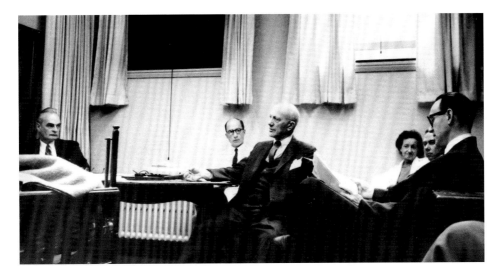

Figure 1.1. The Clinical EEG Conference. Donald McRae, sharp featured, stern faced, the head of neuroradiology, is at the extreme left, next to the patient's bed. Herbert Jasper, of distinguished pate and in shirtsleeves, is next, followed by Penfield, at centre. The photographer has caught Penfield as he is about to make a statement since he has removed his glasses for effect. Next is Brenda Milner, in white lab coat. Jake Hanberry, later head of neurosurgery at Stanford University, is at her left. The distinguished gentleman at the extreme right, impeccably dressed in a dark suit, is Theodore Rasmussen, later to be the second director of the Montreal Neurological Institute. Unseen are the residents and fellows sitting in a neat row of chairs behind the discussants. Montreal Neurological Institute and McGill University.

Preparation for surgery began at eight in the morning as the patient was brought to a small induction room next to the operating room. Her head was washed with a sterile soap solution and shaved, and the scalp incision was outlined on her denuded scalp with a sterile marker. She lay on her right side, her head resting on a circular foam cushion covered by a sterile towel. Her face was uncovered so that the movements of her eyes and twitching of her facial muscles could be observed, and her verbal responses could be heard. She wore a loose-fitting hospital gown, which

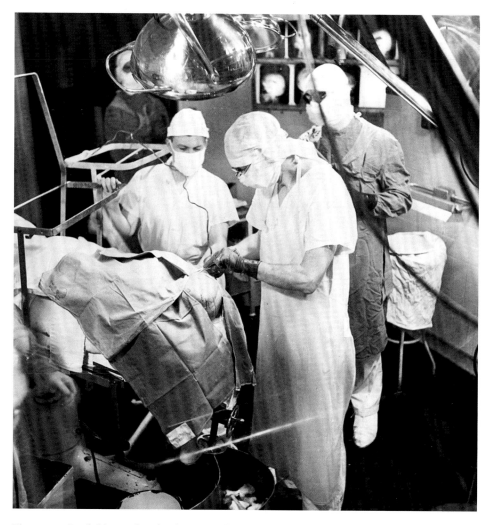

Figure 1.2. Penfield suturing the drapes to the scalp that has been infiltrated with a local anaesthetic in preparation for a left-sided craniotomy. André Pasquet, the anaesthetist, is to Penfield's right, observing the suturing to satisfy himself that the patient feels no discomfort. Montreal Neurological Institute and McGill University.

allowed her limbs to move unimpeded when the motor strip was stimulated with a weak electric current. Her scalp was sterilized with an antiseptic solution. The incision line was infiltrated with a local anaesthetic containing epinephrine to constrict the blood vessels and limit the spread of the anaesthetic and minimize bleeding from the scalp. The first dose of anaesthetic was infiltrated using a short, small-bore needle, raising a weal and blanching the superficial layer of the scalp. The second injection was just within the blanched area so that the needle prick was painless. The process was repeated until the whole of the incision line was anaesthetised, the only discomfort coming with the first injection. A longer, larger-bore needle was then used to infiltrate the deeper layers of the scalp and the periosteum enveloping the skull. Sterile towels were sewn within the anesthetised area along the incision line, to assure that the sterile field would not be compromised if the patient had an intraoperative seizure. She was covered with sterile sheets held above her head and body by interlocking rods and stands rigged up to support a makeshift tent of sterile sheets open to one side. This gave the anaesthetist ready access to assure that she remained comfortable and well, and allowed the effects of electrocortical stimulation of the brain to be observed. The opposite side of the tent was covered with a large double-layered sterile sheet, which separated the surgical assistant and instrument nurse from the patient. The instrument nurse stood on a low platform so that she could access the Mayo tray that rested on supports on top of the tent and that held the instruments that would be needed during the operation.

It had taken six years for patient M.P. to come to this point, awake with her brain exposed to the cool air of Theatre One of the MNI. She had had a seizure during a febrile illness when she was twelve months old. She recovered and was free of seizures until adolescence. But she learned to speak later than her siblings, and she walked in her sleep. She began to have episodic, jerking movements of the right hand and forearm in her mid-teens, and at the age of twenty-one she began to have episodes when she felt as if she had left her body. The first of these episodes occurred when she was riding in a bus one evening when she suddenly saw herself outside the bus looking in. The vision dissolved like a scene from a silent movie, but similar episodes recurred up to twenty or thirty times a month. Sometimes during a conversation, she would feel a spell coming on and hurried to complete her sentence before it began, then stayed quiet until the feeling passed. If she didn't finish her sentence in time, she continued to speak, but her words were unintelligible. Some episodes were more elaborate. On one occasion she walked past her husband without any sense of recognition, her gaze staring ahead as she made her way down the hall to the bedroom and lay down. She had no memory of this occurrence when she came to herself. The nature of the patient's illness was obvious to her neurologist, who diagnosed psychomotor epilepsy on the basis of feelings of unreality, out-of-body experiences, loss of contact with her environment, automatic behaviour, and amnesia for the events that occurred during a spell.[1]

M.P. was twenty-five years old when she was admitted to the MNI, on 7 January 1954. Her case was discussed at the weekly Clinical EEG Conference. (See figure 1.1.) These were attended by Penfield, Herbert Jasper, head of the Department of Neurophysiology and Clinical Electroencephalography, Donald McRea, head of the Department of Neuroradiology, Brenda Milner, head of the newly created Department of Neuropsychology, house staff, research fellows, and visitors to the institute.

The patient's history and the radiological findings were reviewed. The latter showed that the temporal horn of the lateral ventricle was larger on the left than on the right, which indicated that the medial structures of the left temporal lobe were sclerotic and atrophied, and the likely source of her seizures. Brenda Milner had recently joined the staff of the MNI and reported the results of the patient's neuropsychological evaluation. She had scored in the high average range in intelligence, but her verbal memory was poor, which lateralized the seizure focus to the language-dominant hemisphere. The EEG findings were concordant: the epileptic activity originated in the anterior and inferior aspects of the left temporal lobe, and Jasper concluded that the electrographic pattern indicated the presence of a deep left anterior temporal epileptic focus. Penfield concurred and ended the conference by stating, "Operation seems justifiable."

Penfield incised the scalp, reflected the skin, and elevated a bone flap. Five burr holes were placed and a wire saw was passed from one to the next using a flat, malleable saw guide that protected the underlying dura. The skull was sawed through with vigorous too-and-fro movements as Penfield's assistants held the patient's head so that it would not be jarred from its headrest. The bone was cracked while still attached to the temporalis muscle and hinged inferiorly to expose the dura. The dura was incised circumferentially and reflected to one side, exposing the brain. This was often difficult as there could be thick, vascularized adhesions between the undersurface of the dura and the scarred surface of the cortex. A photographer stationed in a cubby underneath the observation gallery took a photograph of the cortex.

"On first inspection," Penfield noted, "the first temporal convolution seemed a little atrophic, and there was some atrophy above the fissure of Sylvius." The atrophy of the anterior temporal lobe was so severe that the frontal operculum had protruded into the middle fossa and abutted against it. A set of recording electrodes was arrayed onto the cortex. The electrodes were affixed to a bar clamped to the skull to prevent them from moving during the recording. The wires emanating from the electrodes were gathered into a cable that coursed from the operating table to the observation gallery, where Herbert Jasper stood over an encephalograph.

Penfield stimulated the cortex with a fine, flexible, blunt-tipped electrode while the EEG recorded cortical activity.[2] Stimulation began at a low voltage that was increased in increments until a response was obtained. In M.P.'s case this was achieved at two volts along the postcentral convolution, which produced quivering of the

Figure 1.3. *Opposite top* Penfield perforating the skull in an awake patient under local anaesthesia. Osler Library of the History of Medicine.

Figure 1.4. *Opposite bottom* Penfield opening the dura. Montreal Neurological Hospital and McGill University.

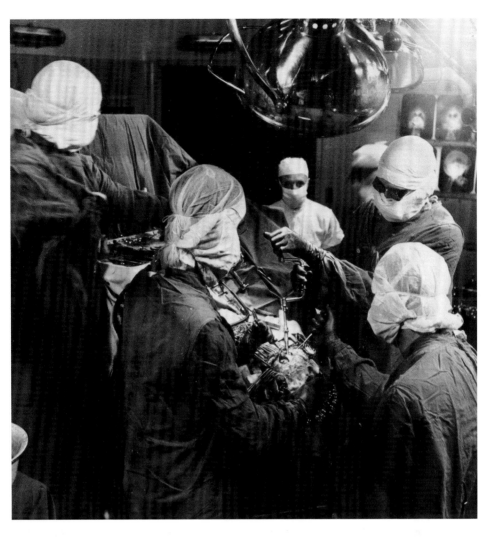

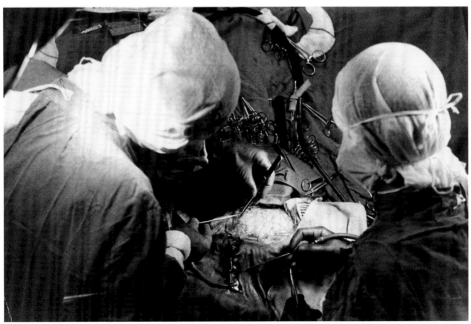

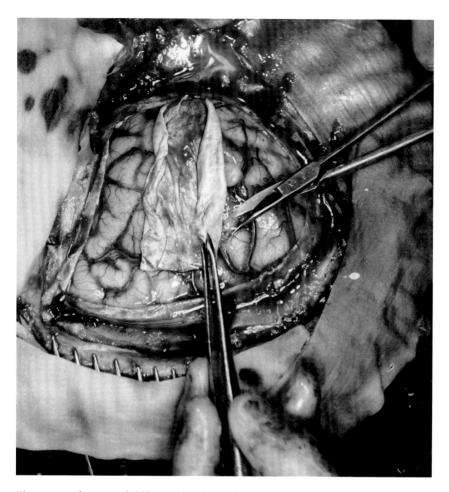

Figure 1.5. *Above* Penfield lysing dural adhesions from the cortex. Montreal Neurological Hospital.

Figure 1.6. *Opposite top left* Operative photograph of another case. The bone flap has been elevated and the temporalis muscle has been retracted by blunted fishhooks attached to heavy silk sutures affixed to the drapes with mosquito clamps. The incised dura has been reflected to the left of the exposure, remaining attached by a pedicle. Dandy clamps are arrayed as a halo along the skin incision as they retract the galea. Montreal Neurological Hospital.

Figure 1.7. *Opposite top right* Operative photograph of the exposed left hemisphere, seen from the anatomical viewpoint. The parietal lobe is to the right and the frontal lobe is to the left. The temporal lobe is at the inferior aspect of the exposure, where the first two temporal convolutions are seen to course almost horizontally. An array of eight electrocorticography electrodes has been applied to the frontal and parietal lobes. An electrocortical stimulator is seen at the left of the operative exposure. Notice the impossibility of identifying the pre- and postcentral gyri by direct vision. Montreal Neurological Hospital, case L.McK., 1947.

Figure 1.8. *Opposite bottom* Penfield annotating the patient's brain map. Herbert Jasper, in the gallery, is analyzing the patient's cortical EEG, as the anaesthetist (foreground) observes the patient. Montreal Neurological Institute and McGill University.

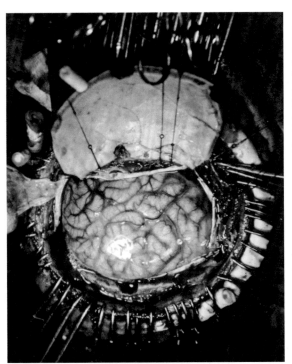
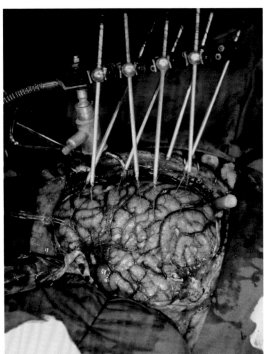
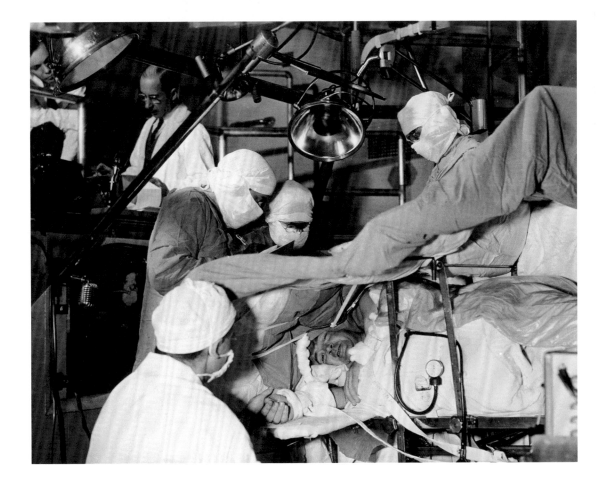

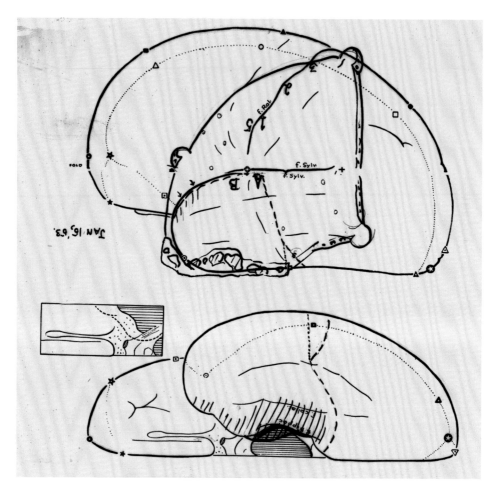

Figure 1.9. M.P.'s brain map seen in the anatomical viewpoint. Numbers 1–3 identify the post-central gyrus. Number 5 is on the precentral gyrus. The small circles indicate points where stimulation had no effect. Epileptic activity was recorded along the first temporal convolution, as indicated by letters A and B. The anterior end of the first temporal convolution, the uncus, and the hippocampus were found to be sclerotic, as indicated by the hatching. The small arrows pointing to the anterior temporal lobe indicate that it was atrophic, which allowed the frontal lobe to protrude downward into the temporal fossa. The darkened area in the lower illustration indicates that the uncus and anterior hippocampus had herniated into the perimesencephalic space. The dotted line indicates the extent of the resection. The small triangular area enclosed in a separate line indicates a cortical area that was also resected. Montreal Neurological Hospital, case M.P., 1953.

right side of the mouth, tingling of the right upper lip, and numbness of the second and third fingers of the right hand. With stimulation of the precentral cortex, "there were tremulous movements of the fingers followed by movements of the forearm and then the arm," and the patient reported, "this is like what my attacks used to be." (See figures 7.3, 7.4.) Stimulation of the inferior aspect of the motor strip and of Broca's area caused pulling of the lips to the right and difficulty speaking. Small, sequentially numbered paper tickets were placed on the cortex where stimulation had produced a response. Blank tickets indicated unresponsive cortex.

Identifying the pre- and postcentral gyri delineated the Rolandic fissure between the frontal and parietal lobes. Penfield followed the Rolandic fissure downward to its junction with the Sylvian fissure and identified the superior aspect of the temporal lobe. The delineation of the Rolandic and Sylvian fissures and of the lobes that they defined allowed Penfield to recognize the convolutions on which he now placed the EEG electrodes. In this case, the cortical EEG revealed epileptic spikes arising from the atrophic first temporal convolution. Letters on small paper tickets identified the sites from which epileptic activity was recorded, and the location of the letters and numbers was drawn onto a brain map for later analysis. In earlier times, before Penfield began using a preprinted map, the operative exposure was hand drawn onto a sterile piece of paper on which numbers and letters corresponding to cortical responses and epileptic areas were drawn in. Now, however, Penfield dictated the patient's every reaction to a secretary in the gallery, who accurately transcribed every word in shorthand. Her notes were later typed and became part of the patient's medical record. A second photograph of the now tagged cortex was taken. The photograph was later used to accurately measure the site of each stimulation point in relation to the Rolandic and Sylvian fissures.

The lateral neocortex was resected *en bloc*, exposing the uncus and hippocampus. These structures were yellow and tough, and Penfield noted "marked incisural sclerosis … and herniation of the hippocampal gyrus inside the incisura of the tentorium." The uncus and hippocampus were resected. The outline of the resected area was added to the brain map and a third photograph was taken. These were used to correlate the extent of resection with the postoperative outcome. The dura, galea, and scalp were closed, and the patient's head was covered with a bulky dressing. She was returned to her ward fully awake, responsive, and undoubtedly relieved that the whole thing was done with.

And it had all started at the Royal Victoria Hospital.

PART ONE

The Royal Victoria Hospital, 1928–34

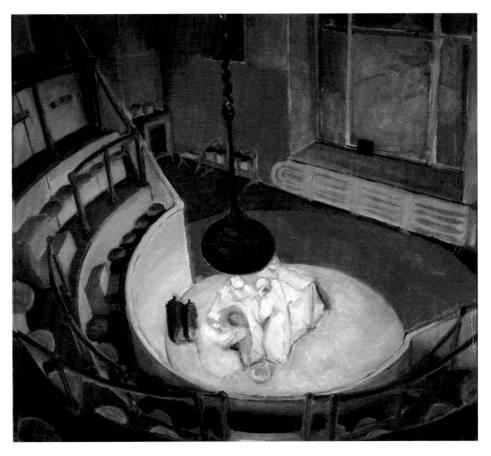

Figure 2.1. The operating room of the Royal Victoria Hospital, 1928.
Norman Bethune, *Night Operating Theatre*. The Royal Victoria Hospital.

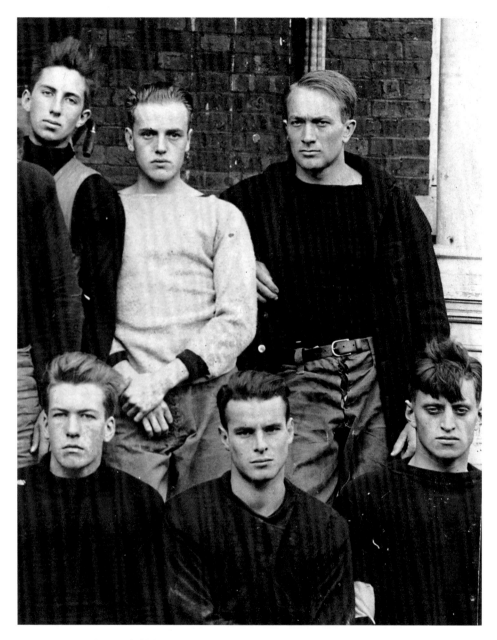

Figure 2.2. Wilder Penfield (upper right) at Princeton University, ca. 1913. Osler Library of the History of Medicine.

The Making of a Neurosurgeon

Brain surgery is a terrible profession –Penfield, 1921

The Royal Victoria Hospital was built through the generosity of Donald Smith (Lord Strathcona), George Stephens (Lord Mount Stephen), and two million dollars in cash and Great Northern Railroad securities. The RVH opened its doors "for the use of the sick and ailing without distinction of race or creed," in 1893. It received its royal appellation in honour of the fiftieth anniversary of Queen Victoria's ascension to the throne.[1] It is a massive structure of grey stone built in what is referred to architecturally as the Scottish Baronial style. The "Vic," as it was known, rose on the southern slope of Mount Royal, the extinguished volcano from which Montreal derives its name. From this vantage point the Vic had a commanding view onto the city and the Saint Lawrence River. When it opened its doors it was the finest and best-equipped hospital on the continent.[2]

Edward Archibald, the head of surgery at McGill University, recruited Wilder Penfield to McGill and the Royal Victoria in 1928, where Penfield practised until the opening of the Montreal Neurological Institute in 1934.[3] Edward Archibald was one of the most prominent surgeons in North America and one of the first to devote himself to the practice of neurosurgery. He graduated from McGill University's Medical School in 1896 and trained in general surgery at the RVH and in Breslau, Germany.[4] Having decided on a neurosurgical career Archibald then travelled to the National Hospital for the Paralyzed and Epileptic at Queen Square, London, where he studied with Sir Victor Horsley, the founder of the discipline of neurosurgery. Archibald published a comprehensive treatise on *Surgical Affections and Wounds of the Head*[5] early in his career and was a founding member of the Society of Neurological Surgeons, with Harvey Cushing and thirteen other pioneers of North American neurosurgery. Archibald's career flourished in Montreal, but he was a firm believer that "advances in surgery could only come from research and familiarity with the basic sciences."[6] He realized that in order to progress, neurosurgery required more than a busy practice and surgical skill. Advances in neuroscience at the time were to come from neurocytology and neuropathology, areas in which Archibald had no training. Penfield, however, had travelled to Madrid to learn the difficult cell-staining techniques for neurons and glial cells devised by Santiago Ramón y

Cajal and Pío del Río Hortega. Penfield returned to America having mastered the Spanish methods, in which no one else on the continent was adept, and applied them to the study of the human brain in health and disease.

THE ROAD TO RHODES

Wilder Penfield was born in Spokane, Washington, on 26 January 1891 to Jean Jefferson and Charles Samuel Penfield, a physician. Charles Penfield was, in Wilder's estimation, "a failure in medicine."[7] The resulting financial strains caused Jean and her three children, Herbert, Wilder, and Ruth, to seek the comfort of the Jefferson family home, in Hudson, Wisconsin. The move was to be temporary, until Charles called for the family to return to Spokane, but the call never came.[8]

As is often the case in such circumstances, Penfield's mother was both parent and confidante. And so it was that, after attending a public lecture by a returning Rhodes Scholar, Jean excitedly told her thirteen-year-old son, "This scholarship is just the thing for you Wide."[9] Penfield later wrote that this was so because, in a house with a single parent, "if I should win it, it would bring me three years in Oxford, England, all expenses paid."[10]

But the road to Oxford's spires and quadrangles was not straight nor was it easily travelled. Nonetheless, it was the prospect of a Rhodes Scholarship that set Penfield's mind on Princeton University: "In those days a Rhodes Scholarship was awarded in each state two years out of three. Since New Jersey, where Princeton is located, is small, I would meet less competition for the scholarship there than at Yale or Harvard."[11] Despite his aspirations, Penfield was an indifferent student. He did, however, try out for the Princeton Tigers football team but he didn't make the cut in his freshman year. Driven by need – athletics was a requirement of the Rhodes scholarship – Penfield persevered, became a reasonable place kicker, and eventually did make the varsity team.

He had less success in the classroom, however, until he took a class with Edwin Grant Conklin, the distinguished professor of biology at Princeton, and a close friend of William Osler. Through Conklin's eyes, Penfield saw "how tiny cells within the living, growing body bud and multiply,"[12] and his aversion to medicine, fuelled by the fear that the same failure that had estranged him from his father, vanished among the specimens and histology slides of Conklin's laboratory. Ultimately, it would be through the microscope that Penfield achieved his first successes in neurobiology.

Penfield's application for the 1913 Rhodes Scholarship was rejected by the New Jersey Rhodes Committee in favour of a candidate from Rutgers University. Undeterred, Penfield was successful in his second attempt, and he was awarded the 1914 Rhodes Scholarship for New Jersey. But fate intervened with the onset of World War I, and Penfield had to abandon hope of taking up his scholarship at Oxford.

America was not yet in the war, and the effect that a European conflict had on Penfield was more personal than patriotic: "For me it meant, as I thought, a personal loss of the money for three years of medical training, and the loss of so much more that I had dreamed of and worked for. I gave up all hope of going to Oxford."[13] Thus, depleting his savings, Penfield registered at the College of Physicians and Surgeons at Columbia University and began his first year of medical school. But things were not as dire at Oxford as Penfield had thought. After six months at Columbia, Penfield received a postcard from Wilburt Davison, a fellow Rhodes Scholar from New York State and later founder of Duke University Medical School,[14] which read, "Medical teaching here is better than ever. Americans are welcome."[15] Penfield thus renewed his application to Merton College, Oxford University. Merton accepted him for admission to the School of Physiology in 1915. Soon after his arrival at Oxford, Penfield reached out to Sir William Osler, the Canadian-born Regius Professor of Medicine and the most prominent physician of his time. Osler had begun his career at McGill University before relocating to Baltimore, where he played a key role in the creation of the medical school at Johns Hopkins University. By the time Penfield met him in 1915, Osler's own son was in the trenches in France, where he died two years later.

After his first term at Merton College, Penfield crossed the English Channel for the first time to serve at a Red Cross hospital in France. On his second trip, in 1916, the ship carrying him to France was torpedoed. It is insightful to read in Penfield's autobiography that he thought, as he was thrown into the air by the blast, "This cannot be the end. My work in the world has only just begun. This cannot be the end."[16] Reflecting on his thoughts towards the end of his life, Penfield shared a candid moment with his readers as he wrote, "You, reader, may laugh at the reasoning that went on in the air. Call it naiveté or colossal egoism. It was naive and, surely egotistical. Nevertheless, it happened that way, and it demonstrated my deep conviction that here was work in the world for me to do. This was in fact, a central concept of my own personal religion. Purpose and a plan in life seemed to me, then, things to cling to. They still do after these many years."[17] Rescued and wounded, Penfield was returned to England for treatment. The Oslers took him in for the period of his convalescence, a kindness that warmed Penfield's heart to the end of his life.

Penfield recovered from his injuries and after two years at Oxford he returned to America in 1917 to finish medical school. Armed with a letter of support from Osler, he was accepted at Johns Hopkins. He graduated in 1918 and took a position as intern at the Peter Bent Brigham Hospital in Boston, where he was exposed to the gargantuan personage that was Harvey Cushing. By all accounts Cushing was impressed by this "very nice gentlemanly fellow" and offered him a position as his resident. Penfield declined, as he wished to return to England to finish the laboratory work necessary to obtain a BSc from Oxford University. Thus, with his third year of the

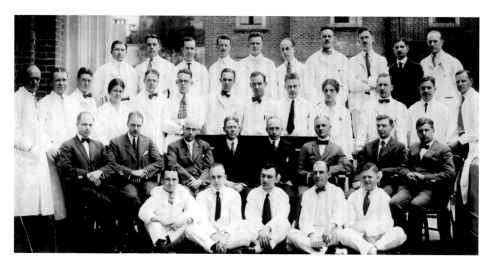

Figure 2.3. Penfield (top row, extreme right) at the Peter Bent Brigham Hospital. Percival Bailey is ninth from the left in the third row. Cushing is seated in the second row, sixth from the left. Montreal Neurological Institute and McGill University.

Rhodes Scholarship still available, Penfield returned to Oxford, to Charles Sherrington's laboratory. Cushing would have been sympathetic to Penfield's wish to work with Sherrington, as Cushing had also come under Sherrington's influence at the turn of the twentieth century, when he helped Sherrington stimulate the motor cortex of the great apes.[18]

Penfield met with Sherrington upon his return to Oxford in 1919. Sherrington, as Penfield recalled, said, "You could perhaps begin by helping me to study a problem that puzzled me in regard to the reflex action of the cat's hind leg."[19] Shortly thereafter, Sherrington was appointed president of the Royal Society, and Penfield's research was reoriented to the microscopic study of the Golgi apparatus following axonal transection,[20] under the supervision of the renowned histologist Harry Montgomery Carleton, and to the study of the decerebrate animal,[21] under the supervision of Cuthbert Bazett. Bazett would later leave Oxford to become the professor of physiology at the University of Pennsylvania. Penfield later reflected on what must at the time have seemed a crushing blow: "Curiously enough, Sherrington's temporary withdrawal from active experimentation did serve my eventual purposes remarkably well. Collaboration with Bazett led to the later study of the function of the human-mechanism related to consciousness. Carlton's studies with the microscope launched me in neurocytology, which was to become my first serious approach to the human brain."[22]

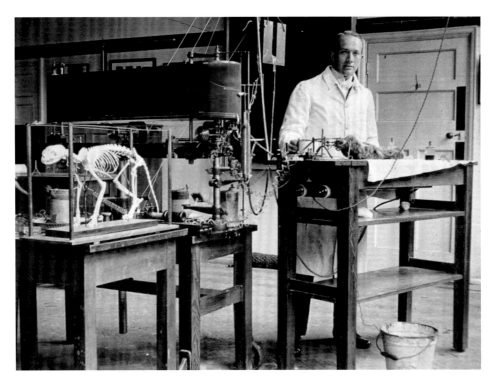

Figure 2.4. Wilder Penfield at Oxford, in Sherrington's laboratory. Osler Library of the History of Medicine.

NEW YORK — "A BRUSHWORK OF NEUROGLIA"

Penfield obtained his BSc from Oxford in 1920, but he wished to remain in England to improve his clinical skills. The financial support from his Rhodes Scholarship having ended, Sherrington secured Penfield a most prestigious Beit Memorial Medical Fellowship, which allowed him to study at the National Hospital, Queen Square. Penfield was thus afforded the opportunity to learn neuropathology with J. Godwin Greenfield, neurology with Gordon Holmes, and neurosurgery as Percy Sargent's assistant. Sargent had succeeded Victor Horsley at Queen Square and was considered Britain's most brilliant neurosurgeon of the postwar period.[23] Penfield, however, was mostly impressed with his technical skills, which, at the time, mainly meant speed of execution:

> A patient came to Mr Sargent for operation with an enormous bony enlargement on the skull. It was like a horn … "This is an endothelioma," said Mr Sargent. "It is really a bony growth. Horsley had a number of cases like this. Under that horn is a soft tumour pressing on the brain." To my joy he asked me to assist him in

the operation. "It will bleed," he said … Sargent made the incision with his scalpel and turned a flap of scalp back from the bony horn, working at top speed … "Now it will bleed," he repeated … "Now it is going to rain"… He made cuts or trenches in the normal bone all the way around the horn. It bled like a suddenly released fountain. But he carried out his excision with a breathless speed and dexterity that I had never seen before. In the hands of a slow operator, that patient would have bled to death. But this one came through it, and did very well.[24]

With Sargent's encouragement, Penfield reviewed Horsley and Sargent's cases and published his first paper on a clinical neurosurgical topic, "Osteogenetic Dural Endothelioma: The True Nature of Hemicraniosis,"[25] a previously unrecognized manifestation of meningioma. This would be characteristic of Penfield's career, the insightful study of individual cases correlated to pathological findings, observed at surgery or in the laboratory.

Penfield would have read the very authoritative textbooks available to him at the time of his apprenticeship in neurosurgery: Archibald's *Surgical Affections and Wounds of the Head*,[26] and *Cushing's Surgery of the Head*,[27] both published in 1908, as well as Fedor Krause's magnificently illustrated, three-volume treatise *Surgery of the Brain and Spinal Cord*, published in its English translation between 1909 and 1912.[28] Penfield would have been especially interested in the second volume of Krause's trilogy in which he deals with the surgical treatment of Jacksonian epilepsy.[29] Krause was one of the first surgeons to devote himself entirely to neurological surgery. He and the renowned neurologist, Hermann Oppenheim, established a centre for neurology and neurological surgery at Augusta Hospital, Berlin, which enjoyed worldwide renown.[30] Krause, like Foerster and Penfield who followed him, determined the epileptogenicity of the cortex about a scar through electrocortical stimulation, using a current which "was so mild that applied to the tongue of an assistant, it was perceived by him as only a mild burning sensation accompanied by a slight acid taste."[31] Despite the low amplitude of the current applied to the cortex, Krause "was enabled on numerous occasions to induce a typical epileptic attack by touching certain foci within the cerebral cortex with the faradic electrode."[32] Krause referred to any such area whose electrical stimulation triggered an attack as the *primary spasming centre*.[33] Resection of this area, even in patients whose seizures had been longstanding, was often beneficial because Krause felt that the sharply demarcated, aseptic scar that resulted from surgery did not produce a new epileptogenic focus.[34] This would be Penfield's rationale for operating on his own epileptic patients.

Penfield left Queen Square as a thirty-year-old neurosurgical assistant with little or no experience in general surgery. Yet, in June 1921 he was on his way up Park Avenue

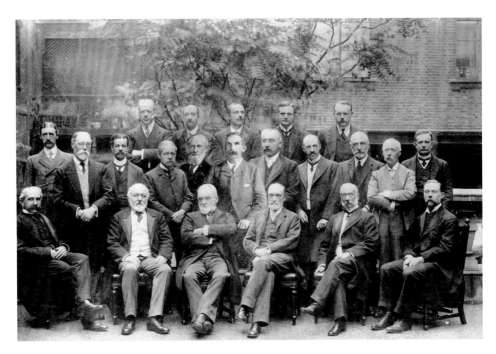

Figure 2.5. Photograph of the staff at the National Hospital for the Paralyzed and Epileptic, Queen Square, 1906. Percy Sargent is in the top row, fourth from the left. Victor Horsley is sixth in the second row. John Huglings Jackson and Charles Ferrier are in the front row, third and fifth from the left, respectively. Montreal Neurological Institute and McGill University.

to meet Allan Whipple, surgeon-in-chief at the Presbyterian Hospital and professor of surgery at Columbia University.

"I'd like to have you join my staff to do the neurological surgery," Whipple said, quickly coming to the point.

"I'm not much of a surgeon," Penfield could only think to reply.

"I know that," Whipple laughed, stating the obvious. "We can teach you surgery. We want you because of your training and your interest in physiology and pathology."[35]

And so, Wilder Penfield joined the staff of the foremost teaching hospital in New York City.[36] Penfield was assigned to the second surgical service at the Presbyterian Hospital and functioned mainly as a general surgeon. Nonetheless, during his apprenticeship in general surgery, he operated on two neurosurgical patients. Both were comatose, one from a brain abscess, the other from a brain tumour, and neither survived the operation. While attending the autopsy of his second case, Penfield lamented to no one in particular, "brain surgery is a terrible profession."[37] Despite this dismal assessment, Penfield took steps to improve his neurosurgical skills, and arranged for a short sabbatical to visit Walter Dandy in Baltimore, Charles Frazier in Philadelphia, and Harvey Cushing in Boston.[38] And so, in November 1923, Whipple informed Penfield that his surgical apprenticeship had come to an end and that he was now the full-time neurosurgeon at the Presbyterian Hospital.

As had been the case with his exposure to Conklin at Princeton, while at Columbia Penfield made the acquaintance of a basic scientist who would have a determining effect on his career. One of Penfield's responsibilities at the medical school was to act as instructor in a course given by William C. Clarke, professor of pathology at Columbia. Clarke looked bemusedly upon Penfield and asked of him,

"What goes on in the brain? ... How does it heal."
   Penfield then realized that there was no answer to Clarke's question.
   "Wouldn't you like to know?" Clarke continued earnestly.
   Then came a moment that again determined Penfield's future:
   "A series of experimental wounds in laboratory animals examined after different intervals of time would make a wonderful addition to our teaching collection ... and you might learn something in the process."[39]

This simple conversation would eventually send Penfield on a four-year journey of exploration and experimentation that led him to the bright, sunlit skies of Madrid and to the plains of Lower Silesia.

Penfield took Clarke's advice in earnest and undertook an overly complex experiment to study the healing process of the injured brain.[40] Experiments involving large bilateral craniotomies were performed to expose both hemispheres of animals, and brain wounds of varying severity were created. The animals were sacrificed at different intervals to evaluate the evolution of the brain's response to injury. Penfield was able to demonstrate a progressively more organized reaction of the traumatized cerebral tissue, which ultimately took on the appearance of a *brushwork of neuroglial fibrils* about the damaged cortex and white matter. Prominently, adhesions formed between the superficial layer of the damaged cortex and the covering dura. For the remainder of his career, every operative report that Penfield wrote would have a comment on the presence or absence of cortical-dural adhesions. Penfield did not yet see another feature of maturing brain wounds, neovascularization, which would be of critical importance to his later studies.

It took Penfield two years to complete these experiments, and he was dissatisfied with the results. Upon review, this is not surprising. The experiments were too complicated, were inadequately controlled, and lacked a standardized lesion to yield anything but preliminary, empiric observations. Penfield, however, felt that the main deficiency of his experiment lay in the deficiency of the stains available to him to adequately study the reactive changes produced by cortical injury. Then, a moment of insight occurred as he recalled that Sherrington had suggested that he use special stains developed by Ramón y Cajal for his study of the Golgi apparatus of the transacted axon. Penfield took his problem to Whipple and explained his dilemma:

> Cajal has gathered a school of Spanish cytologists about him since he received the Nobel award … They have always hidden their work in Spanish journals. But in the drawings published by one of them, Pío del Río Hortega, the cells, which are no more than ghosts in my standard preparations, stand out sharp and clear, each cell body and nucleus and fibre and granule … The Spanish scientists have been studying normal animals. What I want to do is to use their methods to study the brain of man, and then move on to the effects of disease on the brain.[41]

Penfield asked Whipple for a six-month sabbatical to go to Spain and learn the Spanish methods of staining brain cells using gold and silver salts. Whipple enthusiastically agreed and obtained funds from the Rockefeller family for Penfield's sojourn in Madrid. It was not the last time that Penfield would benefit from Rockefeller largesse.

MADRID 1924 – GHOST CELLS

A few months later Penfield was in Madrid where, unannounced, he made his way to Río Hortega's laboratory at la Residencia des Estudiantes – the university student residence, at a time when Cajal and Río Hortega had parted ways because of a difference of opinion on the interpretation of experimental results. Río Hortega had discovered an as yet unidentified structure that was neither neuron nor either of the two neuroglial cells that were known at the time, the astrocyte and the microglia. Río Hortega believed it to be a third type of glial cell, which he called the *oligodendrocyte*. Cajal did not agree. Río Hortega wasted no time and immediately taught Penfield his silver carbonate technique and set him the task of proving him right. After diligent work at the bench, Penfield showed Río Hortega a slide that showed a distinctly clear cluster of cells, which were neither astrocyte nor microglia, but the heretofore elusive oligodendrocyte. The oligidendrocyte, Penfield observed, was more prevalent in the white matter than in the grey. Its nucleus was round or oblong and contained a large amount of chromatin. The cytoplasm was eccentric and granular. Silver stains revealed long, complex, vine-like projections that invested nearby myelin sheets "in a manner analogous to the sheath of Schwann cells about peripheral myelinated fibers."[42] In the grey matter, they tended to cluster as satellites about nearby neurons and blood vessels. Penfield published this finding in *Brain* in 1924,

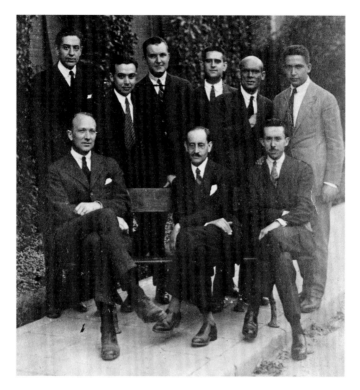

Figure 2.6. *Above* Penfield seated to the right of Pío del Río Hortega. Osler Library of the History of Medicine.

Figure 2.7. *Opposite* Penfield's drawing of oligodendrocytes and their vine-like prolongations. Note the clustering about the cerebral blood vessel in the lower part of the illustration. The large stellate cell at lower right is an astrocyte. Montreal Neurological Institute and McGill University.

under the title of "Oligodendroglia and its relationship to classical neuroglia."[43] In the conclusion of his description of the cell, Penfield hazarded an opinion as to its function, which was later proven to be correct:

> The function of oligodendroglia cells is not settled, but their relation to nerve cells and medullary sheaths corresponds strikingly with the relation of the sub-capsular cells to the neurons of the spinal ganglia, and that of the sheath of Schwann cells to peripheral nerves. Moreover, oligodendroglia cells appear in the central nervous system at the time of maximum myelinization, and contain unusually large cytoplasmic granules, which suggest a secretory function. These facts, as well as the arrangement of the cells along the medullary tubes, make it probable that they have to do with the elaboration and maintenance of myelin.[44]

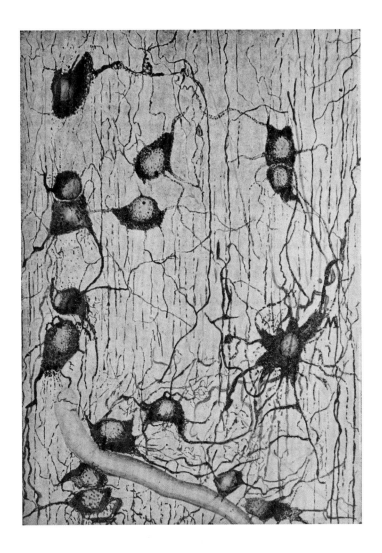

Penfield's identification of the oligodendrocyte, incidental to his quest for a better understanding of cerebral wound healing, was of momentous importance. It led Percival Bailey and Paul Bucy to describe the oligodendroglioma, a previously unknown brain tumour with malignant potential, but, perhaps more importantly, the oligodendrocyte has been the focus of research into multiple sclerosis since its discovery. Penfield, however, saw a more immediate application for the techniques that he had learned with Río Hortega: the study of brain wounds.

Now, under the tutelage of Río Hortega, Penfield undertook a well-controlled experiment using a single, standardized lesion. The experimental design was simple but brutish. A trocar was driven through the skull of a rabbit into its brain. This produced a small, simple lesion ideal for cytological study. Perhaps to Penfield's disappointment, oligodendrocytes did not participate in the reactive, gliotic response to injury. This was limited to microglia – the scavenger cells of the nervous system – that cleared the debris produced by the injury, and to astrocytes, which arrayed themselves about the wound in a radial fashion. Collagen fibres, Penfield observed, were laid down, lined the wound, and caused the newly formed scar to contract. There were no dural adhesions, and no vascular response.[45]

Following this master class in experimental neurobiology and confident in the use of the silver and gold stains, Penfield returned to the Presbyterian Hospital in New York and established the Laboratory of Cytology, where he repeated the experiments that William Clarke had first suggested and that had sent him on his quest for better stains.

The experiments were performed in collaboration with Richard Buckley, from Yale University, and their results were presented to the American Neurological Association in May 1927.[46] The experiments consisted in comparing two groups of experimental animals. In one group an injury was created much as Penfield had done with Río Hortega, by the insertion of a blunt brain needle into the brain. The same procedure was followed in the second experimental group, but a hollow needle was used and brain tissue was removed through aspiration, much as one would do in performing a brain biopsy. The results were striking. The removal of the damaged brain tissue resulted in a well-defined cavity along the needle tract, with minimal gliosis or vascular response – a clean, atraumatic wound with little reactive change and no vascular proliferation. The results in the other group, in which the damaged tissue was not removed, could not have been more different in their complexity and consequences. The persistence of the damaged brain tissue set off a dramatic response characterized by invasion of the wounded area by reactive fibrillary astrocytes, infiltration of fibroblasts, the laying down of a framework of collagen, and the generation of a prominent plexus of reactive blood vessels that anastomosed with the normal cortical arterioles about the wound. With the passage of time, the collagen fibrils within the gliotic scar hypertrophied and contracted, in a process to which Penfield referred as *cicatricial contraction* of the brain.[47] The contraction of the brain and the reactive angiogenesis suggested an etiological mechanism for delayed, posttraumatic epilepsy. As Penfield conjectured, "the slow contraction of such a scar, continuing as it does for years, must produce a constant irritation which may well be the starting point for a nervous discharge resulting in Jacksonian epilepsy."[48]

But at this time, this was only conjecture.

CHAPTER 3

Brain Scars

In such tissue lies hidden the secrets of epilepsy —Penfield, 1921

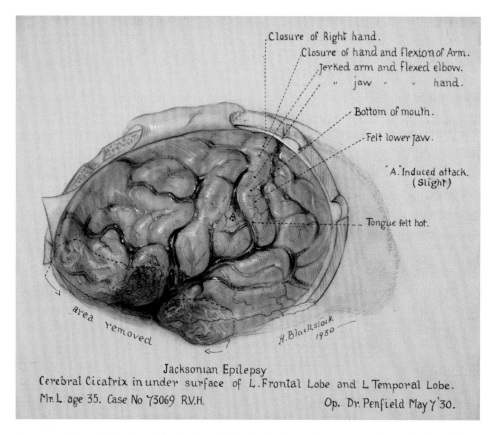

Figure 3.1. Harriet Blackstock's drawing of the brain of a patient operated upon by Penfield at the Royal Victoria Hospital in 1930. Penfield's operative report reads, "There were quite dense adhesions between the arachnoid and the dura over the whole frontal lobe and extending down over the temporal lobe … The under surface of the temporal lobe was somewhat gelatinous and the same was true of the under surface of the frontal lobe." Both scarred areas were resected. Montreal Neurological Hospital, case H.L., 1930.

THE MENINGOCEREBRAL CICATRIX

Penfield's experiment had been confined to animals but it was significant enough to warrant a paper in *Brain*, which Penfield published in 1927, under the title "The Mechanism of Cicatricial Contraction in the Brain."[1] It is the most informative of Penfield's papers on the topic and marks the end of one phase of his career, the search for the etiology of posttraumatic epilepsy, and the beginning of the next, when he applied his findings to its treatment. Penfield's paper unified two elements of the posttraumatic response – the astroglial contracting scar and the angiogenic response – into a single, pathophysiological entity to which he referred as the *meningocerebral cicatrix*. Penfield's brilliant insight came with the realization that two systems invest the whole of the cerebral cortex: a network of astrocytes with their axonal projections, and the cerebral vasculature arborizing throughout the cortical mantle. Penfield recognized that these two systems are interconnected by astrocytic projections, called footplates, which abut on the walls of cortical arteries, creating an anatomical and physiological entity composed of astrocytes, footplates, and cortical vessels, which Penfield termed the *vaso-astral framework*.[2] For Penfield the vaso-astral framework constituted "the supporting framework of the adult nervous system."[3] One might also add that the vaso-astral framework contained all the elements necessary for a neurogenic vasomotor reflex.

The vaso-astral framework was the starting point. A penetrating injury, Penfield had observed, produced connective tissue adhesions intertwined within a plexus of blood vessels that anastomosed with the cortical vessels at its periphery. Penfield was now ready to explain how the meningocerebral cicatrix might lead to epilepto-genesis by stating, simply, "it is of course, characteristic of such connective tissue scars to contract."[4] The contracting scar would then apply traction to the surround-ing cortical vessels.[5] The implication was clear: traction on the arteries of the cortex triggered a vasomotor response that rendered it ischemic and epileptic. This was so in animals, would the same be true in patients whose head injury didn't occur in the sterile environment of the experimental laboratory? It would not be long before the opportunity came to test that hypothesis.

WILLIAM VERNON CONE

William Cone had joined Penfield in the Laboratory of Cytology at the Presbyterian Hospital in 1925, shortly after Penfield's return from Madrid.[6] Their friendship lasted a lifetime before coming to a tragic end with Cone's untimely death in 1959.[7] Cone had attended medical school at the University of Iowa. A short, stout man, he had supported himself financially in his undergraduate years as a boxer and wrestler. Upon graduation, Cone gravitated to the pathology laboratory at the University of

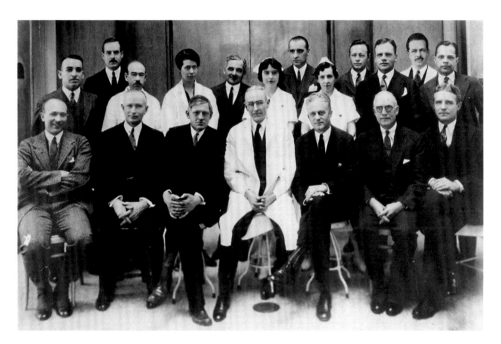

Figure 3.2. The surgical staff at the Columbia Presbyterian Hospital, 1927. Penfield is in the front row at the extreme left. Cone is standing directly behind him in the second row. Whipple is at the centre of the front row, in a white coat. William Clarke, who set Penfield on his research career, is sitting at Whipple's right. Montreal Neurological Institute and McGill University.

Iowa where he soon became a skilled neuropathologist, albeit limited by the staining methods of the day. Cone came to New York in 1924 to apprentice in neurology with Frederick Tilney, professor of neurology at Columbia University and neurologist-in-chief at the Presbyterian Hospital. Cone soon felt the attraction of Whipple's personality, and, as had been the case for Penfield, Whipple and the surgeons at the Presbyterian Hospital tutored him in general surgery.

His surgical apprenticeship ended, Whipple assigned Cone to train in neurosurgery with Penfield. As Penfield later wrote, "He learned fast. Soon, he seemed to double my potential. He became my alter ego throughout the hospital. He acquired the art of neurosurgery and patient care as if by instinct."[8] In the opinion of Sir Geoffrey Jefferson, the distinguished British neurosurgeon, Cone at his peak was the best neurosurgeon in the world.[9] It was at the Presbyterian hospital that the working relationship between Penfield and Cone was established: "While Penfield would break off for a few days to collect his thoughts, finish manuscripts, and regain his drive, Cone did not tire. He rarely turned aside for diversion … Penfield's projects became Cone's projects … Evening hours found him in the hospital, carrying out some kindly act for a patient with the help of the intern, or working in the laboratory."[10]

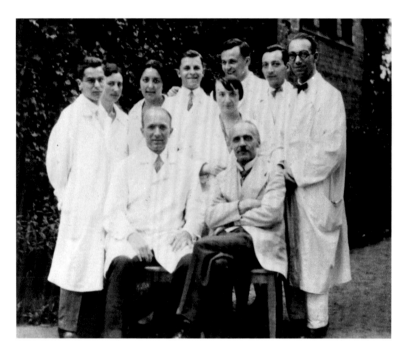

Figure 3.3. Wilder Penfield (sitting, left), Otfrid Foerster (sitting, right), and Foerster's staff, 1928. Montreal Neurological Institute and McGill University.

Neuropathology was at the time as important to the advance of neurology as molecular neurobiology is today. Thus Penfield's mastery of the silver and gold methods of staining normal and pathological cells was in high demand. His relationship with Charles Elsberg, head of neurosurgery at the Neurological Institute of New York, had become strained, and Penfield was not invited to practise at that institution when it became affiliated with the Columbia-Presbyterian Hospital. Thus Penfield saw little chance of advancement in New York. Penfield was therefore receptive to the many offers that came from prominent universities to relocate to their medical institution. None, however, offered resources for scientific work until Edward Archibald came from Montreal to New York with an offer of research facilities and financial support. After some discussion and administrative delays, Penfield accepted Archibald's offer if it also extended to William Cone, a condition which Archibald was all too happy to accept.[11] Penfield, as he had of Whipple, asked Archibald if he could delay taking up his position at the Royal Victoria Hospital to study with Otfrid Foerster, in Breslau, Germany, a request to which Archibald readily agreed.

Foerster had trained in neurology with Jules Dejerine, Pierre Marie, and Joseph Babinski in Paris. From Paris, Foerster had gone to England, where he visited David Ferrier's laboratory at a time when Ferrier was studying the localization of motor

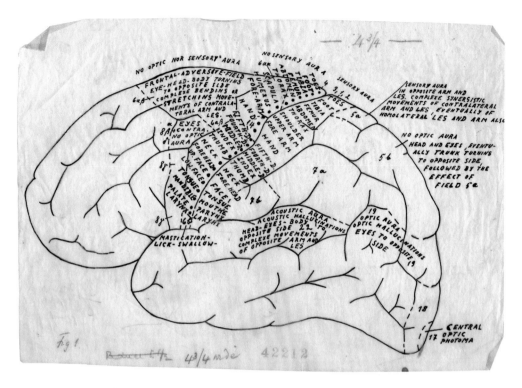

Figure 3.4. Foerster's brain map translated into English by Penfield. The small printed numbers represent somatotopic areas as originally delineated by Cécile and Oskar Vogt in the monkey. Montreal Neurological Institute and McGill University.

function of the brain in a variety of animals. Foerster assisted Karl Wernicke when he returned to Breslau before settling into his neurological practice. Foerster became a neurosurgeon by necessity when, during the Great War, he took up the scalpel due to a shortage of qualified surgeons to operate on soldiers with neurological injuries. Following the war Foerster gained international recognition for the surgical treatment of posttraumatic epilepsy and for his studies on the localization of the sensorimotor functions of the human brain.[12]

Penfield did not go to Breslau unprepared. He was expert in the use of the cutting-edge technology of the day, the Spanish silver and gold methods of staining the cells of the central nervous system. In Breslau, he learned Foerster's approach and technique for the surgical treatment of epilepsy. In return, he studied Foerster's resected specimens to see if the meningocerebral cicatrix that he had discovered in animals also occurred in man. And so, on 22 April 1928, Penfield wrote to his mother,

Last Sunday came a telegram from Foerster to say he would operate on a case that I would be interested in, the next day. He did a splendid operation removing a 16-year-old gunshot wound scar from the brain … He made it possible to get hold of some chemicals and I took the specimen for examination. During the next three or four days I worked hard at the tissue and succeeded in getting some very pretty stains of different kinds of glia cells. *In such tissue lies hidden some of the secrets of epilepsy.*[13]

The case in question was that of a German World War I veteran who had been shot in the left side of the head in the opening days of hostilities.[14] The injury was to the parietal area, and it had left him with loss of sensation and a tremor of the right arm. The patient later developed focal motor seizures and was eventually admitted to Foerster's service. A pneumoencephalogram (PEG), a procedure in which air is insufflate into the lumbar subarachnoid space through a lumbar puncture and

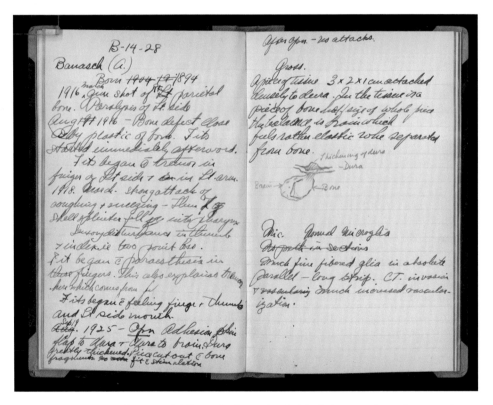

Figure 3.5. Two pages from Penfield's Breslau's case book. The left page relates the case of patient upon whom Foerster operated. The right page contains a gross, macroscopic description and a drawing of the resected specimen, and a description of its microscopic features. The text reads: "Gross. A piece of tissue 3 x 2 x 1 cm attached diffusely to dura. In the tissue is a piece of bone half size of whole piece the balance is brain, which feels rather elastic [when] separated from bone. Mic[roscopy]. Normal microglia. [Crossed out] Much fine fibered glia in absolute parallel – long strip. CT [cortex] invasion [crossed out] much increased vascularization." The drawing is an illustration of the meningocerebral cicatrix. The dura is the thick, longitudinal structure on the surface of the specimen. The scar continues under the dura and is composed of three elements: sclerotic brain tissue making up the mass of the scar, a fragment of bone (dotted) embedded within the scar, and parallel glial fibres. McGill University, William Feindel Fond.

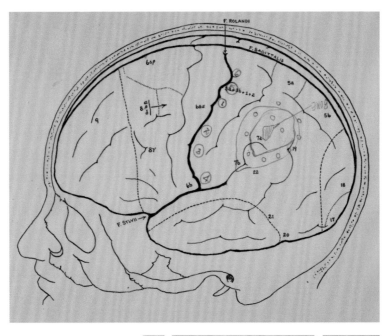

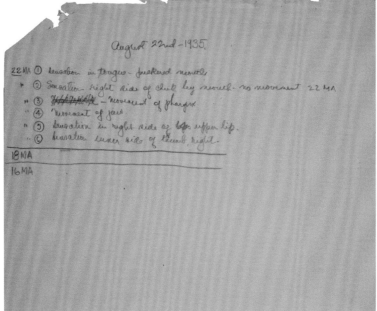

Figure 3.6. *Top*. Penfield's operative map of a patient with a meningocerebral cicatrix from a penetrating head injury. The operative findings are recorded on Foerster's transcription of the Vogts' simian brain map that Penfield had begun to use to illustrate his operative findings. The meningocerebral cicatrix is outlined as the smaller circle within the larger circle that represents the area to be resected. The encircled numbers represent the results of cortical stimulation and identify the postcentral gyrus. The small, open circles about and within the cicatrix indicate points where electrical stimulation had no effect. *Bottom*. The results of cortical stimulation were recorded on the verso of the map. Stimulation produced: 1. sensation in the tongue and puckering of the mouth, 2. sensation in the right side of the cheek, 3. movement of the pharynx, 4. movement of the jaw, 5. sensation of the right upper lip, 6. sensation of the inner side of the right thumb. Montreal Neurological Hospital, case C.G., 1935.

makes its way into the ventricles of the brain, showed that the left lateral ventricle was enlarged and displaced towards the site of injury – a finding to which Foerster referred as "the wandering ventricle," and a term that Penfield adopted in his early writings. Based on the clinical aspects of the patient's seizures and the radiological findings, Foerster decided to operate. Foerster, operating under local anaesthesia, did not raise a bone flap as we would today, but rather he chipped away, bit by bit, at the skull until an opening of adequate size was created. Proceeding in this way, he eventually uncovered the dura and found it to be adherent to an underlying, cystic cortical scar. With the aid of a stimulating electrode Foerster found that the scar was immediately behind the cortical area responsible for movements of the fingers.[15] The lesion was removed, avoiding encroachment on the motor strip, and the patient was relieved of his seizures. Penfield studied the resected specimen and found that

> A bit of bone was embedded in the cicatrix and bands of fibrous tissue could be seen passing downward into the brain. Microscopic examination shows the connective tissue to be entering the brain scar in more or less parallel lines. Closer examination shows these bands to be made up of blood vessels and sturdy collagen fibres. When stained so as to demonstrate both collagen fibres and neuroglia fibres, it is seen that the two types of fibres are more or less intermingled and parallel as though they were strands in a rope. Deeper in the brain neuroglia fibres are found lying in parallel lines, pointing upwards towards the meningo-cerebral adhesion.

As Penfield further observed, the associated cortex was thinned and gliotic, and nerve cells were few, if present. The "outstanding feature of all of these scars," he wrote, "was the rich plexus of newly formed vessels in and about the cicatrix."[16] With this last observation, what had been suggested by the animal studies now became a fully formed hypothesis on the aetiology of posttraumatic epilepsy in man. Penfield conceived of two possible explanations for the cause of posttraumatic epilepsy: damage to the cortical nerve cells from the initial trauma or the vascular reaction in response to it.[17] "But," Penfield reasoned, "if cellular damage was the cause, the attacks should start shortly after the injury."[18] This, however, was not the case. Epilepsy following a penetrating injury of the brain often appeared months or even years after the event. Another mechanism had to be sought to account for the delayed development of the epileptogenic focus. The gradual maturation of the cicatricial vascular plexus, of its anastomosis with the arteries at the periphery of the scar, and the gradual contraction of the cicatrix, Penfield thought, could account for the delay.[19]

Penfield published two papers in rapid succession on the surgical treatment of epilepsy upon his return from Breslau to Montreal: a long paper coauthored with Foerster in which they described the meningocerebral cicatrix and the results of its resection, and another, shorter paper, entitled "The Radical Treatment of Traumatic Epilepsy and its Rationale,"[20] in which Penfield reported for the first time his own experience with the surgical treatment of epilepsy. In it he described the semiology of epilepsy arising from different parts of the brain and how the offending scar can be localized by PEG. This was followed by a description of surgery performed under local anaesthesia aided by electricocortical stimulation, as he had learned from Foerster. Penfield ended his paper with a description of the meningocerebral cicatrix and the statement that the "*radical, clean excision of a contracting scar does not result in scar reformation,*"[21] as Krause had surmised two decades before.

THE CORTICAL CICATRIX:
A CAREFULLY CONSIDERED HYPOTHESIS[22]

Penfield considered the meningocerebral cicatrix as a clinical-pathological entity produced by a *penetrating* wound to the head. In contradistinction, a *cortical cicatrix* resulted from a panoply of causes in which the calverium was not breached. These included intra-uterine complications, difficult labour and birth injury, meningo-encephalitis, cerebral abscesses, and nonpenetrating cranio-cerebral trauma. In the latter case the sudden impact of the blow can damage the neurons, glial cells, and small superficial blood vessels of the cortex and white matter, creating a local contusion. The damaged, nonviable cells are scavenged by microglia, and fibrous astrocytes invade the contused area, which becomes atrophic and gliotic. The atrophic area takes on a yellowish hue as the extravasated blood cells degenerate and discolour the cortex. Although not as florid as a meningocerebral cicatrix, a cortical scar can be highly epileptogenic as it matures over time. If the blow is more severe, frank hemorrhage can ensue within the contused area and the subjacent white matter. In that circumstance, the scar can become cystic as the blood and necrotic brain are resorbed and liquefy and can even act as a mass lesion, much like a tumour, as the hemorrhagic cyst slowly expands. The clinical syndrome produced by a cortical cicatrix is identical to that resulting from a meningocerebral cicatrix, but the cortical scar can be more difficult to localize, as there are often no external signs of trauma. If this was the case, Penfield relied on the clinical history, on the physical examination, and on the PEG to localize the offending lesion.

Penfield's approach to the investigation of a patient with focal epilepsy began with a detailed history designed to bring out any antecedent that might have contributed to its onset. Penfield then obtained a detailed description of the seizures from the patient and from his or her family. Clues obtained by history that were suggestive of the location of the seizure focus were few, as the semiology of epilepsy was poorly defined at the time. Head and eye turning and a Jacksonian march were useful in lateralizing the epileptic focus to the right or left hemisphere and in localizing the

focus to the frontal lobe and central area. Any asymmetry in the physical examination – a facial droop, weakness of one hand, a Babinski sign – could also point to
the hemisphere involved, if not to the site of the offending lesion. The presence of
calcification seen on plain skull X-ray was a useful if infrequent finding, which
helped to localize the site of a calcified scar, tumour, or vascular malformation.[23]
The PEG was a mainstay of ancillary examinations.[24] Simple in concept, it was a
dreaded procedure for both practitioner and patient. It consisted of removing cerebrospinal fluid through a lumbar puncture and the insufflation of a like volume of
air into the subarachnoid space. The air then made its way up through the subarachnoid space around the spinal cord and entered the cerebral ventricles. Air, being less
dense than the skull and the substance of the brain, outlined the ventricles on an
X-ray plate and demonstrated any change in their configuration that might indicate
the presence of a scar or tumour. The PEG was especially useful in cases of temporal
lobe epilepsy when focal enlargement of the temporal horn of the lateral ventricle
was demonstrated.[25]

A typical procedure is described from a patient's chart:

Sitting position. Initial pressure 250 mms of water. Very free flow of spinal fluid
under increased pressure. Exchange carried out in 5 cc. amounts rather rapidly.
The first two amounts of 10 cc. were exchanged for 5. When 60 cc. of air had been
injected patient commenced to get faint and spinal fluid pressure was low. Pressure was raised and air exchange continued until 100 cc. of air had been injected
and 105 cc. of fluid withdrawn. Patient had a fair amount of reaction from the
injection, with some vomiting and pain over the right orbit.[26]

The vomiting and head pain were caused by the irritating effect of the air inside
the cavities of the brain, and it might take several days for the air to be absorbed
and the discomfort to abate. Ventriculography was another diagnostic procedure
that was sometimes used. It consisted of puncturing the brain with a blunt needle
through a burr hole placed in the skull and insufflating air directly into the ven-
tricular system. Ventriculography provided more detailed and reliable images than
PEG but, because of its inherent risk, it was reserved for cases that were more difficult to diagnose.[27]

Craniotomy was undertaken on the basis of the concordance of history, clinical
signs, and radiological findings. Later, EEG recordings were added to the diagnostic
armamentarium, but it took some time after its introduction at the MNI before Penfield relied on it in the absence of a structural lesion demonstrated by PEG or uncovered at surgery. On occasion, the EEG would fail to reveal the source of a patient's
epilepsy. In this circumstance, the epileptogenic focus could be uncovered by having
the patient hyperventilate or by injecting the stimulant drug metrazol, which caused

the patient to have an epileptic attack while the EEG was being recorded. The patient's case and its diagnostic findings were discussed at the Clinical EEG Conference, where a decision on the advisability of surgery was made.

By necessity, the craniotomy was large, so as to expose as much of the brain as possible to identify any abnormality and to allow electrocortical stimulation of the cerebral convolutions. The exposed cortex might display adhesions to the overlying dura mater and discolouration of one or more gyri if the causative lesion had been haemorrhagic. Thin convolutions were seen if an atrophic process, such as a scar, was the offending agent, and multiple, small gyri were seen with polymicrogyria. Alternatively, the gyri might be flat and wide and the sulci shallow and drained of CSF if a tumour or cyst was hidden in the subcortical white matter and pressing upward, compressing the cortex. Gentle palpation with the index finger was then a useful tool, revealing the soft necrotic centre of a cystic lesion and its hardened edges, roughly delineating its limits. Conversely, a uniformly firm area indicated a subcortical tumour. Cortical stimulation was necessary to identify motor, sensory, or speech areas before any resection could be undertaken in order to avoid encroaching upon it during the resection of the epileptic area.[28] This was performed by applying a gentle current to a point on the cortex using a handheld electrode connected to an electrical generator by a sterile wire.

Penfield recorded all cortical responses and the associated pathology by sketching the exposed area of brain onto a sterilized sheet of paper using a blunt-point, sterilized pencil. Sometimes the blunt-tipped pencil did double duty and served as a pointer. Especially interesting cases were also professionally rendered by a medial illustrator. Later, a preprinted brain map was used to record the effects of stimulation and the epileptic areas. The initial type of brain map used by Penfield at the Royal Victoria Hospital indicated the somatotopic areas as originally delineated by Cécile and Oskar Vogt in the monkey and which Foerster adapted to the human brain.[29]

After Penfield and Cone moved to the MNI, in addition to drawing the exposed brain, photographs were taken through an ingenious array of lenses and mirrors, before and after stimulation and resection.[30] The collaboration between the Vogts at the Kaiser Wilhelm Institute in Berlin and Foerster in Breslau was well described by Igor Klatzo, who worked with the Vogts before coming to the MNI after the Second World War:

Although all their data was limited to animal experimentation, in which primates were mostly used, the Vogts were full of anticipation that their experimental findings could be substantiated by observations in man. It came soon to happen, when Otfried [*sic*] Foerster, the prominent neurosurgeon from Breslau, started to use cortical electrical stimulation to facilitate the localization of an epileptogenic focus in patients suffering from seizures. This opened the opportunity to

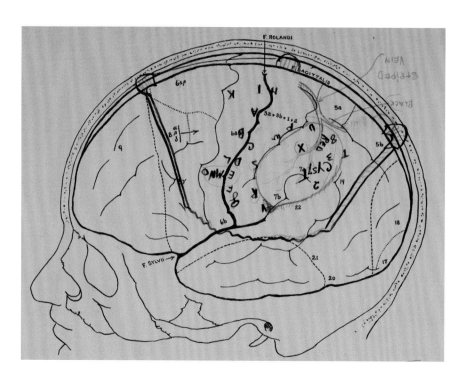

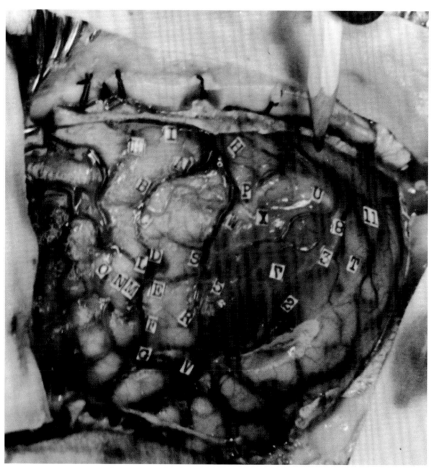

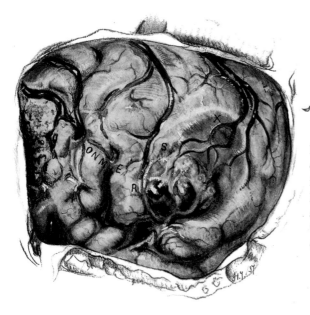

Figure 3.9. Artistic representation of the phenomenon illustrated in the previous two figures. Montreal Neurological Institute and McGill University. Penfield, "The Cerebral Cortex and Consciousness."

verify in human brains the close interrelationship between cyroarchitectonic features and physiological responses, as observed in experimental animals. A triumphant point of collaboration between the Vogts and Foerster on this subject was reached when, on the same day, they mailed from Berlin and Breslau separately accumulated charts containing marked points of cortical stimulation with description of observed physiological responses in primate and human brains, respectively. The comparisons of these independently obtained observations revealed a striking similarity between man and monkeys regarding the topographic patterns and close association between cytoarchitectonic substrate and type of an elicited response.[31]

The extraordinary success of neurosurgery and neuroscience when applied to a common problem as exemplified by Foerster and the Vogts was not lost on Penfield when he conceived of the Montreal Neurological Institute.

Figure 3.7. *Opposite top* Operative sketch of a patient with focal epilepsy from a posttraumatic, cystic scar. After a seizure produced by electrical stimulation at point X, the vein emanating from the cyst contained oxygenated blood and appeared red. The topmost arrow is pointing at a vein draining the cyst, which contained an admixture of venous and arterial blood. Montreal Neurological Hospital.

Figure 3.8. *Opposite bottom* Intraoperative photograph of the exposed hemisphere in the same patient as in the preceding figure. The pencil tip is pointing at the vein containing an admixture of arterialized and venous blood. Montreal Neurological Hospital.

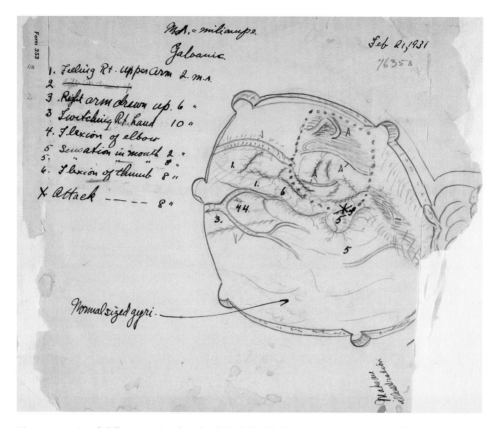

Figure 3.10. Penfield's operative sketch of the left-sided craniotomy performed in case W.S. The orientation of the illustrated operative field is unconventional. Turning the sketch 45 degrees to the right provides the anatomical view. The Y-shaped vein at the left of the illustration between the numbers 3 and 44 represents the Rolandic vein as it courses towards the superior sagittal sinus at the vertex of the head. The area of cortical scarring and two prominent arteries mentioned in Penfield's operative report are in the parietal lobe. They are contained within the dotted lines and are identified by the letter "A." The dotted lines also indicate the extent of the resection. Stimulation at the point indicated by the letter "X" produced a focal seizure, which was followed by a generalized convulsion. The text at left indicates that galvanic stimulation was performed at 2 to 10 milliamperes and reads as follows: 1. Feeling in the right upper arm, 2. illegible, crossed out, 3. right arm drawn up, 3. Twitching of the right hand, 4. flexion of the elbow, 5. sensation in the mouth, [the ditto marks indicate the same response], 6. flexion of the thumb. Montreal Neurological Hospital, case W.S., 1931.

Penfield's approach to the resection of a simple posttraumatic cortical cicatrix was similar to Foerster's and is illustrated by the case of patient W.S. This case also illustrates that, although the scar might be simple, intracranial surgery never is.

W.S. sustained a cerebral contusion when he was nine years old and fell from his bicycle onto the left side of his head. He later developed focal motor seizures of the right arm, which were sometimes heralded by a sensory aura. He was admitted to the MNI in 1931, at the age of twenty-two. Examination revealed a scar on the scalp overlying the left parietal region and weakness of the right arm. The clinical findings and the description of the seizures clearly identified a left central epileptic focus, and it was decided not to submit the patient to the discomfort of a PEG. The patient underwent a large, left parietal osteoplastic craniotomy. Reflection of the dura revealed that the sulci between the exposed convolutions were widened, which indicated that the initial trauma had produced a more extensive injury than had been appreciated and had resulted in diffuse cortical atrophy. This was all the more evident at the level of the Sylvian fissure, which was appreciably wider and deeper than is usually seen in a person of the patient's age. The inferior aspect of the parietal lobe was markedly atrophic and was traversed by two large arteries. Cortical stimulation indicated that the atrophic, scarred area lay within the postcentral gyrus. A seizure was produced as Penfield was exploring the area about the scar with the stimulating electrode. The seizure was focal and consisted of movement of the right side of the face and turning of the head and eyes to the left. Penfield observed that the arteries traversing the scar lost all pulsation for the duration of the attack but that arteries in other parts of the exposed brain remained pulsatile. As the pulse returned in the affected arteries, the patient's seizure became generalized. At this time, as Penfield noted in his operative report, "The venous pressure rose enormously and haemorrhage from numerous veins was profuse." Tamponading the bleeding points with cotton sponges controlled the bleeding, and it abated at the end of the seizure. The bleeding now under control, the scar was removed, along with the two reactive arteries. The area excised measured some seven centimetres in diameter. Bleeding from a large dural vein draining into the superior sagittal sinus was incurred with closing of the dura. Packing the area with a small piece of muscle harvested from the temporalis muscle and the hypotension from blood loss eventually arrested the bleeding. Despite the heart-stopping intraoperative complications, Penfield dispassionately noted in his operative report, "the fact that the arteries in this area stopped pulsating during the focal seizure is excellent evidence that there is a local vasomotor phenomenon associated with these seizures." William Cone examined the resected specimen and observed, "The tissue is of tough consistency in one area containing a core of dull grey scar tissue of great tensile strength, through which may be seen small blood vessels. The rest of the tissue is diffusely scarred to a lesser but very definite extent. On section it is glossy grey in areas, with whitish parallel strands coursing perpendicularly to the cortex."

Penfield's observation on the changing appearance of the arteries within the scar in response to focal and generalized seizures, and Cone's histological observations, added support to Penfield's vascular theory of epileptogenesis, which he would continue to explore as he and Cone relocated across University Street to the Montreal Neurological Institute.

CHAPTER 4

Conjectures and Refutations

DARK CONJECTURE

*Watching the brain during the epileptic seizures demonstrated to us
phenomena associated with epilepsy, which before were no more than
dark conjecture* –Penfield[1]

The description of the meningocerebral cicatrix was one of Penfield's first contributions to epileptology. Using gold and silver stains, Penfield observed that the meningocerebral cicatrix is composed of radially arranged strands of fibrous tissue. Abnormal blood vessels invade the region as the collagenous core thickens, solidifies, and contracts. Penfield stressed that the meshwork of blood vessels entrapped within the cicatricial core anastomosed with the blood vessels of the cortex at the periphery of the scar. The vascular constituent of the meningocerebral cicatrix suggested to Penfield that the vessels encased in the scar exerted a progressive traction on the normal cortical vessels with which they anastomosed. The relative ischemia that resulted, he surmised, would render the cortex epileptogenic. Thus, Penfield concluded, "the hypothesis at once suggests itself that a *vasomotor reflex* secondary to this traction is responsible for the initiation of the convulsive seizures."[2] This, however, was not a new notion.

THE VASCULAR HYPOTHESIS

Broadly stated, the vascular hypothesis of epileptogenesis held that epileptic seizures are triggered by cortical ischemia resulting from reflex constriction of cerebral arteries.[3] The vascular hypothesis was based on Claude Bernard's 1851 discovery that transection of the cervical sympathetic chain caused increased blood flow in a rabbit's ear and elevated the temperature of its brain. These phenomena were reversed when he stimulated the distal end of the sympathetic chain with an electrical current.[4] Bernard concluded from these experiments that the intracranial circulation

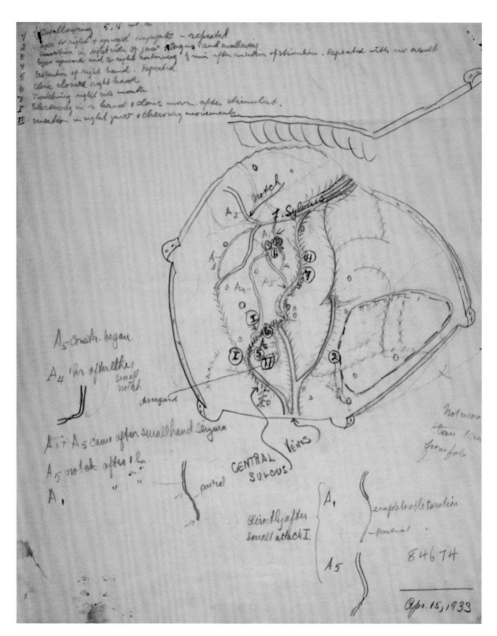

Figure 4.1. Brain map, surgeon's viewpoint, of a patient operated upon for left frontal lobe epilepsy, illustrating various severities of arterial constriction. Such findings led Penfield to believe that epileptic seizures were triggered by a vaso-constrictive reflex and ischemia. Montreal Neurological Hospital, case D.S., 1933.

is under the influence of the sympathetic nervous system, which produced vaso-constriction, and of another, as yet unspecified system, which produced vasodilation. Penfield and his research fellow, Jerzy Choróbski, would discover the parasympathetic nature of this system and its pathway from the medulla oblongata to the intracranial arteries in the early 1930s.[5]

Adolf Kaussmaul and Adolf Tenner observed in 1857 that electrical stimulation of the cervical sympathetic system of rabbits, in which a circumscribed area of the skull had been replaced with a watch glass, produced constriction of the cortical arteries and convulsive attacks. These experiments led them to conclude, *"epileptic convulsions can be brought about by contraction of blood vessels induced by vasomotor nerves."*[6] Jacobus van der Kolk, a highly influential anatamo-histologist and contemporary of Kaussmaul, shared this opinion and located the epileptogenic focus, whose irritation led to "spasm upon the cerebral vessels" and triggered an epileptic seizure, within the ganglion cells of the medulla oblongata.[7] Evidence that seizures originate from the cerebral convolutions was lacking until the experiments of Gustav Fritsch and Eduard Hitzig on the cortex of the dog in 1870. Fritsch and Hitzig observed that, in some of their dogs, cortical stimulation of the motor cortex produced focal motor seizures.[8] John Hughlings Jackson situated the "discharging lesion" at the origin of focal epileptic attacks within the convolutions of the brain and proposed that vasoconstriction was at the origin of epileptic seizures and their propagation along the motor strip.[9] Jackson considered that each functional area of the motor cortex – the face, the arm, the leg – had its own, distinct vascular supply and conceived that an epileptic discharge, once begun, "leads to further and further discharges in the vascular region in which the unstable nerve tissue lies."[10] And there the vascular hypothesis lay, until surgeons began performing exploratory craniotomies and observed cortical vessels directly as epileptic seizures were triggered by electrocortical stimulation.[11]

While Penfield was at Queen Square assisting him in the operating room, Percy Sargent was preparing a brilliant address with the deceptively simple title of "Some Observations on Epilepsy," which he delivered to the Royal Society of Medicine on 13 October 1921.[12] Predictably, Sargent's address dealt with the contributions that neurosurgery could make to the treatment of focal epilepsy. But, Sargent told his audience, "surgical procedures for the treatment of epilepsy … *are greatly hampered by the obscurity which still exists as to the essential factors that underlie convulsive attacks in general.*" Of utmost importance, therefore, was "the desirability of searching in every case for the physical basis which forms the starting point of the convulsive seizures."[13] The starting point, Sargent thought, was cerebral ischemia:

during the frequent opportunities which I have had of viewing the living brain, under both normal and abnormal conditions, I have been greatly impressed by the striking rapidity with which visible circulatory changes may occur in response to various disturbing causes. I cannot help feeling that sufficient importance is not attached to the possible effects upon cerebral function of what may perhaps be called minor and transitory circulatory disturbances. It is not upon the congestion or anaemia of the brain as a whole that I would lay stress, but upon the local variations and abnormalities which can be observed in connection with tumours and various traumatic lesions. It seems to me that the only local influence which an operation can have upon an epileptogenous area … must be exercised through the medium of the local circulation. If there is a fundamental precipitating cause for all convulsive attacks, any hypothesis which does not take into account the pathogenesis of fits originating in the neighbourhood of a gross lesion must fail to touch that essential point.[14]

Sargent gave a telling example of how such a synergy might trigger an epileptic fit in patients who had sustained a gunshot wound to the head – of which he saw many as the consulting neurosurgeon to the British Expeditionary Force during the First World War. Sargent had observed that penetrating head injuries often produced a dense collagenous scar that extended from the cortex to the subcutaneous layers of the scalp through the cranial defect created by the injury. In these cases, he proposed that changes in position of the head might cause a vascular reflex leading to transient ischemia about the scar, which resulted in a focal epileptic attack. Thus, Sargent devised an operation, which he performed on some 200 patients, in which the scar was removed and the adhesions were lyzed.

When a brain, attached to the scalp by adhesions, attempts to move in response to a change of posture, it is prevented from doing so from a pull at the point of anchorage; this pull either mechanically or, possibly, by causing a reflex vasoconstriction, may well produce a momentary local anemia in the damaged brain, and so initiate a fit … We now possess a good deal of evidence to show that the fits can in many cases be either abolished, or very considerably reduced in number and severity, by an operation which succeeds in removing or at least modifying, the local exciting cause.[15]

A vascular mechanism was not limited to posttraumatic scars, but, in Sargent's view, it was also applicable to epilepsy caused by other structural lesions, such as a brain tumour, as he had observed, "In the immediate neighbourhood of many of these lesions the appearances are such as to suggest that rapid or sudden alterations of vascularity could readily take place."[16]

Percy Sargent's influence on Penfield's career has not previously been seen in its true light. It is as Sargent's assistant that Penfield acquired his first practical experience in operative neurosurgery, which led to his appointment as the designated neuro-surgeon at the Presbyterian Hospital in New York. Just as importantly, Sargent's "Some Observations on Epilepsy" raised the putative role of vasomotor reflexes in the generation and propagation of epileptic seizures, a hypothesis that Penfield embraced and which guided his clinical and basic research for more than a decade. But most of all, Penfield took this from Percy Sargent: "I am convinced that, in properly selected cases, surgical treatment [of focal epilepsy] can be of great value in lessening the task demanded of medicinal and other therapeutic measures."[17]

The vascular hypothesis was based on uncontrolled, intra-operative observations. Less anecdotal evidence in support of the hypothesis came form Walther Spielmeyer's microscopic studies of epileptic brains. Walther Spielmeyer was a notable figure in the history of twentieth-century neurology, and, as director of the Kaiser Wilhelm Institute of Neuropathology, he was an early visitor to the MNI. Spielmeyer gave a highly influential address to the Association for Research in Nervous and Mental Disease in New York City in 1929, in which he suggested that recurrent vasospasm was a factor in initiating epileptic attacks.[18] Spielmeyer based this opinion on the microscopic changes that he had observed in epileptic cortex, which he thought were characteristic of ischemia. This led Spielmeyer to conclude, "that vasomotor disturbances are effective in the mechanism of the epileptic attack."[19] Undoubtedly spurred by Spielmeyer's address, Penfield reviewed his surgical cases for evidence of vasoconstriction in the cortices that he had exposed at surgery by reviewing his brain maps and operative reports. He found twenty-six cases in which he had observed unusual reactions of cortical arteries that were concurrent with the beginning or end of a spontaneous or electrically induced seizure. Penfield reported his observations in a paper entitled "The Evidence for a Cerebral Vascular Mechanism in Epilepsy," which he read before the American College of Physicians when it met in Montreal in 1933.[20]

The vascular changes that Penfield observed in association with epileptic seizures were varied, but they were initiated in most cases by constriction or occlusion of large cortical arteries in which blood flow either took on a bluish, venous hue or stopped completely. In some cases, the radial pulse was lost. This suggested to Penfield that there might have been a generalized sympathetic discharge associated with the seizure. In most cases, however, the phenomenon was restricted to the brain. As a result of his analysis Penfield concluded that, "from a purely morphologic point of view, intracerebral vasomotor reflexes are possible."[21] Whatever the mechanism, Penfield noted, "very little blood is passing through the capillary bed of the brain during the actual seizure."[22] As the epileptic attack abated, the arteries in which pulsation had stopped now began to pulsate anew, rapidly and vigorously, and the blood that they carried became bright red. The arterial circulation was so enhanced that in some cases even the veins took on a reddish appearance, a phenomenon that Penfield thought to be the result of post-ictal shunting of arterial blood through a newly dilated capillary bed.[23]

In contradistinction to the dramatic effects of post-ictal arterial dilatation, Penfield had also observed that *spasmodic closure of large arteries*[24] sometimes followed the epileptic attack, at least in some patients. This was characterized by "constriction of one or more pial arteries, a constriction which shut off the vessel completely. It may be at one point or it may extend a long distance, or there may be multiple constrictions."[25] The cortical areas irrigated by these arteries appeared blanched as they became anaemic. A dramatic demonstration of this occurrence is exemplified by the case of patient M.B.

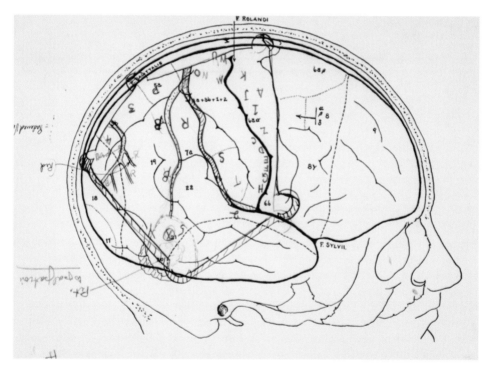

Figure 4.2. Brain map of a patient who had suffered from right otitis media as a child, and focal motor and sensory seizures involving the left side of the body. There was "a rather marked area of softening so that the finger went into the brain there as it did not do elsewhere" in the posterior aspect of the second temporal convolution as it joined the angular gyrus, where stimulation produced an epileptic seizure. "After the production of a seizure by stimulation at X it was gradually observed that the veins draining that particular area were carrying oxygenated blood and not quite as bright red as I had seen in other cases but definitely much brighter than in the other dark veins." Montreal Neurological Hospital, case J.R., 1937.

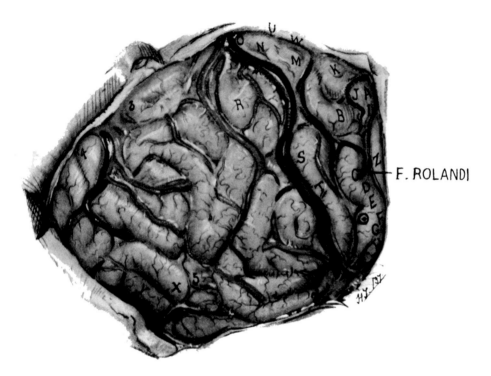

F. ROLANDI

Figure 4.3. *Above* Illustration of the red cerebral veins observed in the previous figure. Penfield concluded that red, oxygenated blood in veins draining an epileptogenic cortical area were the reflection of a hypermetabolic state associated with a cerebral seizure. Montreal Neurological Institute and McGill University, case J.R., 1937, Penfield, "The Cerebral Cortex and Consciousness."

Figure 4.4. *Opposite* Penfield's operative sketch drawn from the surgeon's viewpoint. The top of the head is at the lowermost aspect of the drawing, where the midline of the skull is indicated by the words "MID LINE" and where the reflected dura is folded upon itself. The prominent line just to the left of centre indicates the Rolandic fissure, which is labelled as the "central sulcus." The Y-shaped structure that parallels it to the right is the Rolandic vein, which is seen entering the superior sagittal sinus under the folded dura. The results of cortical stimulation are numbered and recorded on the map: 1. flexion of the right wrist, 2. extension of the right wrist and flexion of the fingers, 3. numbness of the mouth, 4. clonic movements of the muscles of the whole right arm. The star (*) indicates the point where stimulation of the cortex "inaugurated" a convulsion. The dotted line represents the pallor of the cortex that followed the first convulsion, which Penfield ascribed to vasoconstriction of the artery (A-2) supplying the epileptogenic area. The area encircled by the dashed line illustrates a blanched area resulting from the constriction of artery A-1, which appeared after the second convulsion. The X at the end of the curving arrow indicates the site of constriction of the artery A-1. The constriction of this artery is faintly reproduced and enlarged at the bottom of the page. Montreal Neurological hospital, case M.B., 1930.

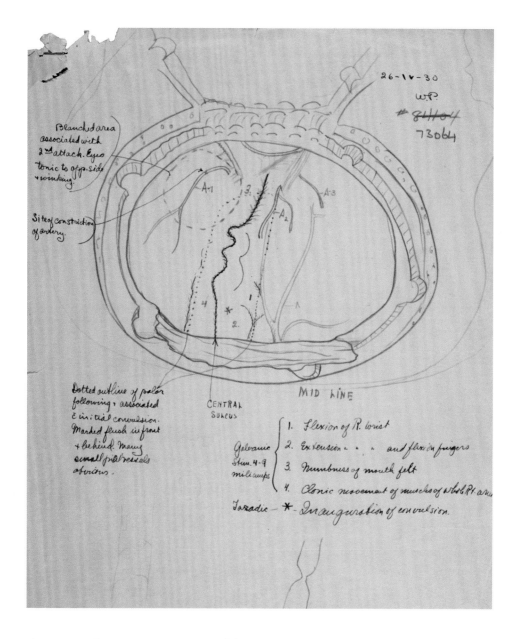

A strange phenomenon was noted[26]

M.B. was nine months old in 1918 when his parents first observed uncontrolled shaking of his right arm. By the time he was three years old he was having one or two episodes per week. He was free of seizures from ages four to eleven, when his attacks recurred and became progressively more frequent. He was admitted to the MNI in 1930 when he was thirteen years old. A craniotomy was performed with the expectation that a focal, structural lesion would be uncovered, but none was obvious within the large cortical area exposed at surgery. Cortical stimulation identified the

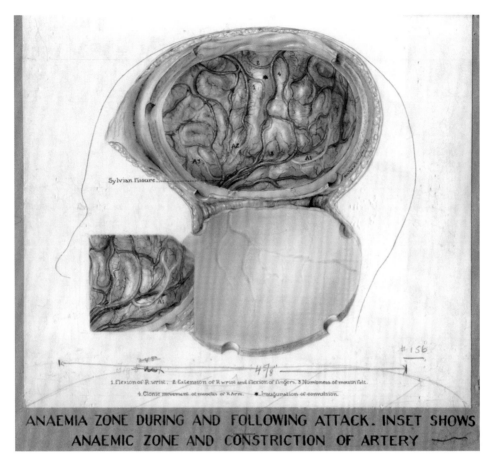

ANAEMIA ZONE DURING AND FOLLOWING ATTACK. INSET SHOWS
ANAEMIC ZONE AND CONSTRICTION OF ARTERY

Figure 4.5. Harriett Blackstock's depiction of Penfield's operative sketch, rendered in the anatomical view. Montreal Neurological Institute and McGill University, case M.B.

hand and arm regions within the pre- and postcentral gyri. As Penfield applied the stimulating electrode to the inferior aspect of the motor strip a "strange phenomenon was noted": a prolonged convulsion ensued coincident with the constriction of a prominent cortical artery, and the pre- and postcentral gyri changed "from a good color to blanching … in the almost imperceptible way that a cloud shadow may be seen to cross the landscape on a sunny day."[27] The remainder of the cortex remained suffused with a reddish tinge. As the convulsion subsided, the previously constricted artery began to pulsate violently and the pale areas began to display their normal, reddish hue. This and similar cases led Penfield to conclude that

the vasomotor spasms and changes seen so characteristically in the cerebral cortex of epileptics are due to vasomotor reflexes but reflexes that are probably not subserved by autonomic neurones placed outside of the cranial cavity. They seem to be subserved by such nerve cells upon the blood vessels of the brain and by a local vascular nerve plexus, which I believe from histological studies to be significantly increased at least in some cases. Where such a lesion exists, excision of a focal scar with its vascular plexus is at present the most effective way of abolishing these malignant local reflexes.[28]

No resection was performed, and M.B. subsequently underwent a sympathectomy, to no avail.[29]

Arterial ligation

But what if there was no scar? In some cases, as that of M.B., Penfield observed one or more prominent arteries supplying an epileptogenic area that had been identified by cortical stimulation. The epileptogenic area, however, appeared unremarkable to inspection and normal to gentle palpation. The thought occurred to Penfield that excising or ligating these arteries might interrupt the reflex arc that caused their constriction. Penfield first did this in a patient from New York that he had met in Foerster's clinic and who later sought his counsel in Montreal.

The patient was a young man, William Ottman,[30] who had been born after a difficult, prolonged labour. William began having epileptic attacks when he was thirteen years old, and his mother had sought consultation with Foerster three years later, in August 1928, when Penfield was in Breslau. Foerster recommended a ventriculogram to identify a putative epileptogenic lesion, but William's mother, Madeleine Ottmann, wavered when the procedure was described to her, and she asked for Penfield's advice. Under the circumstances Penfield could do little until he was free to consult on the patient in his own clinic.[31] This occasion arose in March 1929, when William was admitted to Penfield's service at the Royal Victoria Hospital. A ventriculogram was performed and showed evidence of a long-standing, atrophic process involving the left hemisphere, undoubtedly the result of a birth injury. Despite this lateralizing finding, a focal lesion could not be localized. Electroencephalography was not available at the time and, as William did not have a seizure during his hospitalization, Penfield could not deduce the origin of the attacks. Surgery could not, therefore, be confidently recommended. Nonetheless, Madeleine Ottmann made a substantial gift to the MNI in gratitude for Penfield's solicitude, which allowed Penfield to pursue his research activities and to fund a fellowship program in epilepsy. It was the first gift that the MNI had received without solicitation.[32] William was readmitted to the MNI in January 1930, as his seizures had worsened. By this time, it was apparent that his attacks originated near the hand region and Penfield was prepared to undertake exploratory surgery. However, since the ventriculogram had not demonstrated a scar, Penfield called upon Walter Spielmeyer to come from Munich to be present at the operation, to offer whatever insight he could on any pathology that might be exposed at surgery. Penfield also asked Stanley Cobb, one of his closest friends and a neurologist at Boston City Hospital, to join Spielmeyer. Cone would assist.

Exposure of the cortex confirmed the findings of the PEG: all of the exposed convolutions were atrophic, without any one appearing more affected than another. But Penfield also observed an unusually large branch of the middle cerebral artery emerging from the Sylvian fissure, which coursed toward the pre- and postcentral gyri.[33] Electrocortical stimulation identified the motor strip, but further stimulation to delineate Broca's area produced a violent generalized seizure. The violence of the seizure caused venous engorgement and bleeding from many small cortical veins. As Penfield and Cone busied themselves with controlling the venous bleeding, Penfield noticed that, as the seizure abated, "snowy white patches" appeared on the crowns of the convolutions in the area that was supplied by the unusually large artery. The snowy patches formed a triangle whose apex was at the point from which the artery appeared from the Sylvian fissure, indicating that it supplied the area that had been rendered anaemic. Penfield concluded that the large artery had first caused increased blood flow to the epileptic area with the onset of the seizure and that secondary reflex vasoconstriction caused the cortex to blanch as the seizure abated. Surprisingly, Penfield suggested that the artery should be excised, presumably to interfere with the mechanism that he felt was the cause of the seizure. Spielmeyer and Cobb enthusiastically agreed. Cone, undoubtedly thinking that a hypothesis should not be tested on an exposed brain after a violent convulsion, disagreed. Penfield proceeded to resect the artery despite Cone's dissenting voice, and William suddenly stopped talking and was unable to move his right arm. Both the aphasia and paralysis gradually cleared, however, proving the old surgical adage that it is better to be lucky than good. As for William, he remained seizure-free for the rest of his life.[34] Buoyed by this success, Penfield resected "Ottman's artery" in three more cases without success, and abandoned the procedure.

CEREBROVASCULAR INNERVATION

Clinical observation of cortical arteries during the chaos of an epileptic seizure was not enough to confirm that they played a role in initiating, propagating, or stopping an epileptic attack. A mechanism other than traction on cortical arteries was needed to explain the triggering of a vasomotor reflex; this required the presence of nerve fibres supplying cerebral blood vessels. Penfield took to the laboratory and, using a novel staining technique devised by his technician, Edward Dockrill, was able to show that the arteries supplying the cortex and their penetrating branches are, indeed, innervated but, surprisingly, not by sympathetic nerves.[35] This Penfield determined when he observed that only a minority of the nerves were lost after

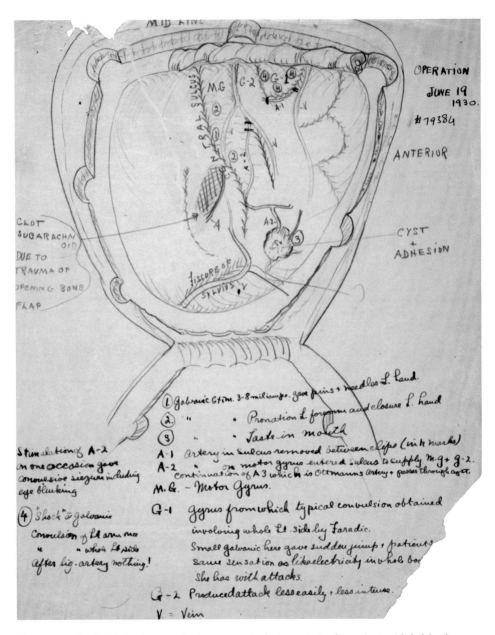

Figure 4.6. Penfield's brain map, in the anatomical viewpoint, of a patient with left body Jacksonian motor seizures, which became generalized. Craniotomy revealed a small cystic area in front of the motor strip to which coursed two arteries that appeared to be abnormal (A-1, A-2). Artery A-2 corresponds to the artery that Penfield had ligated in another patient, William Ottman, with beneficial effect and to which he referred as "Ottman's artery." Ligation of A-1 and A-2 in this case, however, was ineffectual, and the patient underwent the resection of the cystic area that had been supplied by these arteries eighteen months later. Montreal Neurological Hospital, case V.R., 1930.

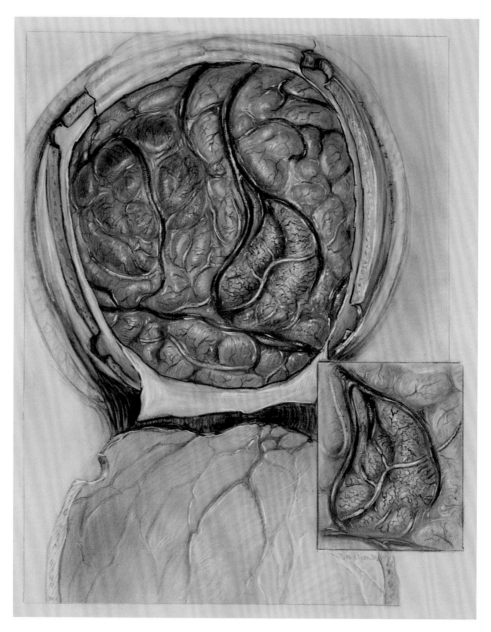

Figure 4.7. Harriet Blackstock's drawing of a blanched and focally constricted "Ottman's artery," a prominent cortical branch of the middle cerebral artery coursing over the right frontal operculum to supply the precentral gyrus. Penfield thought that ligating or resecting this artery would have a favourable effect on Jacksonian motor seizures. Although this procedure had been successful in the first patient in whom it had been attempted, it ultimately proved to be ineffectual and was abandoned. Montreal Neurological Hospital, case M.DeV., 1933.

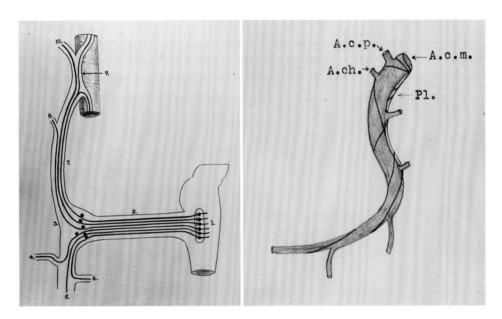

Figure 4.8. *Left.* Schematic drawing of parasympathetic neurovascular fibres from their origin in the brain stem (1) to the geniculate ganglion (3), and along the great superficial petrosal nerve (7) to the carotid plexus (9). *Right.* Neural plexus (P1) on the middle cerebral artery. Penfield thought that parasympathetic innervation of cortical arteries could counteract the vasoconstrictive effects of the sympathetic nervous system. Montreal Neurological Institute and McGill University, Choróbski, 1931–32.

sympathectomy.[36] The nerves, Penfield concluded, were therefore parasympathetic. The minor role that sympathetic innervation plays in the arteries of the epileptic brain was confirmed by Penfield's research fellow, Lyle Gage, who demonstrated that sympathetic stimulation did not significantly lower the epileptic threshold in animals in whom he had produced a cortical wound.[37] Nonetheless, Penfield concluded, "from a purely morphologic point of view, intracerebral vasomotor reflexes are possible," and added, "the origin of these intracerebral vascular nerves forms the subject of an unfinished study."[38] Penfield entrusted this study to Jerzy Choróbski, whose research was funded by Madeleine Ottman.[39]

Jerzy Choróbski had come to the MNI in 1930 as an Ottmann Research Fellow in Epilepsy, after studying psychiatry with Eugen Bleuler, neurology with George Guillain and Joseph Babinski, and neurosurgery with Thierry de Martel and Clovis Vincent, a who's who in continental neurology and neurosurgery. Choróbski's first task at the MNI was to study cerebrovascular innervation.[40] He found that in primates, fibres originating in the geniculate ganglion attached to the internal carotid artery and its intracranial branches, and that stimulation of these fibres produced dilatation of cortical arteries.

Choróbski's work had been undertaken as part of a collaborative project on cerebral innervation between Penfield and Stanley Cobb. The experiments began at the MNI, where Choróbski and Penfield performed a sympathectomy in five monkeys. The monkeys were transported across a porous border from Montreal to Stanley Cobb's laboratory at the Boston City Hospital, where they were implanted with a "Forbes window." The Forbes window was similar in concept to the watch glass used by Kussmaul and Tenner, but it was more air and water tight, which assured the maintenance of the intracranial pressure. With the animal's head firmly fixed in a head clamp, it allowed precision photography through which the effects of neural stimulation on the diameter of pial arteries and veins could be photographed, measured, and compared to the resting state.[41] These experiments led to two landmark papers on the nerve supply of the intracranial arteries,[42] in which Penfield, Cobb, and their collaborators demonstrated that cerebral arteries deprived of their sympathetic input nevertheless remained reactive and capable of dilating. This suggested, as Claude Bernard had deduced, that two antagonistic neural systems, one constrictive – the sympathetic – and the other relaxing – the parasympathetic – influenced cerebral blood flow by their antagonistic effects on the diameter of intracranial arteries, just as they did elsewhere in the body. Epileptic seizures, it was implied, resulted from an imbalance of the two systems.

Sympathectomy

Penfield had taken the opportunity during his sojourn with Foerster to visit René Leriche, chair of surgery at the University of Strasbourg. Leriche was the most prominent surgeon of his day, and his influence was felt throughout Europe and America.[43] Leriche had dedicated himself to the treatment of pain, often of a lower limb, caused by insufficient circulation. The procedure that he performed, a sympathectomy, consisted of denuding the arteries that supplied the ischemic limb of their constrictive, sympathetic innervation, thus improving blood flow and relieving pain.[44] Penfield was much taken with Leriche's sophistication and elegance,[45] his surgical dexterity, and his innovative spirit.[46] Inspired by Leriche's approach Penfield had hoped to improve blood flow to the epileptic brain by removing the sympathetic ganglions at the carotid bifurcation. The rationale was simple: "such an operation may alter the functional activity of the brain of the epileptic person, perhaps by means of improved circulation, and may greatly decrease the number and severity of seizures."[47] Such an operation would be considered bold by any neurosurgeon, then and now, and Penfield himself considered it experimental, although William Alexander, a surgeon in Liverpool, England, had performed it in the 1880s.[48] The first patient to be considered for the procedure was referred to Penfield by Stanley Cobb, who had been impressed with Penfield's boldness in treating William Ottman. Resection of "Ottman's artery" was not an option in Cobb's patient because his seizures were generalized. Penfield thus proposed resecting the sympathetic ganglion at the level of the carotid bifurcation in the neck on one side and, depending upon the results, perhaps on the other side also. "So," Penfield wrote, "[Cobb] and I explained the plan to the parents. Since they were desperate, they approved gratefully."[49] The first operation was successful in stopping seizures arising from the hemisphere on the side of the sympathectomy. The same operation was therefore performed on the opposite side, with similar success. The procedures were beneficial to Penfield as well as to the patient, who was the son of a trustee of the Rockefeller Foundation, which later funded the creation of the MNI.[50] Spurred by this first success, Penfield continued to perform sympathectomies late into the 1930s, most often with little, if any, impact on a patient's seizures. One such instance was in the case of patient C.Y., whose craniotomy demonstrated vascular constriction but no epileptogenic lesion, and who later underwent a unilateral sympathectomy:

Name: C.Y.   4th Floor.   Date: December 18th, 1937.

Operator: Dr. Penfield.

Anaes: Avertin, Ether.   Sterilization: Green Soap & Water, Alcohol, Ether & Iodine.

Provisional diagnosis: Epilepsy.

Final diagnosis: The same.

Operation: Left sinu-carotid neurectomy.

Objective findings: There was a heavy reddened bit of tissue at the bifurcation which might quite well be a large carotid body. The sheath itself was not unusually thick anterior to the common carotid but on the mesial aspect and posteriorly it was really quite thick and made a heavy covering. This passed upward on both external and internal carotids. The arteries themselves were not of unusual size. There was no evidence of any inflammatory process.

Procedure: An oblique incision was made. A complete removal of sheath of common carotid and internal and external carotids was made; removal of body also made and section of carotid nerve. Closure was made in layers by Dr. Reeves.

WGP/HO

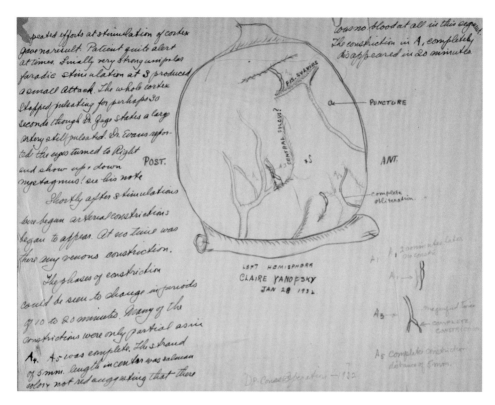

Figure 4.9. Brain map of the surgically exposed left hemisphere in a patient with right-sided, focal motor seizures and secondary generalization, seen from the surgeon's viewpoint. The operation was performed by William Cone. The text reads in part: "very strong unipolar faradic stimulation at S produced a small attack … Shortly after stimulations there began arterial constrictions began to appear [sic] … Many of the constrictions were only partial as in A4. A5 was complete. The strand of 5 mm length in center was salmon color not red suggesting that there was no blood at all in this segment. The constriction in A1 completely disappeared in 20 minutes." The circle indicates where the brain was punctured with a biopsy needle. As there was no obvious lesion, no resection was performed, and Cone limited the procedure to a temporal decompression. Penfield performed a sympathectomy in 1937, with no beneficial effect. Montreal Neurological Hospital, case C.Y., 1932.

Patient C.Y. received no benefit from either procedure, and Penfield eventually abandoned sympathectomy as he had abandoned arterial ligation, as neither procedure was successful in alleviating seizures.[51]

Penfield was clearly at sea. With one procedure, arterial resection, he strived to decrease blood flow to an epileptic area by cutting of its blood supply; with another he endeavoured to increase it by interfering with vasoconstriction. Both phenomena could not be synchronous but they could, conceivably, be sequential. But Penfield had done all that could be accomplished with simple observation. The issue could only be resolved by experimentation.

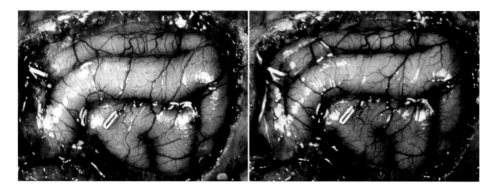

Figure 4.10. Left hemisphere of the cat under normal conditions (left) and after the induction of vasospasm (right). The arteries coursing over the convolution in the middle of the exposed hemisphere (the supra-Sylvian gyrus) are no longer apparent, and the convolution appears blanched. Histological examination of the cortex subjected to vasospasm revealed ischemic changes. Penfield took this as supportive evidence of the vascular hypothesis of focal epilepsy. Montreal Neurological Institute and McGill University, Echlin, "Cerebral Ischemia and Its Relation to Epilepsy."

Cerebral vasospasm

Planning for the Montreal Neurological Institute put increasing demands on Penfield's time, and he set aside the investigation of the vascular hypothesis. With the opening of the institute in 1934, Penfield's priority was to analyze the results of cortical stimulations, which eventually led to the iconic motor and sensory homunculus. As these tasks were completed, Penfield's attention turned once again to the vascular hypothesis, which he approached from two complementary directions. Francis Echlin would confirm Spielmeyer's observation that vasospasm could produce ischemic changes in the cortex, and Theodore Erickson would measure cerebral blood flow in animals subject to epileptic seizures from an experimentally created epileptic scar.

Francis Asbury Echlin graduated from McGill Medical School in 1931. After studies in neurology, neurosurgery, and neurophysiology in the United States, France, and England, Echlin joined the house staff of the MNI as a research fellow in 1937. His task was to determine if experimentally induced, prolonged constriction of cortical arteries could produce the histologically verified ischemic changes that Spielmeyer had observed in epileptic brains.[52] To do so, Echlin turned large craniotomies to expose the cerebral hemispheres in cats. He then caused vasospasm of the cortical arteries by gently stroking them with a glass rod, by stimulating them with a low electrical current, or by stretching them with a small thread looped around them.[53]

Echlin's model owed much to one developed by Howard Florey in Sherrington's laboratory a decade earlier.[54] Echlin found that spasm of a cortical artery resulted in a triangular area of cortical ischemia, much as Spielmeyer had observed. Echlin's most significant observation, however, was unappreciated at the time. Echlin mentions the occurrence of prolonged vasospasm following subarachnoid haemorrhage produced by inadvertent bleeding from a cortical artery. The significant mortality and morbidity associated with vasospasm as a consequence of subarachnoid haemorrhage would not be recognized until decades later.[55]

REFUTATION

The history of science is the history of technology

Everything seemed to be in place to test the vascular hypothesis. The essential element, the innervation of cerebral blood vessels, had been demonstrated, the reactivity of cortical arteries had been established, and prolonged vasoconstriction had been shown to produce cortical ischemia. All that remained to support the vascular theory was to confirm that experimentally created cortical scars could trigger seizures by altering cerebral blood flow. Penfield assigned this task to Theodore Erickson, a talented experimentalist and one of the most accomplished physician-scientists to train at the MNI. Erickson obtained his MD degree from the University of Minnesota in 1931 and trained in neurosurgery with Charles Frazier and Francis Grant, two early pioneers of the discipline. Theodor Erickson is remembered today for his co-authorship with Penfield of the landmark book *Epilepsy and Cerebral Localization*.[56] Erickson came to the MNI in 1933 to pursue research and he was awarded a doctorate for his studies on the role of the cerebral circulation in epileptogenesis and on the spread of epileptic seizures across the corpus callosum.[57] Surprisingly, Erickson's experimental model was based on Ivan Pavlov's experimental studies of half a century earlier, to which he applied the newly described thermoelectric method for assessing cerebral blood flow.

Pavlov's classic treatise on the conditioned reflex was published in English translation in 1926.[58] It is comprised of twenty-three lectures that Pavlov had given at the Military Medical Academy in Petrograd in 1924, although Pavlov had performed the experiments to which I refer in 1906. Lecture nineteen, entitled "Pathological Disturbances of the Cortex, Result of Surgical Interference," was instrumental in Penfield's investigation of the role of vascular reflexes in the genesis of posttraumatic epilepsy.[59] Pavlov had been worried that the extensive surgery necessary to expose the brain of his dogs would result in so much blood loss that his experiments on the cerebral cortex would be invalidated. Thus, he performed surgery in two stages so that the animal could renew its blood volume between the first and second operations. Consequently, the first stage of Pavlov's operation was to incise the scalp, excise the temporalis muscle, remove a bone flap, and close the scalp incision over the dura. Unforeseen by Pavlov, however, the animals became subject to epileptic attacks. These were relatively minor when they began but became more frequent and more severe with the passage of time. This evolution mimicked posttraumatic epilepsy in humans. When the second operation was performed, Pavlov observed that dense adhesions had formed between a thick cortical scar and the subcutaneous layers of the scalp. Furthermore, Pavlov noted that resecting the scar often caused the animal's seizures to disappear.[60] Erickson hoped that by using Pavlov's model he could create an epileptogenic scar that would trigger epileptic seizures and that he could demonstrate that these resulted from decreased blood flow in the scarred region of the cortex. Erickson produced cortical scars by a myriad of cortical insults, which included inserting skin, hair, and bone fragments into the wound that he created by cortical excision. Erickson even went to the lengths of operating without gloves in an unsterile environment to cause an infection in the scar or of applying carcinogenic substances to the wound. Alterations in blood flow were assessed using a thermocouple device.[61]

Erickson's disappointment is palpable as he writes in his dissertation that none of the eighteen macaque monkeys and only five of the thirty-eight cats operated upon developed convulsions. Three of these cats died before they could be experimented upon, and of the two remaining animals, reproducible data could be obtained only in one. But one is all that it took. Although the poor beast suffered many convulsions, the blood flow in or about the scar was not altered in any way. As Erickson wrote, "The spontaneous fluctuations in blood flow … were exactly the same in the cicatricial and juxta-cicatricial portions of the brain as they were in the normal portions of the grey matter. This was so clear and was repeated so many times that it is strong evidence against there being any local qualitative alteration of vascular function by the presence of a cerebral cicatrix."[62] Erickson's conclusion with regard to the vascular hypothesis was brief: "The theory that cerebral cicatrices may induce epileptiform fits by causing abnormal local variability in blood flow … has not received any support from the results of the present series of experiments."[63] William Bridgers, also a MNI fellow at the time, struck a similarly dissonant note in his histological study of posttraumatic epileptogenic scars that Penfield had resected. Bridgers found circumscribed areas of progressive neuronal loss in the vicinity of the scars, which he ascribed to focal arterial spasm. Similar changes, however, were seen in patients who had sustained severe head trauma but were not epileptic. This led Bridgers to question the role of vascular spasm in the initiation of epileptic seizures.[64]

A black swan[65]

Penfield reviewed the topic of the circulation of the epileptic brain in a symposium on the cerebral circulation in 1937.[66] The introduction to his address is startling: "Speculation and fragmentary observations have led to the assumption that an

epileptic seizure was immediately preceded or accompanied by widespread constriction of the cerebral vessels. This conception must now be abandoned in the
light of greater familiarity with the vascular alterations associated with epileptic
seizures." What brought this change was the introduction of the Gibbs thermocouple
device, which allowed the *qualitative* assessment of the cerebral hemodynamics by
measuring temperature changes produced by alterations in cerebral blood flow.[67]
This method is based on the principle that the temperature of a needle inserted
into vascularized tissue varies inversely with blood flow: increased blood flow cools
the needle, decreased flow warms it. Gibbs first measured blood flow in cats using
a needle placed into its cortex through a burr hole and recorded the temperature
before and after pharmacologically induced seizures.[68] Gibbs observed that the
needle cooled during the convulsion, indicating increased blood flow. Gibbs and
his collaborators then performed similar measurements in epileptic patients using
a needle inserted into an internal jugular vein, which was left in place until a seizure
occurred.[69] There was no reduction in blood flow with the onset of a seizure in these
unfortunate patients. Gibbs's measurements, however, referred to global intracranial
blood flow in patients with generalized seizures and no structural lesion. Would the
same be true in patients with focal seizures from a discreet structural lesion?

And so, Penfield and two exceptionally imaginative MNI researchers, Kalman von
Santha and André Cipriani, applied the thermoelectric method in patients with
focal epilepsy. Von Santha and Cipriani had come to the MNI in 1936 and helped
Herbert Jasper establish the Department of Clinical Electrophysiology at the institute. Von Santha was a Rockefeller Fellow from Budapest, who pioneered in the development of neurology and neurosurgery in Hungary after leaving the MNI.[70]
André Cipriani was a brilliant biophysicist and engineer. He built the first EEG apparatus at the MNI and the thermocouple devise that Erickson and others[71] had used
to measure cerebral blood flow in the laboratory.[72] Von Santha and Cipriani stimulated the motor strip in dogs to produce a simple motor response, and using a
thermocouple device, they observed that the movement of the animal's limb resulted
in increased cerebral blood.[73] Inspired by these results, Penfield, von Santha, and
Cipriani, in an exceptionally far-reaching paper descriptively entitled "Cerebral
Blood Flow during Induced Epileptiform Seizures in Animals and Man," reported
the results of their use of the thermoelectric method to measure blood flow in the
epileptic brain.[74] Cipriani modified a thermocouple device for use in the exposed
cerebral cortex, which Penfield used during the resection of a cerebral, epileptogenic
scar.[75] A fine thermocouple wire was inserted near the structural lesion before and
after Penfield induced a seizure by electrocortical stimulation. The brain map of a
patient, operated upon in the presence of the influential neurophysiologist John
Fulton, is published here for the first time.

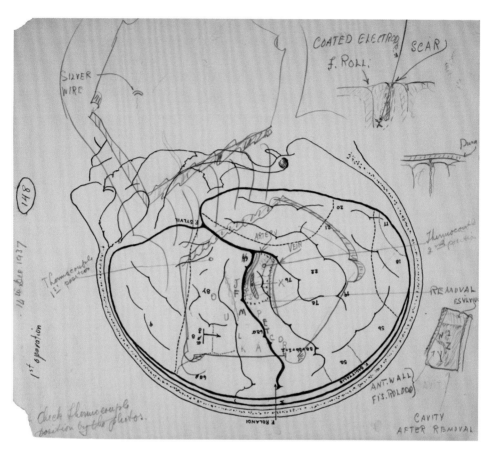

Figure 4.11. Penfield's brain map of a patient operated for focal motor seizures involving the left side of the body that led to generalized convulsions. Fine adhesions between the dura and the postcentral gyrus led to "an elongated crevasse in which there was soft gelatinous tissue." (Detail at middle right.) An insulated, unipolar electrode was passed through the cortex into the underlying scar and surrounding brain at point "X," where stimulation produced the patient's typical attack. (Detail at top right.) A thermocouple probe was placed near the scar and in the frontal lobe. Such studies showed that, rather than vasoconstriction and ischemia, there was increased blood flow in the epileptogenic area during a seizure, thus falsifying the vascular hypothesis. Increased cerebral blood flow is now recognized as a feature of focal epileptic seizures. Montreal Neurological Hospital, case B.K.-C., 1937.

Penfield's matter-of-fact description of the effects of seizures on the local cerebral blood flow in these patients belies the significance of his conclusions: "During the seizure there is an increase in circulation within the circumscribed area of cortex which is involved in the 'discharge' that produces the fit. This increase begins within the first minute *after* the precipitating stimulus with no preliminary decrease in flow and it outlasts the clinical evidence of the seizure. More distant areas of cortex may show no alteration in blood flow."[76] With these observations the vascular hypothesis was no longer tenable: focal epileptic seizures are not triggered by reflex vasoconstriction, and Penfield was compelled to echo Erickson and state, "The evidence of our present communication indicates that vasospasm plays no role during a seizure nor is there evidence of widespread anemia following it. Vascular spasms and anemias [sic] may be concerned in the pathological background of epilepsy but at all events they play no role in the actual mechanism during a seizure." Penfield, having tested the vascular hypothesis with a critical experiment, had found it wanting and rejected it.

Hemodynamic-metabolic coupling

Penfield's investigation of the vascular hypothesis shows the weakness of a hypothesis based on inductive reasoning: it can be falsified by a single counterexample.[77] But these experiments did more than falsify a tenuous hypothesis. They brought to light a basic neurophysiological principle: that cerebral blood flow is coupled to the metabolic demands of the brain. The full significance of this discovery was not apparent until the early 1980s when blood flow measurements performed with positron emission tomography confirmed von Santha and Cipriani's observations of the coupling of cerebral metabolism and cerebral blood flow. This became the founding principle of functional brain imaging as it is used today throughout the world and which has brought new understanding to cerebral function in normal and pathological states. As for focal epilepsy and cerebral blood flow, Penfield, von Santha, and Cipriani's observation has been confirmed by thermal diffusion flowmetry – the modern successor of the thermometric method – and modern imaging methods, such as single photon emission tomography and positron emission tomography: focal epileptic seizures do trigger a vasomotor reflex, but this results in hyperperfusion, not ischemia, as Penfield had thought. Penfield reflected upon his research in blood flow and epilepsy, and concluded, "Those who would come upon the truth should elaborate their incomplete hypotheses, keeping always clear in mind what is proven fact and what is fancy. You never know which, if any, of your theories will be verified in your lifetime."[78]

EPILEPSY AND SURGICAL THERAPY 1928–33

The scar being carefully removed, the convulsion did not recur –Ivan Pavlov[79]

Penfield presented the first systematic analysis of his results of the surgical treatment of epilepsy in July 1935, at the Second International Neurological Congress in London, in an address entitled "Epilepsy and Surgical Therapy."[80] His series consisted of seventy-seven patients upon whom he and Cone had operated between 1928, when they first arrived at the Royal Victoria Hospital, and 1933 when the cornerstone of the MNI was laid. Patients whose epilepsy was secondary to a cerebral neoplasm were excluded from analysis. The patients had undergone the resection of a meningocerebral cicatrix or of a cortical scar without the benefit of preoperative EEG, as this method of investigating epileptic patients was not yet available. The major flaw in Penfield's analysis was the short period of observation following surgery, a fact that he confronted directly by stating, "The period during which these patients have been followed is short, and nothing less than a lifetime is altogether satisfactory."[81] In fact, many of the patients included in the study had been operated upon less than a year before Penfield read his paper. Another failing of the study was Penfield's arbitrariness in characterizing the outcomes of surgery.

Penfield considered his results in three categories, "Cured" if the patient was seizure-free since surgery; "Improved" if the seizures were less frequent or less severe after operation; and "Failure" if there was no postoperative improvement. Only forty-four of the seventy-seven patients had a cortical resection, and twenty-four had no resection at all since no lesion was found at surgery. Penfield considered the latter as a control group. A full three-quarters of the forty-four patients who had undergone the resection of a cerebral scar were cured or improved. These results, however, must be looked at quizzically, since one-fifth of the patients whose craniotomy was purely exploratory also had a similar result!

Table 4.1
Results of the operative treatment of focal epilepsy, 1928–33

Procedure	No. of patients	"Cured"	Improved	Failure
Excision of a meningocerebral cicatrix	22	10	7	5
Excision of cortical scar	22	9	7	6
Arterial ligation	4	1	0	3
Evacuation of subdural fluid	3	1	1	1
Exploration without excision	24	2	3	19
Deaths	2			

CHAPTER 5

A Bird in an Aviary

In such tissue lies hidden the secrets of epilepsy –Penfield, 1921

The proportion of exploratory operations in which no structural lesion or epilep-togenic focus were found was a stark reminder that familiarity with the clinical manifestations of focal epilepsy and the blunt instrument that was PEG were not entirely reliable in deciding on whom to operate. It was hoped that the arrival of Herbert Jasper and electroencephalography would enhance the ability to select patients for surgery and to identify an epileptic focus intra-operatively.

Herbert Henri Jasper was born in La Grande, Oregon, in 1906. After his post-graduate studies at the University of Iowa, Jasper studied axonal excitability at La Sorbonne, in Paris.[1] Upon his return from France in 1932 he established an EEG laboratory at Brown University in Providence, Rhode Island. From this laboratory came the first publication on the human EEG to originate from North America.[2]

Jasper first met Penfield in the autumn of 1937 when Penfield was invited to Brown to give a seminar on cortical stimulation of the brain. Jasper, in his memoirs,[3] gives a vivid account of their encounter:

Dr Penfield's lecture was most exciting indeed and was attended by many members of the medical community in Providence, as well as the staff and students of the psychology department. His colored slides of the large exposed cortical surface, marked with tickets showing the sites of various sensory and motor responses to electrical stimulation were beautiful and most impressive. I thought immediately of the wonderful opportunity this would provide to record electrical potentials directly from the cortical surface in conscious man. The following day Dr Penfield came out to our laboratories in East Providence to see our work with electroencephalography. I had told him the day before that I could localize an epileptic focus in epileptic patients by recording from electrodes placed on the surface of the scalp. He was quite skeptical but he came to see what we were doing nevertheless.

As Jasper later recalled, Penfield found him, "moving about like a bird in an aviary," in a cage made of chicken wire, which shielded the EEG apparatus from electrical interference. Nonetheless, Jasper continues,

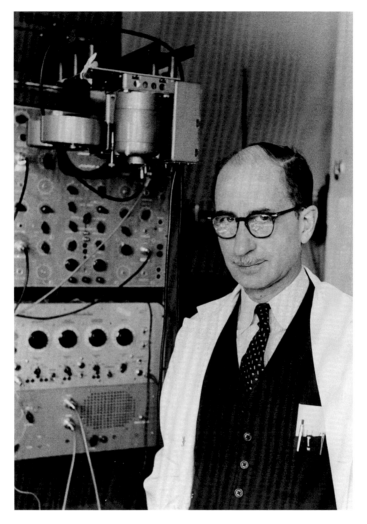

Figure 5.1. Herbert Jasper. Montreal Neurological Institute and McGill University.

We were able to demonstrate the normal EEG, using myself as a subject for I knew I had good alpha waves. We then recorded from one of the epileptic patients in the Bradley Hospital. He was a 12 year old Italian boy by the name of [S.C.] who was also a severe behavior problem. He had fallen to the floor in infancy resulting in a fractured skull and injury to the right hemisphere with paresis of the left arm. He then developed frequent epileptic seizures beginning with a sensory aura in the left hand and arm, proceeding to convulsive movements of the left side followed by generalized convulsions with loss of consciousness. We found a spike focus localized to the right central area and slow waves extending into the right fronto-temporal lesion.

Penfield was impressed but still skeptical. I asked him if he would be willing to put our findings to a test by operating on some of our patients after we had determined the EEG focus. He finally agreed providing the seizure pattern and the pneumoencephalogram were consistent with the EEG findings.

After discussion with Dr Bradley and the parents we agreed to take [S.C.] to Montreal to be the first patient to be operated upon by Dr Penfield with localization guided by the preoperative EEG examination. There was a second patient, a young lady by the name of [E.C.], who had seizures since childhood and showed a consistent focus of spikes in the right frontal region. She agreed to come to Montreal with S.C. They arrived in Montreal in November of 1937.

Since we wanted to be able to record from the surface of the exposed cortex. Howard Andrews assembled a portable two-channel amplifier which could be readily transported in my car, together with some piezoelectric ink writing pen recorders we had recently acquired from Frank Offner in Chicago. By the time this could be arranged in late November winter had already come to Montreal. I packed the apparatus into my big Oldsmobile car with my skis on the top since I wanted to sample the skiing as well as the scientific climate in Montreal. S.C. and E.C. had already arrived at the Neurological Institute for preliminary clinical and pneumoencephalographic studies in order to make sure that Dr. Penfield would agree to the operation.

I set out to Montreal on Friday afternoon and arrived safely at the Canadian border about midnight but had some trouble at the Canadian Customs with the EEG apparatus. The officer could not find it in his book so was rather suspicious. I told him I was going to use it to record brain waves for Dr Penfield, the famed neurosurgeon, in Montreal. I showed him a letter from Penfield and asked him to call Penfield to confirm my story. He finally decided to take a chance and call it "electrical brain testing equipment" which was not far from the truth …

I arrived in Montreal by daybreak on Saturday and was shown to a bed on the eight floor of the Institute by a nurse who had been informed that I was coming. S.C. had come the week before to have a work up before my arrival. He was raising hell on the children's ward. Nurse Goldie [later Mrs Jasper] who was in charge, had learned to handle him, with the help of some of the patients. She admitted he was a "little hellion" but they seemed to be becoming friends just the same. E.C. had also arrived and was well established on the third floor. I was informed that both patients had been studied by Dr Penfield and his staff and he had agreed to operate.

Penfield had organized a ski trip to the Laurentians over the weekend, as he had the habit of doing with his staff and fellows throughout the winter … We returned to Montreal on the ski train looking forward to the operation on my patients during the week. I was very anxious that they be successful since I thought my future at the Institute was hanging in the balance depending upon the accuracy of my EEG localization. On Monday morning I attended the weekly grand round held in the Hughlings Jackson Amphitheatre where my two patients were presented for general discussion. The clinical and the pneumoencephalographic findings were satisfactory and consistent with the EEG localization so that all agreed that both patients qualified for operation since they were not controlled by anticonvulsant medication.

I was then taken on a tour of the Institute by André Cipriani whom I had met on our ski trip. He also helped me install the EEG recording equipment in the operating room for the operation which was scheduled for Tuesday morning.

After a brief tour of orientation, we took my EEG apparatus to No. 1 operating theater to see if it would be suitable for EEG recording. I had misgivings about artifacts from all the unshielded apparatus already in the OR as well as the absence of shielding or even grounding in the OR itself. My fears proved to be well founded for when we first turned on my amplifiers with the recording electrodes attached we heard the local broadcasting station loud and clear. There was also much 60 cycle artifact which we failed to suppress during the operation. What a disappointment. Cipriani agreed to help me correct the situation before we attempted to record during the other operation. The operation itself was reasonably successful since an obvious cicatrix and area of atrophy was found in the postcentral gyrus corresponding well with our preoperative EEG localization and the sensory aura in his left hand …

With the help of Andy Cipriani we were able to improve the grounding of equipment and the operating room table itself before the second operation to be carried out on E.C. the following Thursday. This was much more satisfactory since we were able to record without general anesthesia and with a minimum of electrical artifact. An excision was made in the right frontal region guided by the abnormalities in the electrocoticogram since there was little objective evidence of a lesion, although her typical aversive seizure was reproduced by electrical stimulation during the operative exploration. Penfield seemed well pleased with the results.

Although E.C. was the first patient in whom an electrocorticogram (ECOG) was successfully performed at the MNI, Jasper and Penfield had been preceded by Foerster and the physiologist Hans Altenburger, who recorded an ECOG in 1935.[4] Foerster's work in the electrophysiology of the epileptic brain was curtailed by the death of Altenberger at the beginning of the Second World War, which Foerster himself did not survive.

Jasper accepted Penfield's invitation to relocate to Montreal, and plans were drawn for a small extension to the basement of the institute to house the Laboratory of

Electrophysiology, which was fully operational in 1939. The EEG apparatus at the time was able to record from four electrodes at once. The electrodes were moved from one area of the scalp to another in a prescribed pattern to record the electrical activity from both hemispheres of the brain. However, recording and interpreting the electrical activity generated by the deeper midline structures, such as the medial aspects of the frontal and temporal lobes, was difficult. The apparatus was quickly modified so as to record from the exposed cortex during surgery to help localize the epileptogenic area around a cerebral scar.

EXTRA-TEMPORAL EPILEPSY

The frontal lobe – The best electrogram taken in the operating room

Patient J.T.[5] was not the first MNI patient to benefit from ECOG at the MNI, but, as Jasper wrote in his intraoperative report, his was "the best electrogram taken in the operating room of the … epileptiform spikes from a meningiocerebral cicatrix."

The patient was eleven years old in 1925 when he fell and struck his head on a rock, sustaining a compound, depressed fracture of the left frontal bone. The fracture was elevated, a bone fragment was removed, and an abscess was drained four days later.[6] J.T. began having generalized seizures four years later, which led to his admission to the MNI in 1939. An EEG was performed and recorded "an exquisitely focal epileptiform discharge … on the left frontal lobe just over the former opening for drainage [of the abscess]," and the patient underwent a left frontal craniotomy. A dense and extensive dural scar was uncovered as the bone flap was elevated and an EEG was performed with the electrodes placed upon the dural scar. The epileptic activity was widespread and, although confirming the presence of epileptic activity originating from the underlying cortex, it had no precise localizing value. The dura was incised and reflected, revealing a gelatinous scar that penetrated downward directly into the brain, to a depth of about three centimetres.

Stimulation behind and immediately below the scar produced interference with speech, but the responses were more confusing than enlightening, as they produced crude vocalization, slowing of speech, or speech arrest when the same point was repeatedly stimulated.

Penfield was in a quandary. Although the scar was obvious, it appeared to lie close to eloquent cortex. Under other circumstances Penfield would have performed a wide resection of the cortex about the scar, but the proximity of eloquent cortex precluded this approach. Prior to the introduction of ECOG, the operation might have ended at this point, without resecting the scar for fear of damaging the speech area. Now, however, the ECOG was repeated, this time not from the dura but from the exposed cortex, and epileptic spikes were recorded at the anterior and lateral edges of the scar, that is, in an area anterior to where verbal responses had been

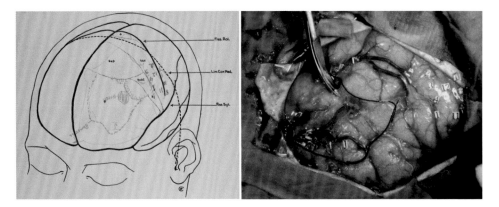

Figure 5.2. *Left.* Penfield's brain map. *Right.* Operative photograph. The black thread outlines the planned resection margin. The density of the collagenous response about the scar is indicated by the recourse to sharp dissection with fine scissors. The resection spared the area from which verbal responses were obtained. Despite this precaution, there occurred a delayed, transient postoperative aphasia, which was likely the result of postoperative edema. Montreal Neurological Hospital, case J.T., 1939.

obtained. The cortical scar was so dense that Penfield needed fine scissor to resect it. The use of sharp dissection, rather than the usual silk suture method, minimized the chance of damaging the speech area. Microscopic examination of the specimen revealed a meningo-cerebral cicatrix.[7]

The patient developed delayed but transient aphasia from cerebral edema in the postoperative period, which illustrates Penfield's acumen in avoiding resection of the cortex posterior to the scar. The patient stayed in contact with Penfield and later with Theodore Rasmussen, Penfield's successor at the MNI, for the next thirty-two years and reported only the occasional seizure. Ultimately, J.T.'s case stands out because, coming so early after Jasper's arrival at the MNI, it proved to Penfield that ECOG recordings could help in his treatment of epileptic patients.

PARIETAL LOBE EPILEPSY

It soon became apparent to Penfield that the outcome of surgery depended largely on the location of the offending scar, which in turn determined how completely it could be excised. The best outcomes were obtained from the resection of a frontal scar that excluded the motor strip. The worst outcomes were in patients whose scar resided within the pre- or postcentral gyri or within the parietal lobe.[8]

The first difficulty encountered when considering parietal epilepsy is nomenclature. For the purpose of analyzing the outcome of surgery, Penfield considered that the pre- and postcentral gyri constituted a distinct functional unit separate from the remainders of the frontal and parietal lobes. Thus, when Penfield wrote of the parietal lobe in the context of epilepsy, he was referring to the part that resides be-tween the postcentral gyrus and the occipital lobe.[9] Further, because of its proximity to the central region, the manifestations of seizures originating in the parietal lobe can be difficult to discern since sensory-motor symptoms and signs may accompany them. Similarly, because of its proximity to the occipital lobe, parietal lobe seizures can include visual phenomenon. The latter became obvious in an early case operated upon by William Cone.

The parietal lobe and the visual associative area

E.B. was twenty-two years old when he was hit on the head with a hammer and sustained a depressed skull fracture. Six months later he saw a flash of light and fell into convulsions. His seizures persisted and were sometimes heralded by seeing a vaporous form rise within his left visual field. He was admitted to the RVH in 1932, two year after his injury, under the care of William Cone. Cone turned a large pari-eto-occipital craniotomy centreed on the site of the fracture. He observed that "the dura had been torn and spicules of bone penetrated the brain. The surrounding brain showed a definite cicatrix … [which was] at a considerable distance from the motor area at about the region where one usually expects to find the supramarginal gyrus." Cone localized the scar by first identifying the postcentral convolution through cortical stimulation, which defined the Rolandic fissure. Following the Rolandic fissure downwards led him to the Sylvian fissure, and, proceeding back-ward to its termination, he arrived at the supramarginal gyrus.

Electrical stimulation around the scar was as striking as it was unexpected: "Faradic stimulation at various points about the cicatrix produced contralateral col-orless dancing lights and 'quivering' before both eyes with lights to the left." An ex-planation was required to explain effects that would be expected from stimulation of the occipital lobe originating, incongruously, within the parietal lobe. Or, as Penfield put it when he commented on this case, "It seems unlikely that the current could have escaped from this area all the way to the calcarine cortex." This led Penfield to the "conclusion that neuronal discharge in the region of the supra-marginal gyrus, and possibly extending into [Brodmann] areas 19 and 22, may pro-duce a sensation of light."[10] Brodmann area 22 corresponds to the first temporal convolution, which ends at the angular gyrus. Brodmann area 19 is behind the an-gular gyrus and within the occipital lobe, but far from the calcarine cortex. We now know that Brodmann area 19 is part of the visual associative system and is referred to a "V3" in current neurobiological nomenclature. Like other visual association areas, area V3 is felt to be a way station between the reception of light images from the calcarine cortex and the formed images that we see in the mind's eye. But this was unknown to Penfield, who reverted to the prevailing paradigm, the conditioned

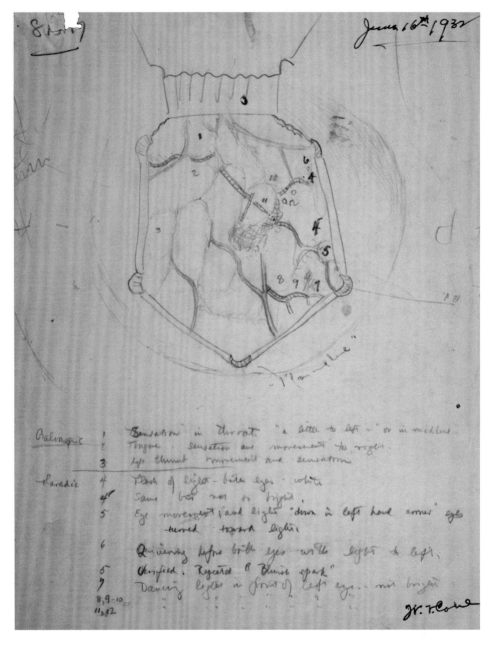

Figure 5.3. William Cone's operative sketch of the right parietal lobe drawn from the surgeon's viewpoint. The postcentral gyrus is indicated by sensory responses obtained from stimulation at points 1–3. Cone identifies the scar, indicted by the crosshatched area, to be within the supramarginal gyrus. Visual responses were elicited by stimulation of points 4–9 in the posterior aspect of the parietal lobe, which was later discovered to be a visual associative area. Montreal Neurological Hospital, case E.B., 1932.

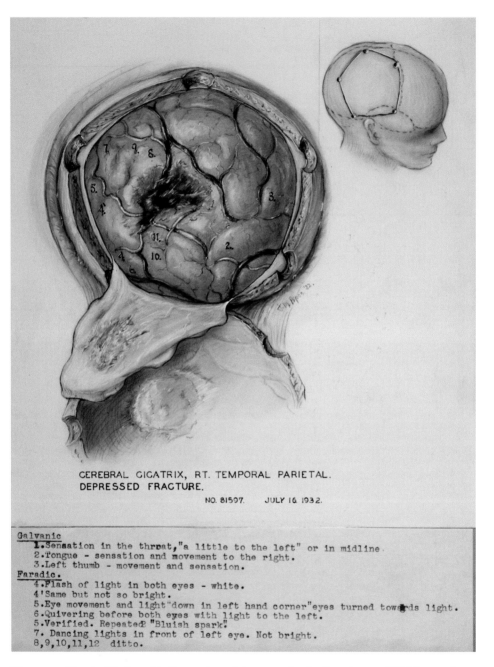

Figure 5.4. Harriet Blackstock's illustration of the operative findings in case E.B. Montreal Neurological Hospital, case E.B., 1932.

reflex, to explain visual phenomena originating from what he understood to be nonvisual cortex: "An habitual seizure, by virtue of its frequent repetition, may eventually establish a complicated neurone pattern, so functionally organized that it may be stimulated electrically although no such complicated response could be obtained from stimulation of the normal brain." This occurred, Penfield thought, through "a pattern of neuronal connections established by the conditioning influence of previous individual experience."[11] Penfield would later invoke the same mechanism to explain the acquisition of memory and the construction of the experiential phenomenon.[12]

Parietal lobe epilepsy and the central region

Extensive cortical scarring within the parietal associative area can also extend to its anterior border with the postcentral gyrus, which can add sensory-motor manifestations to parietal lobe seizures. Such was the case with patient V.D., who struck his head after a fall at the age of two and a half years. His seizures began two years later and occurred in three patterns, sometimes consecutively, sometimes in combination. They consisted of a feeling of dizziness and the appearance of brightly flashing, coloured lights, which was sometimes followed by the elevation of the left arm and jerking movements of the left hand. On other occasions, he fell unconscious onto his face without warning and exhibited jerking movements of the left arm. The patient was admitted to the MNI in 1947, when he was nineteen years old. Sensation and rapid alternating movements were diminished in the left upper extremity, and the deep tendon reflexes were accentuated. Epileptic discharges were recorded over the temporal, parietal, and postcentral regions, and PEG showed that the right lateral ventricle was enlarged. Thus, there was concordance of clinical, electrophysiological, and radiological findings, and a craniotomy was performed, exposing the central and parietal regions of the right hemisphere. Scattered adhesions were noted between the dura and arachnoid in the inferior parietal region, which overlay a yellowish, though tenacious, scar. There were two atrophic gyri behind the scar, from which epileptic activity was recorded. Resection included the scarred area and extended to the central fissure anteriorly and to the Sylvian fissure inferiorly. Two cysts were encountered in the white matter in the depth of the resection, the result of a remote haemorrhagic contusion. The cysts were evacuated and marsupialized so as to drain into the subarachnoid space. The fluid that the residual lining of the cysts might generate would then be absorbed with the cerebro-spinal fluid. As is often the case in parietal lobe epilepsy, the prognosis was guarded. Despite the extensive resection of the scar and evacuation of the cysts, the resection was only partial as the scar extended well into the central region.

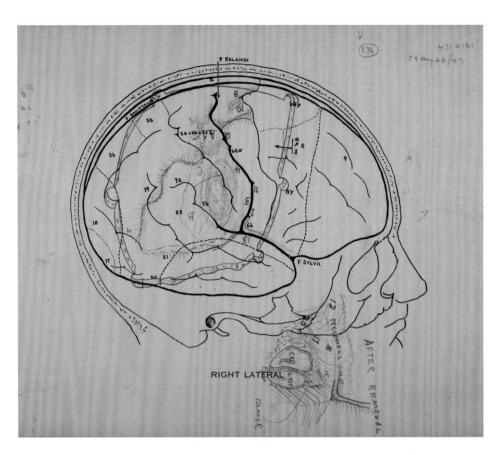

RIGHT LATERAL

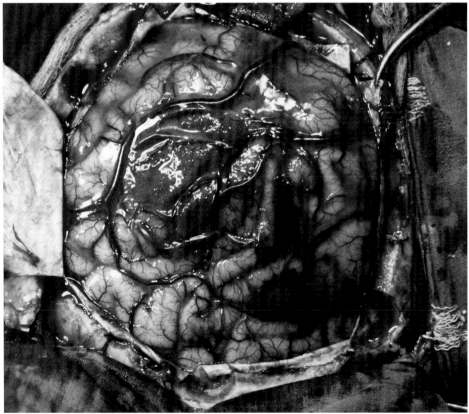

THE OCCIPITAL LOBE

The colours dreadful

It would seem that epileptic seizures arising from the occipital lobe should be easily recognized. Its function is well defined and its structure is well delineated. In reality, however, diagnosis is difficult and localization is uncertain. Penfield operated on few patients with occipital lobe seizures, but the information gleaned from their treatment did much to clarify their complex and often false-localizing manifestations.[13] When Penfield first addressed the topic, in 1932,[14] he could only refer to single case studies from nineteenth-century neurologists as his points of reference. John Hughlings Jackson had reported the case of a woman who had focal sensory seizures that affected the right thumb and that progressed to the upper arm, face, and tongue. At other times she experienced "the colours dreadful" – violet, white, and orange – in her right eye.[15] Another of Jackson's patients described "a throbbing light of various colours, green, yellow, and red, in the right eye ... which takes my sight and senses away, and then I go into a fit [in which] I am very much convulsed."[16] Jackson, in commenting on this case, wrote, "I believe that the colour first developed in epileptics, when colour is the first symptom, is usually red."[17]

This was the case in one of Penfield's patients who had sustained a skull fracture during childbirth. The injury resulted in paralysis of his right side and, twelve years later, convulsive seizures. The convulsions were severe, frequent, and heralded by bright, rotating, coloured lights. He was eighteen years old when he was admitted to the MNI. His right limbs were atrophied, hypertonic, and hyperreflexic, and he was blind in the left eye, all of which attested to a severely damaged left cerebral hemisphere. Skull x-ray and PEG findings were limited to a smaller left hemicranium. Epileptic activity was recorded from the left occipital region, which led Penfield to conclude that "the origin of the attacks was obviously in the left occipital lobe," despite the lack of radiological findings suggestive of a focal, atrophic lesion.

Despite the absence of a visible lesion, Penfield proceeded with cortical stimulation. The latter produced striking results when the electrode was applied to the occipital pole, as the patient reported seeing ill-defined red and blue colours, flashing

Figure 5.5. *Opposite top* Operative drawing seen from the anatomical viewpoint. Numbers 1, 3, 4, 5, 8, 10–12, 15, 18, and 20 produced sensory and motor responses, identifying the pre- and postcentral gyri. A whistling sound was heard in the left ear, and stars and lights were seen in the left visual field, as a result of stimulation at numbers 13 and 14, respectively. The two deep posthaemorrhagic cysts and the results of stimulation of the posterior bank of the precentral gyrus are also illustrated. Montreal Neurological Hospital, case V.D., 1947.

Figure 5.6. *Opposite bottom* Intraoperative photograph of the same case as in the previous figure, demonstrating the discoloured, scarred area and the atrophic gyri behind it. Montreal Neurological Hospital, case V.D., 1947.

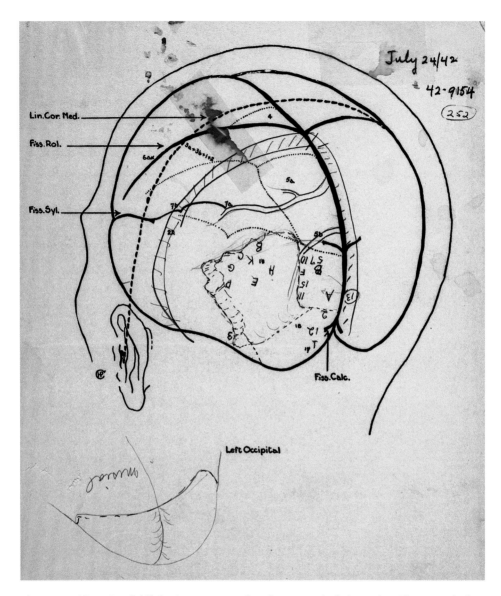

Figure 5.7. *Above* Penfield's brain map rotated to the anatomical viewpoint. Electrocortical stimulation produced a variety of visual phenomena, consisting of ill-defined red and blue colours at number 1; flashing lights at 3; tiny, moving, coloured lights at 4; and long white marks and large white spots at numbers 5 and 7. Epileptic spikes were recorded at letter A, near the occipital pole, and electrographic seizures were recorded at B, at the lateral aspect of the anterior occipital lobe. Stimulation at letter C produced an epileptic discharge and the patient's usual seizure. Montreal Neurological Hospital, case C.J., 1942.

Figure 5.8. *Opposite* Penfield's map of the right hemisphere of a patient with left homonymous hemianopia and whose central vision was spared. The presence of adhesions between the dura and cortex, and the line of resection are indicated. As Penfield noted in his operative report, "The area for sensation in the thumb and index finger was mapped out, but no further exploration was done because of bleeding." Montreal Neurological Hospital archives, case C.F., 1934.

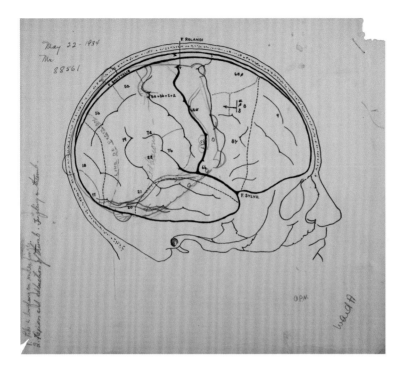

lights, and large white spots. Epileptic spikes were recorded near the occipital pole and at the border of the occipital and temporal lobes. Penfield resected these areas despite the absence of a structural lesion. Penfield's faith in the reliability of electrophysiology in the absence of a structural lesion was, however, limited, and he concluded his operative report by stating that the patient's prognosis was "quite guarded." Penfield's prognosis was overly pessimistic. The patient's seizure abated to one or two per year after surgery, and he then became seizure-free.

Macular sparing

Penfield's first papers in which he discussed the occipital lobes were concerned with discovering the visual pathway of the optic radiations in man as revealed by the effects of resection of the temporal, parietal, and occipital lobes.[18] Penfield was especially interested in the unusual phenomenon known as macular sparing, in which an occipital lesion produces a hemianopia yet spares central, macular vision, a phenomenon that is still poorly understood. The opportunity to study macular sparing came early in Penfield's surgical experience.

The case was that of an eleven-year-old boy who developed epileptic seizures three years after a fall from his bicycle.[19] The attacks were preceded by a sensation in the eyes "as if a dark curtain were being pulled across the left visual field," as his head turned to the left. Convulsive movements began in the left little finger, spread to the left hand, and then became generalized. Sometimes the attack consisted of the visual phenomenon alone. The patient was admitted to the MNI in April 1934, when he was eighteen years old. His examination was unremarkable, except for a

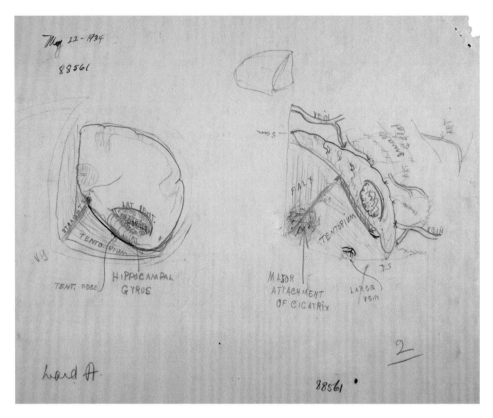

Figure 5.9. *Above* Intraoperative sketches drawn after the resection of the left occipital pole. Both illustrations show the falx cerebri, which separates both hemispheres, and the tentorium cerebelli, which separates the cerebral hemispheres from the underlying cerebellum. The site where the scar was attached to the dura is indicated, as well as prominent veins that drained the scarred area and its surrounding cortex. The occipital horn of the left lateral ventricle has been breached and the choroid plexus is visible through the opening. Montreal Neurological Hospital archives, case C.F., 1934.

Figure 5.10. *Opposite* Hortense Douglas's drawing of the operative sketch. Osler Library of the History of Medicine. Montreal Neurological Hospital, case C.F., 1934.

left homonymous hemianopia with sparing of the central vision. A PEG showed that the occipital horn of the right lateral ventricle was markedly enlarged, attesting to an atrophic process in the right occipital pole. A craniotomy was elevated so as to expose the posterior parietal area and the occipital lobe. Penfield's interest in this singular case is reflected by his operative report, which is one of his most anatomically precise, by the detailed operative sketches, and by the expert drawing of the results of operation that he commissioned. As Penfield noted,

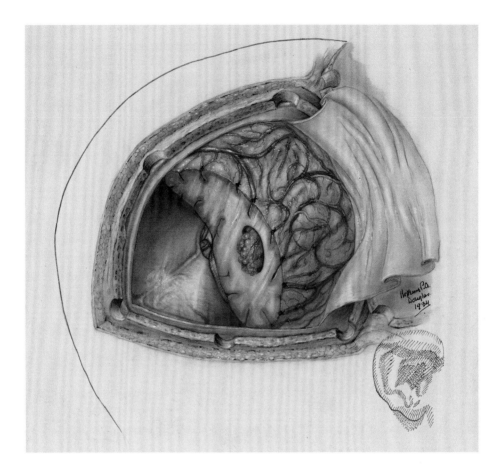

A large occipital bone flap was turned forward by Dr Choróbski. The dura was then opened and dissected free from the pia. A large amount of bleeding was encountered from the horizontal sinus especially [at the site of] the reflected bone flap. The area for sensation in the thumb and index finger was mapped out but no further exploration was done because of bleeding … There were dense adhesions between pia and dura over the external aspect of the occipital lobe. These adhesions became more dense at the tip of the occipital pole where they were replaced by a very dense scar, which passed inward beneath the occipital lobe. The ventricle extended backward into a cyst, which presented on the surface of the brain at the junction between the falx and the tentorium. When the fluid was allowed to escape from the cyst there appeared an excavation, so that it seemed to me that the whole calcarine area had been destroyed. This destruction passed forward and downward to the hippocampal gyrus, where it seemed to stop short abruptly. The convolutions of the occipital lobe seemed a little small and were somewhat flattened … The occipital pole was then removed in a block by silk sutures. The removal passed perpendicularly downward to the posterior end of the corpus callosum. The measured distance from the torcula forward along the falx was 5 centimeters. The measured distance for the line of removal from the torcula lateralwards along the horizontal sinus was 5½ centimetres. The removal followed the hippocampal gyrus below and exposed the edge of the tentorium from the midline outward until it disappeared passing forward. No medial surface of the occipital pole was left behind, if the pole be considered to be that part of the brain which is behind the vein of Galen. I do not think there is any of the calcarine fissure left.

The patient's convalescence was unremarkable, save for the postoperative visual field, which no longer revealed sparing of macular vision in the left visual hemifield.

Penfield's interest in this case resided in a fine point of neuroanatomy. Penfield believed that macular sparing was due to collateral fibres crossing from the right optic tract to the left calcarine fissure via the splenium of the corpus callosum.[20] Thus, Penfield followed the resected specimen into the pathology laboratory and personally examined its microscopic appearance. The final histopathological diagnosis was of a cerebral cicatrix, and, as noted in William Cone's pathology report, "the blocks were reviewed by Dr Penfield and he felt that there was definitely a small trace of calcarine cortex, whether functioning or not could not be said." Penfield chose to believe that the residual calcarine tissue had not been functional and that his operation had interrupted a putative collateral, visual pathway, which has yet to be demonstrated.

These considerations aside, the operation was a great success, the patient reporting no seizures after forty years of follow up.

CHAPTER 6

Brain Tumours

Perhaps the most trying part of a neurosurgeon's work –Cushing

ENCAPSULATED TUMOURS

Wilder Penfield returned to the Presbyterian Hospital after his apprenticeship with Percy Sargent and dedicated the first years of his career to neuro-oncology. His first foray into the field consisted of a report of Victor Horsley and Percy Sargent's cases of osteogenic dural endotheliomas, which we now call meningiomas, benign tumours of the membrane covering the brain.[1] Penfield reviewed 420 cases of brain tumours from the archives at Queen Square in the spring of 1921 and found ten in which cranial hyperostosis, the laying down of bone in the skull in reaction to a meningioma, was a feature. The paper was published in 1923, and, while illustrating Penfield's flair for descriptive neurology – the tumours underlying the hyperostosis were "tender on pressure"[2] – it added to our understanding of the natural history of meningiomas. Penfield's later contribution to the characterization of these benign, encapsulated neoplasms was to elaborate on their microscopic structure and cell of origin.[3] Penfield's opinion on these issues was solicited in both the United States and England, and sketches were drawn and photographs were taken to illustrate addresses and papers on the nature and microscopic appearance of meningiomas. But it is with his studies of the other benign, encapsulated tumours of the nervous system, those that affect the peripheral and the intracranial nerves, the neurofibroma and the Schwannoma, that Penfield had a significant and enduring impact.[4]

Penfield's discovery of the oligodendrocyte[5] and his expertise in the use of the metallic stains were widely recognized and well respected, and it was to learn these techniques that the first research fellows came to his laboratory at the RVH. And it was as a neuropathologist that Penfield published his first substantial paper after his arrival in Montreal.[6] The case was tragic, that of a young woman with von Recklinghausen's disease on whom Penfield was called upon to perform an autopsy.

The patient, A.G., was twenty-one years old when she was first admitted to the RVH in August 1928 because of headache and dizziness, loss of vision, deafness of the left ear, and unsteadiness on her feet. These symptoms and signs had developed

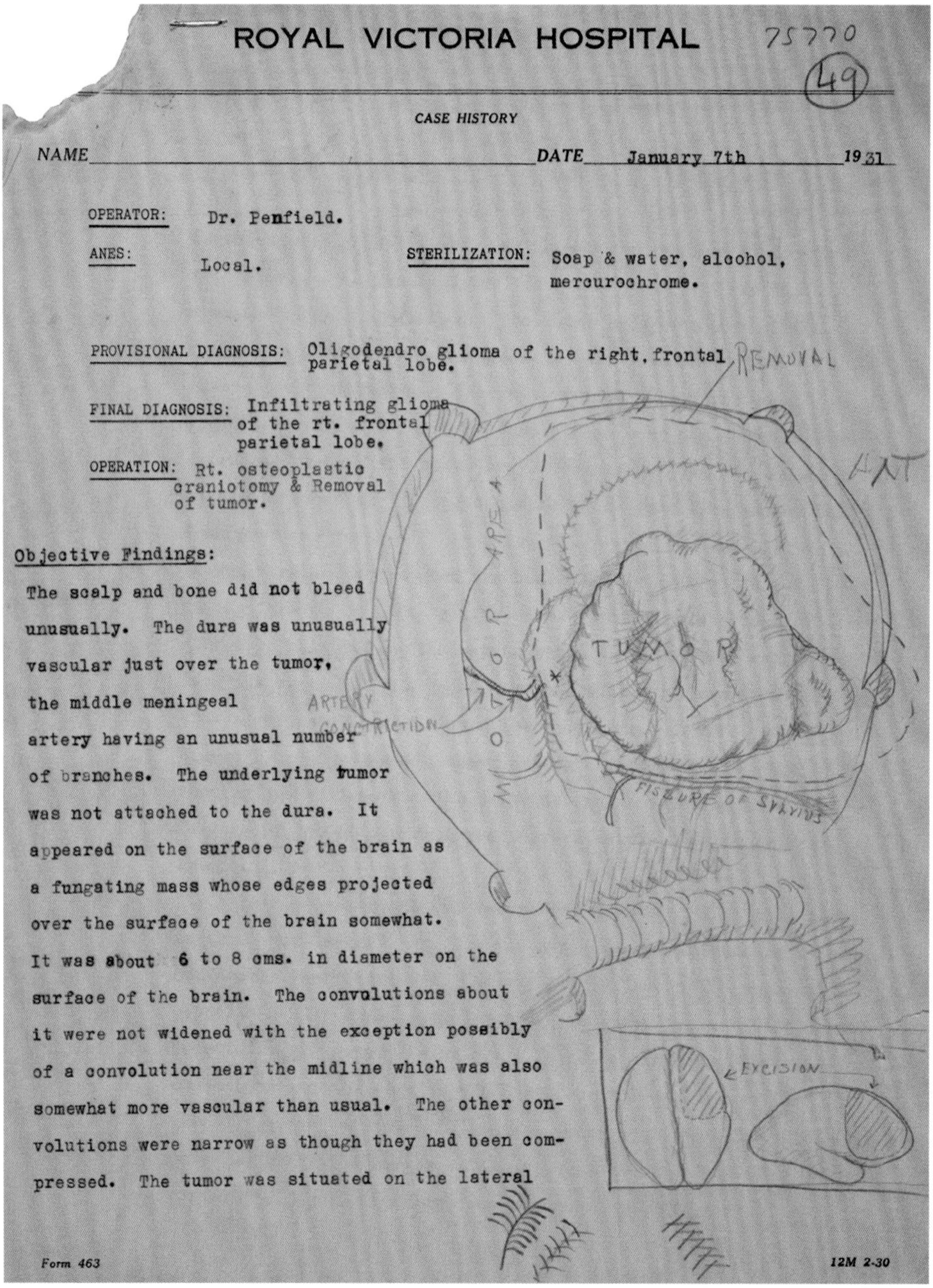

75770
(49)

CASE HISTORY

NAME_____ DATE___ January 7th _____ 19 31

OPERATOR: Dr. Penfield.

ANES: Local.

STERILIZATION: Soap & water, alcohol, mercurochrome.

PROVISIONAL DIAGNOSIS: Oligodendro glioma of the right, frontal parietal lobe.

FINAL DIAGNOSIS: Infiltrating glioma of the rt. frontal parietal lobe.

OPERATION: Rt. osteoplastic craniotomy & Removal of tumor.

Objective Findings:

The scalp and bone did not bleed unusually. The dura was unusually vascular just over the tumor, the middle meningeal artery having an unusual number of branches. The underlying tumor was not attached to the dura. It appeared on the surface of the brain as a fungating mass whose edges projected over the surface of the brain somewhat. It was about 6 to 8 cms. in diameter on the surface of the brain. The convolutions about it were not widened with the exception possibly of a convolution near the midline which was also somewhat more vascular than usual. The other convolutions were narrow as though they had been compressed. The tumor was situated on the lateral

Form 463   12M 2-30

Figure 6.1. Penfield's operative sketch, from the anatomical viewpoint, of a brain tumour occupying the right frontal lobe. The curvilinear indentations represent burr holes in the skull, and the inferior aspect of the main drawing represents the reflected temporal muscle attached to the osteoplastic bone flap. The operative report is typed around the illustration. The precentral gyrus, labelled "motor area," and the Sylvian fissure are indicated. The tumour is seen as it breaches the cortex. The faint line indicates the subcortical extent of the tumour. The thicker, dashed line indicates the area resected, which extends from the frontal pole to the precentral gyrus posteriorly and to the Sylvian fissure inferiorly. The extent of the resection is also indicated in the smaller drawing at lower right. Montreal Neurological Hospital, case H.H., 1931.

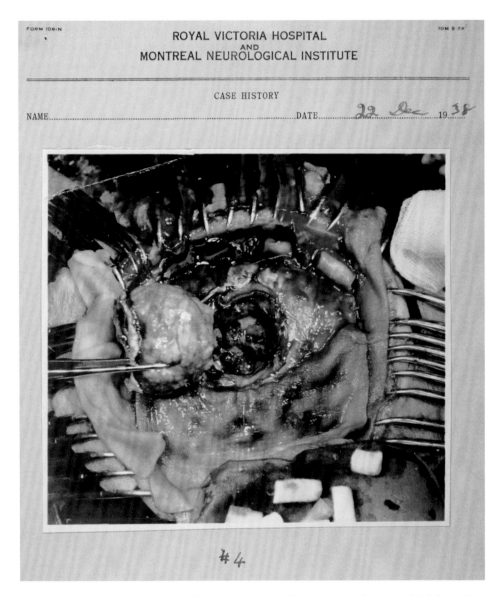

ROYAL VICTORIA HOSPITAL
AND
MONTREAL NEUROLOGICAL INSTITUTE

CASE HISTORY

NAME..DATE............22 Dec 19 38

4

Figure 6.2. Operative photograph, from the anatomical viewpoint, of a resected left frontal lobe meningioma performed in December 1938. The patient was fifty-five years old and had recurrent episodes of unconsciousness preceded by aphasia and twitching of the right eye. The partially calcified meningioma had invaded the inner table of the skull. "The dura was incised just around the tumour. A central core was then removed from the tumour itself by means of the electrocautery. After this the [electrocautery] loop was used to make a further removal out as far as the calcified zone. The tumour was then taken out with great care to preserve the pia over the adjacent brain." Montreal Neurological Hospital, case V.P., 1938.

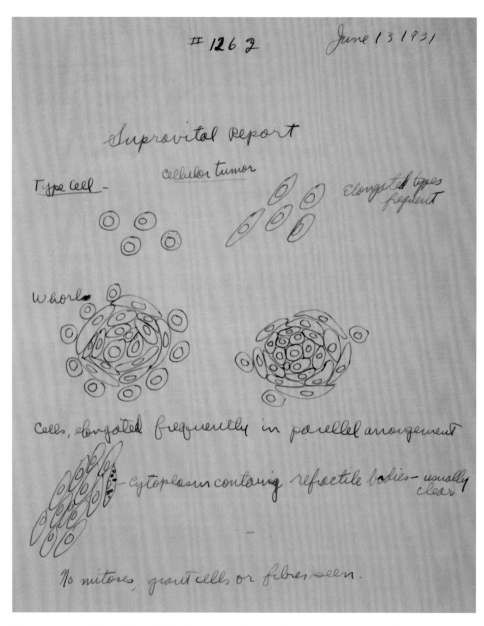

Figure 6.3. Drawing of the cellular elements of a typical meningioma as described by William Cone: "The tumour is quite cellular, its cells being moderately large, round or oval or elongated, containing abundant cytoplasm which in some cases appears rather finely granulated … The cells are arranged in whorls, eddies or more rarely parallel fashion. The whorl pattern is predominant." The whorls are illustrated in the middle of the sketch. Montreal Neurological Hospital, case H.A., 1931.

gradually and had progressed relentlessly over the preceding seven years. Her condition continued to decline while she was in hospital: hearing in the right ear became affected, her vision, previously diminished, now became blurred, and her speech became slurred. The diagnosis of a lesion affecting the cerebellum and brain stem was made, and, in the face of her relentless deterioration, the decision was made to operate. William Cone was consulted on her case, but Francis Scrimger, a general surgeon, performed the surgery. Francis Alexander Caron Scrimger had graduated from McGill University Medical School in 1905 and had served as a medical officer in World War I. He was awarded the Victoria Cross for heroism in protecting his wounded under fire.[7] Scrimger performed a decompressive craniectomy by removing the skull overlying the cerebellum but thought it prudent not to open the dura, which would have caused the cerebellum to herniate from its confines, a situation which surgeons were ill equipped to manage at the time. To everyone's dismay but to no one's surprise, the patient died shortly after surgery.

It has largely been forgotten that Penfield was the first to distinguish between neurofibroma and Schwannoma, the tumours that define von Recklinghausen's disease.[8] Through his mastery of cytological techniques, Penfield reported the characteristic findings that distinguish one tumour from the other: "In the case of von Recklinghausen's disease, nerve fibres will be found to enter each tumour [neurofibroma] with few exceptions, while in solitary perineural fibroblastomata [Schwannoma] the comparatively normal nerve is invariably applied to the capsule of the tumour without penetrating it."[9]

Penfield's paper had been published in 1927 in a very widely read journal,[10] and it was natural that he would be called upon to perform the poor girl's autopsy. Penfield found neurofibromas of the peripheral nerves and spinal nerve roots, an ependymoma of the spinal cord, multiple meningiomas, an astrocytoma of the brain, and Schwannomas of cranial nerves III, V, VII, VIII, and of the lower cranial nerves. The extent and variety of central and peripheral nervous system tumours in this case were brought to the attention of the American Neurological Association in Atlantic City, in 1929,[11] and Penfield published her case the following year in the *Archives of Neurology and Psychiatry*.[12] Of particular interest was the extensive tumoural involvement of the cranial nerves, which he described as he viewed the undersurface of the brain:

a large, firm and encapsulated tumour attached to the left auditory nerve … measuring 5.5 by 3.5 cm. It compressed and distorted the pons, medulla and cerebellum. On section, it was observed to have the consistency of a raw potato. It had irregular areas of fibrous tissue and contained smaller areas of old haemorrhages. A large blood vessel was seen to course through the tumour. The corresponding internal auditory meatus was widened to measure 1.5 by 0.8 cm. A smaller tumour,

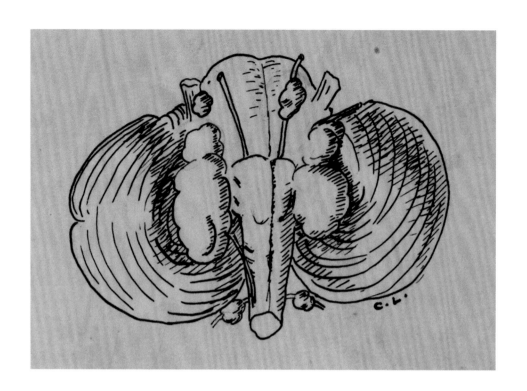

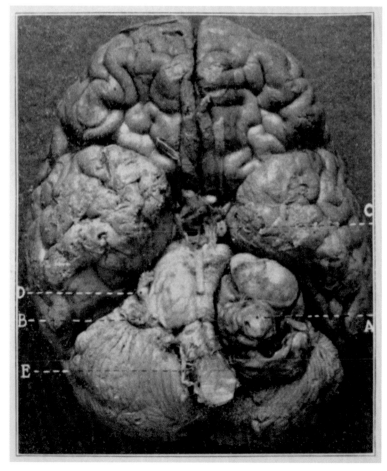

the size of a split pea and well encapsulated, was seen in the right cerebellopontile angle arising from the right auditory nerve about 1 cm. from its exit. The right facial nerve was attached to this tumour. A small tumour was attached to the left oculomotor nerve just after its exit from the mid-brain; it lay below the left posterior cerebral artery. A smaller tumour in the substance of the right trigeminal nerve was present just after the nerve made its exit from the pons. The left trigeminal nerve had an irregular nodular thickening immediately beyond the gasserian ganglion. Pinhead-sized tumours were seen along the glossopharyngeal, the vagus, the spinal accessory and the hypoglossal nerves. Thus, all the cranial nerves were involved with the exception of the first, second and fourth.

Penfield drew a sketch illustrating these tumours and the mass effect on the pons for the pathological report, and a photograph was taken for publication. The paper still stands as one of the best-documented cases of von Recklinghausen's disease.

GLIOMAS

Gliomas are the most common primary brain tumours, but their appellation is a misnomer. When the brain was first submitted to microscopy, the neurons were readily apparent as punctate structures within a sea of amorphous tissue, which the early microscopists believed to be the glue, or *glia*, that supported the neurons. The work of Camillo Golgi, Ramón y Cajal, and Pío del Río Hortega – and Penfield – revealed that the glia is in fact composed of three characteristic cells, which are named for their appearance under the microscope. These are the astrocyte, with its star-like projections, the plump oligodendrocyte, and the small microcyte. Primary brain tumours most commonly arise from the astrocyte and are referred to as *astrocytomas*. The most common form of brain tumour is the *glioblastoma multiforme* – known as GBM – an especially aggressive type of astrocytoma.

Penfield foresaw that the characterization of brain tumours was necessary to make neurosurgery a viable discipline. As he said in his 1930 address to the British Medical Association, "Tumour classification based on histological similarities must serve to

Figure 6.4. *Opposite top* Sketch of the ventral surface of the brain illustrating tumorous lesions of cranial nerves III, V, and VII-XII. Montreal Neurological Hospital.

Figure 6.5. *Opposite bottom* Postmortem photograph of the brain illustrated in the previous figure, showing a tumour of the left and right auditory nerves (A, B), of the left oculomotor nerve (C), of the right trigeminal nerve (D), and tumours of the glossopharyngeal and vagus nerves (E). Montreal Neurological Institute and Hospital, Penfield and Young, "The Nature of von Recklinghausen's Disease."

separate out groups of neoplasms whose biological behaviour is likewise similar …
It makes neurosurgery more discriminating, and it serves as a basis for treatment,
for prognosis, and for analysis."[13] He applied his expertise in the use of the Spanish
gold and silver stains to gliomas and rapidly became an authority on their origin,
classification, treatment, and prognosis.[14] Thus, when he asked outstanding figures
in neuropathology to contribute to the landmark, three-volume *Cytology and
Cellular Pathology of the Nervous System*[15] under his editorial direction, all agreed.
Penfield naturally assigned himself the section on neurofibromatosis,[16] as well as
the chapter on gliomas.[17]

Penfield's academic interest in brain tumours was matched by his clinical activities in his early days at the Royal Victoria Hospital, where he performed more
craniotomies for brain tumours than for posttraumatic epilepsy. Penfield's surgical
approach for the resection of brain tumours was the same as for posttraumatic
scars. First he tried to localize the lesion as precisely as possible from his patient's
history and physical examination, and with pneumoencephalography. This could
be a dangerous examination when performed in patients suspected of having a
brain tumour because the removal of CSF in patients with a brain tumour could
case the cerebellar tonsils to herniate downward, resulting in coma and death.

Once the tumour had been localized, Penfield proceeded as he did in epilepsy
cases. He performed a large craniotomy under local anaesthesia and identified the
motor strip by cortical stimulation so as to avoid encroaching on eloquent areas,
which might lead to paralysis or aphasia. Sometimes, however, the tumour had become large enough to cause a significant rise in intracranial pressure. In such cases
resection had to proceed expeditiously, and cortical mapping might not have been
as detailed as it would have been in a less precarious situation. Such was the case of
Penfield's sister Ruth Inglis.

It is one of the great ironies of Penfield's life that the cell he discovered caused his
sister's death. Ruth had had epileptic seizures since she was nineteen years old. It
took twenty years for her seizures to become disabling, and she was referred to Colin
Russel, the MNI's first neurologist-in-chief. Russel observed swelling of the optic
nerves as he examined the fundus of Ruth's eyes, an indication that the intracranial
pressure was severely elevated, and he found that the left side of the body was
weak, indicating a lesion of the right side of the brain. She was admitted to the Royal
Victoria Hospital, where skull x-rays demonstrated calcification within the right
frontal lobe, a frequent finding in oligodendrogliomas. Penfield operated upon Ruth
on 11 December 1928, a few weeks after arriving in Montreal. It is perhaps not surprising that Penfield would operate on Ruth. After Cushing in Boston, he and Cone
were the ablest neurosurgeons at the time, but the elevated intracranial pressure
made travel to Boston dangerous and surgery was needed urgently. Further, the pressure exerted on Penfield by family and colleagues was insurmountable, and he

agreed to proceed. Penfield, assisted by Cone, turned a large right osteoplastic bone flap under local anaesthesia.

> The presence of the tumour betrayed itself on the surface only by an increased vascularity. The pattern of the convolutions was maintained. On making an incision into the suspected area greyish-brown neoplasm was encountered[18] … We worked for hours, taking that tumour out and trying to leave the untouched brain so normal that there would be no more epileptic seizures. At last we had carried the removal of the frontal lobe back to the motor gyrus. To make sure, I touched the gyrus with an electrode. It caused the hand to move. We could go no further on the surface … But, to my dismay, the growth was not all out. It extended underneath … on the floor of the skull. Enormous veins came up through the tissue … I stopped and looked at Bill Cone. He shook his head. "Don't chance it Wide" … I passed a heavy thread across the mass and pushed the thread down with one finger, forming a surgeon's knot. I tightened it gently, the thread began to cut the growth from the base … I tightened the knot of my thread, little by little, cutting the mass of tumour gradually free from the dura at the base, and hoping that the grip of the thread would close off all of those enormous veins. But suddenly, just as I thought I had succeeded, there came a rush of blood swirling up from the base of the skull and hiding everything in a rapidly deepening pool of blood. I reached in with my gloved fingers and removed the remnant of the tumour mass … The patient's condition now became quite critical and the pulse weak. She was transfused three times in succession and saline solution kept running into the vein of the arm slowly between transfusions[19] … She left the operating room conscious and in fairly satisfactory condition. Three weeks after operation she left the hospital feeling well.[20]

Percival Bailey and Paul Bucy, at the University of Chicago, had recently described tumours arising from the oligodendrocyte,[21] but Penfield, surprisingly, had been sceptical that such a tumour existed. Ruth's case changed his mind, as he recounted in a discussion of oligodendrogliomas at the annual meeting of the American Neurological Association in 1929: "I was doubtful about the oligodendrogliomas at first. I have since had a chance to study Dr Bailey's specimens, and this fall I removed a similar specimen from a patient seen in association with Dr Colin Russel. The patient gave a history of nineteen years duration: the tumour was calcified, and occupied the whole right frontal lobe. I would agree now that there is a type of slowly growing tumour that may be called oligodendroglioma."[22]

Penfield next referred to his sister's case at the annual meeting of the British Medical Association, in Winnipeg, in 1930.[23] Commenting on her case, Penfield reported that there had been "complete absence of any immediate mental symptoms

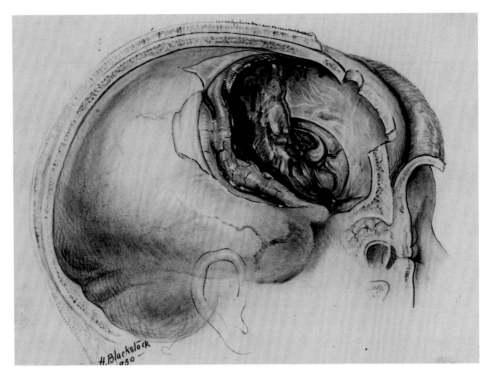

Figure 6.6. Harriet Blackstock's draft illustration of the extent of resection in Ruth Inglis's case: "Amputation was carried back to within a centimetre of the motor gyrus all the way down to the lowest frontal gyrus. From this line it passed across cleanly to the mid-line so that the septum pellucidum and the anterior two or three centimetres of the sectioned corpus callosum were visible after the removal." Osler Library of the History of Medicine.

attributable to the removal of the right frontal lobe" and that in view of the tumorous nature of the lesion, "a secondary removal may have to be undertaken any time within the next ten years."[24] Ten years were too much to hope for. Her seizures recurred as the residual tumour enlarged, and a few weeks after her case had been consigned to the pages of the *British Medical Journal*, Ruth was referred to Harvey Cushing for reoperation. She died six months later from haemorrhage into the residual tumour. Her brain was removed at autopsy and two photographs of it, one from the top and one from the bottom, were used to illustrate an address that Penfield gave at a meeting of the Association for Research in Nervous and Mental Disease in 1932.[25] Her case was also included in a small series of frontal lobe resections that Penfield published in *Brain* in 1935.[26] In this paper, however, Penfield changed his opinion of his sister's postoperative course: "the loss of the right frontal lobe had resulted in an important defect. The defect produced was a lack of capacity for planned administration. Perhaps the element which made such administration almost impossible was the loss of power of initiative."[27] Seeing firsthand the effects

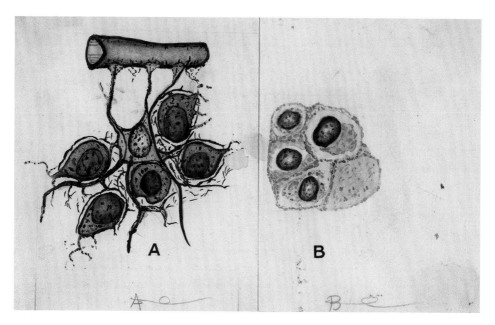

Figure 6.7. Draft drawing of the microscopic structure of Ruth Inglis's oligodendroglioma. "With most staining methods the rounded, even nuclei stain well but the cytoplasm almost not at all, often giving to the nuclei a sort of halo resembling the appearance of swollen oligodendrocytes. The cells are placed closely together like pavement and seem in characteristic area [*sic*] to be separated into groups by the expansions of scattered astrocytes which, in fact form stroma for this tumour." Osler Library of the History of Medicine.

of frontal lobectomy is undoubtedly one of the reasons why Penfield did not perform or endorse prefrontal lobotomy for the treatment of psychotic disorders.

Penfield last referred to his sister's case in 1938, in a masterful treatise on cerebral tumours, in which a drawing of the microscopic appearance of her tumour illustrates the histopathology of the oligodendroglioma.[28]

Penfield operated on his sister under local anaesthesia and with the aid of cortical mapping to identify the motor strip. The mapping was limited in her case because the raised intracranial pressure mandated an expedient resection. In many circumstances, however, seizures were an early sign of an intracranial tumour, and the lesion was still relatively small when it was diagnosed. This allowed more extensive cortical mapping and greater confidence in localizing the Rolandic and Sylvian fissures. The results of electrocortical stimulation in brain tumour patients were recorded as an annotated, intraoperative sketch for later study just as was done for epilepsy patients. One of the sketches reproduced here illustrates the extent of cortical stimulation that could be performed in such cases. The results of stimulation in this case were recorded on a hand-drawn brain map. Once the MNI opened, the

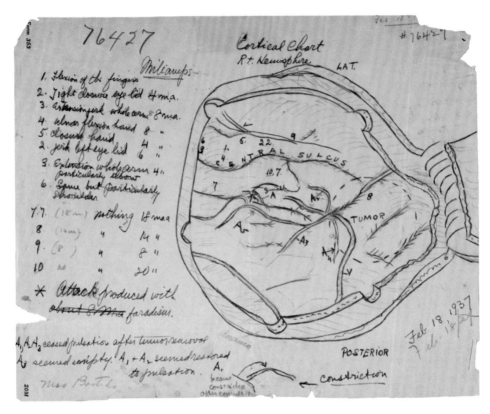

Figure 6.8. Penfield's sketch of the right cerebral hemisphere exposed at surgery. In this orientation the frontal lobe is above the Rolandic fissure, which is labelled "central sulcus," and the parietal lobe is below it. The circular dashed line outlines the temporal tumour, which extends into the supra-Sylvian region and behind the vein of Labbé, labelled V. The results of cortical stimulation are recorded at left and indicated by corresponding numbers in the sketch. An epileptic seizure was triggered by stimulation at the point indicated by the star (between letters A and A5). Montreal Neurological Hospital, case A.B.

results of stimulation were dictated verbatim to a secretary in the gallery, and pre- and poststimulation and resection photographs were taken. The dictated notes, brain map, and operative photographs were included in the patient's chart and were used for the study of the structure–function relationship of the of the cortex.

By 1932, Penfield also used preprinted brain maps to record his operative findings. The map that Penfield first used had been designed by Cécile and Oskar Vogt and was based on their map of the cyto-tectonic areas of the monkey brain. Otfrid Foerster transposed the Vogts' map to a human brain, and Penfield adopted the latter for his own use.[29] Although lacking the immediacy of the hand-drawn sketches, the preprinted map provided a standardized method of recording the results of stimulation and the extent of resection of a tumour or of an epileptic scar. The maps delineated

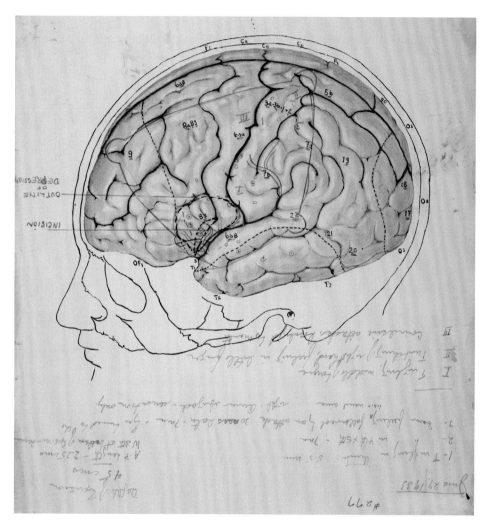

Figure 6.9. Penfield's brain map recording the effects of cortical stimulation and the relationship of the tumour to the surrounding brain. The point of entry into the subcortical neoplasm and the extent of the resection are indicated. Montreal Neurological Hospital, case D.H., 1932.

the somatotopic areas as described by the Vogts, the frontal, squamous, and lamb-doid sutures, and thick black, sinusoidal lines represented the Sylvian and Rolandic fissures. Individual convolutions were rendered in grey-scale to give them a three-dimensional appearance, but this was achieved at the expense of clarity. Although stimulation points could now be recorded in relationship to the fixed, easily recognizable fissures of Sylvius and Rolando, the stimulation points were difficult to discern against the busy grey background. Penfield later switched to a similar map in black and white against which stimulation points stood out more clearly.[30]

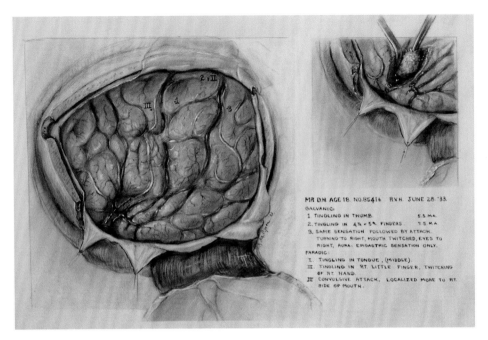

Figure 6.10. Artist's rendering of Penfield's brain map from the preceding figure. The results of cortical stimulation are recorded in relationship to the fissures of Sylvius and Rolando, and the pathological lesion and its resection are clearly illustrated in the inset. Montreal Neurological Hospital, case D.H., 1932.

Patient D.H. was one of the patients in which the first version of the preprinted map was used, and in whom a medical illustrator, Harriett Blackstock, rendered the operative findings.[31] D.H. is also one of the first patients in whom Penfield resected a tumour in close proximity to Broca's area.

D.H. was eighteen years old when he was admitted to the Royal Victoria Hospital in 1933, suffering from focal seizures involving the right arm, following which he was unable to speak for a short time. A skull x-ray showed an area of calcification within the inferior and posterior aspect of the left frontal lobe. A large fronto-temporal craniotomy was elevated and a three-centimetre, depressed, and softened area, limited inferiorly by the Sylvian fissure and posteriorly by the fissure of Rolando, was discovered in the left frontal lobe. This is the classically described location of Broca's area, and as expected, stimulation about the lesion produced aphasic responses.

A small cortical incision centreed on the softened area exposed two calcified nodules surrounded by a well-demarcated accumulation of brownish, gelatinous material. "Passing through the incision the tumour was removed partially by suction. The calcified nodules were rolled out with a spatula … Throughout the procedure the patient talked quite well. There was at no time any evidence of aphasia."[32] The

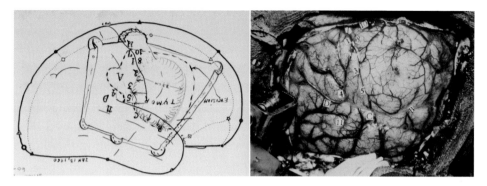

Figure 6.11. *Left*. Operative sketch of a right frontal brain tumour. The arrows within the tumour indicate that the tumour had displaced the Sylvian fissure inferiorly and the central fissure posteriorly. Stimulations at 1 and 2 produced sensations in the tongue and at 3–7 produced sensations in the left side of the face. The mouth opened at 8. Tonic alternating movements and weakness of the left face were produced by stimulation at 10, and stimulation at 12 produced movement of the hand. Number 12 is at the upper extent of the surgical exposure, just outside the resection margin. Rhythmic sharp waves were recorded at A, and electrographic discharges were recorded at B–D, concurrently with a sensation that the patient reported as "the regular feeling of an attack." *Right*. Preresection operative photograph showing the tumour and its relationship to the surrounding brain. The instrument partially visible at mid-left is the lower part of the cortical electrode holder. Montreal Neurological Hospital, case P.O., 1960.

resection of tumours near eloquent areas performed under local anaesthesia and aided by cortical mapping continues to be performed at the MNI to this day.

Penfield published a study entitled "Relations of Intracranial Tumours and Symptomatic Epilepsy" in 1940. It is one of the first studies to address this issue. Penfield and his coworkers, Theodore Erickson and Isadore Tarlov,[33] analyzed the incidence of epilepsy in patients with intracranial tumours and their prevalence by site and tissue type. They found that the occurrence of seizures largely depended on the site of the tumour. Thirty-two percent of patients with a tumour of the occipital lobe had one or more epileptic seizures during the course of their illness. This figure rose to 48% in patients with a temporal lobe tumour. The frequency of seizures in patients with frontal and parietal lobe tumours was 53% and 68%, respectively, the frequency increasing the closer the tumour was to the motor and sensory strips. The relatively low frequency of seizures in patients with a temporal lobe tumour may have been due to the lack of recognition of psychomotor epilepsy at the time, with seizures misdiagnosed as hysteria or mental deficiency.

The prevalence of seizures was also related to the rapidity with which the tumour progressed. Thus, more than 90% of patients with an oligodendroglioma, a very slow growing tumour, developed seizures during the course of their illness. The lowest prevalence of seizures, 39%, was seen in patients with the very rapidly growing glioblastoma multiforme. This led Penfield to bemoan, "slowly growing neoplasms have a higher incidence of secondary epilepsy than the rapidly growing tumours, probably because death terminates the history sooner in cases of the latter type."[34]

Despite the dismal prognosis for patients afflicted with a brain tumour at the time, Penfield's attempts to alleviate their suffering through surgery aided by cortical mapping contributed to the elaboration of the structure–function relationship of the brain and the birth of the homunculus.

PART TWO

The Montreal Neurological Institute, 1934–76

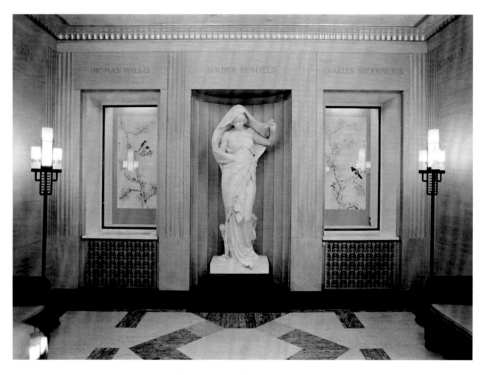

Figure 7.1. Montreal Neurological Institute lobby. *Nature Unveiling Herself before Science.* Montreal Neurological Institute and McGill University.

SECTION ONE

The Structure–Function Relationship of the Brain

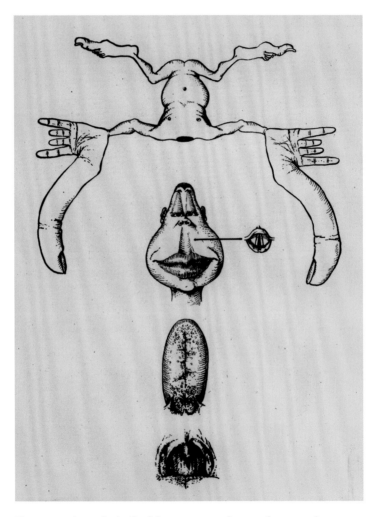

Figure 7.2. An early draft of the sensory and motor homunculus. Hortense Cantile. Osler Library of the History of Medicine.

CHAPTER 7

The Homunculus

I would kill the damn thing if I could –Penfield, 1946[1]

The governor general of Canada, the 9th Earl of Bessborough, laid the cornerstone of the Montreal Neurological Institute on 6 October 1933, and Sir Edward Beatty, chancellor of McGill University, declared the institute open on 27 September 1934. The MNI is on the eastern rise of Mount Royal, the extinct volcano that overlooks the city of Montreal and the Saint Lawrence River. Mount Royal was the source of the grey stone with which the MNI was erected, and so the institute appears to rise from the mountain itself. An elegant, enclosed stone bridge arched over University Street and joined the institute to the Royal Victoria Hospital. A sculptured plaque on the front facade, bordered on either side by representations of the brain and spinal cord, and surmounted by the rising sun, stated the mission of the institute: *Dedicated to relief of sickness and pain and to the study of neurology.* A few steps up from the sidewalk lead to the MNI foyer, which is dominated by a sculpture of un-blemished white marble representing *Nature Revealing Herself before Science.*[2] The foyer's ceiling is adorned with the drawing of a ram's head, the astrological symbol of the brain, surrounded by a ribbon that states, "But I have seen the wounded brain healed." This stunning pronouncement is an annotation discovered in Galen's copy of Hippocratic aphorisms, in which Hippocrates said "a wound to the head is always fatal." Penfield of course sided with Galen, the ancient Greek physician, not the least because, in his treatment of posttraumatic epilepsy, he had seen the wounded brain healed.

The original building was small. The foyer led to clinical offices on the first floor where neurologists and neurosurgeons saw patients in consultation. An auditorium, later named in honour of John Hughlings Jackson, served as the venue for lectures, case presentations, and addresses for visiting speakers. Over the years the latter have included a multitude of Nobel laureates and other leading figures of every aspect of neuroscience. Clinical wards were located on the second, third, and fourth floors. The x-ray department and the operating rooms were on the fifth floor, where they remain today. The sixth floor accommodated research laboratories. Animal quarters were on the seventh floor, and a squash court occupied a small room on the eight floor. In this building of rough, grey stone the homunculus was born.

CORTICAL LOCALIZATION AFTER BROCA[3]

It can be argued that the significant contributions of nineteenth-century neurology can be distilled to three observations: the consistency of the great fissures of Sylvius and Rolando and the delineation of the lobes and convolutions of the brain by Pierre Gratiolet, the discovery of the laminar structure of the cerebral cortex by Jules Baillarger,[4] and the localization of articulate language to the third left frontal convolution by Paul Broca.[5] Further progress in establishing the structure–function relationship of the human brain depended on the clinico-pathological method. This method consists of correlating a distinct neurological deficit to a specific area of the brain, identified at the postmortem examination of the patient. It is also referred to as "lesion analysis." Following Broca in their application of the clinico-pathological method, Theodor Meynert[6] and Carl Wernicke[7] localized the receptive aspects of spoken language to the first and second temporal convolutions of the left hemisphere, and Jules Dejerine localized the inability to understand and express written language to the left angular gyrus.[8] The use of the clinico-pathological method to localize brain function reached its apogee in France, where Jean Martin Charcot and his student Albert Pitres published a catalogue of well-studied, autopsied cases to localize specific sensory-motor functions – those of the face, the hand, the arm, the foot, and the leg – to the pre- and postcentral convolutions in man.[9] However, lesion analysis is limited in its applications. It is hampered by its reliance on the segregation of a single sign or symptom from what might be a panoply of clinical manifestations and correlating it to a specific part of a widely damaged region of the brain. Indeed, the damage in Broca's first patients far exceeded the third frontal convolution.[10] A more specific method consisted of applying a mild electrical current to a point on the cerebral cortex of animals and observing its effects on the body. Gustav Fritsch and Eduard Hitzig used this method in 1870 and demonstrated that motor responses could be elicited from the *gyrus sigmoideus* of the dog, which is the canine equivalent of the human precentral gyrus.[11] Fritsch and Hitzig then resected the stimulated cortex, which caused paralysis of the muscles that had reacted to stimulation. David Ferrier at the West Riding Lunatic Asylum in Yorkshire, England, undertook the systematic localization of cortical function by electrical stimulation and resection in a variety of animals, including subhuman primates.[12] Charles Sherrington elaborated upon Ferrier's work in the great apes and reached the limit of what could be accomplished by stimulation and lesion analysis in animals.

   The localization of functions to the human brain was taken up at the end of the nineteenth century and the beginning of the twentieth by Fedor Krause in Berlin,[13] Harvey Cushing in Boston,[14] Victor Horsley in London,[15] and Otfrid Foerster in

Breslau.[16] These neurological surgeons localized the motor and sensory functions in man by cortical stimulation of the pre- and postcentral convolutions of patients upon whom they operated under local anaesthesia.[17] Krause deserves special mention. He operated upon patients suffering from posttraumatic epilepsy under local anaesthesia and was the first to use cortical stimulation to map the motor strip.[18] Three physicians were present in Krause's operating room to document the effect of cortical stimulations, one to observe the face, the other two to observe the upper and lower extremities. They dictated their observations to a secretary, and Krause noted the points on the cortex from which each response had been generated. In this way Krause not only identified the epileptic focus and motor responses in individual patients, which allowed him to safely resect an epileptic focus or a tumour, he also published the first detailed human brain map localizing the motor strip to the precentral gyrus, in 1908:[19]

> The anterior central convolution contains all the [motor] foci located. Their arrangement on the cortical surface is such that the centres for the lower extremity occupy the uppermost portion of the convolution near the sinus longitudinalis … the lower extremity engages as its locus approximately the upper one-fourth of the central convolution. About one-half of the middle portion responds to stimuli with contralateral muscular contractions of the upper extremity, from the shoulders down to the fingers. The lower one-third of the convolution discloses, upon irritation, the foci of the muscles of the face and those of mastication. Here should also be found the centres of the muscles of the larynx, the platysma myoides, and the muscles of the tongue.[20]

Harvey Cushing published the first results obtained from stimulation of the postcentral gyrus, establishing its role in the perception of somatic sensation,[21] as well as confirming Krause's findings on the function of the precentral convolution.[22] Otfrid Foerster also produced a brain map based on his experience in the operating room, which Penfield transcribed for publication in English in 1930.[23]

PENFIELD AND HIS PATIENTS

Penfield took up the stimulating electrode from Foerster,[24] and in 1937 he published his own brain maps with his coauthor Edwin Boldrey.[25] A distinct parallel can be made between Charcot's clinico-pathological method and Penfield's method of electrocortical stimulation of the brain. As Charcot had done with lesion analysis, Penfield correlated specific sensory and motor responses produced by cortical

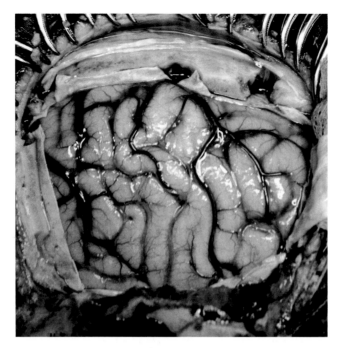

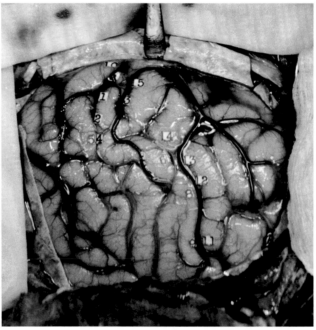

Figure 7.3. *Top* Operative photograph of the right hemisphere of the brain. The pre- and postcentral gyri are indistinguishable. Montreal Neurological Hospital.

Figure 7.4. *Bottom* Same case as in the preceding figure, following electrocortical stimulation. The postcentral gyrus was first identified, as indicated by numbers 1, 2, 4, 6, 8, 9. The precentral, motor, gyrus is identified by numbers 11–15. Montreal Neurological Hospital.

stimulation to specific areas of the cortex of the cerebral hemispheres. This method resulted in a probabilistic map of the structure–function relationship exemplified by the iconic "Penfield homunculus."

Penfield approached the surgery of epileptic patients as a scientist approaches an experiment. Thus, his famous statement that the operating room was his laboratory. By this he meant that the decision to operate was based on the formulation of a well-grounded, evidence-based hypothesis with regard to the site and nature of the pathology responsible for each individual patient's seizures. Each hypothesis was based on a detailed analysis of a patient's seizure pattern and on a meticulous neurological examination. This resulted in a preliminary localization of the epileptic lesion, which, if confirmed by electrographic and radiological findings, led to a decision to operate. As Penfield noted, "The surgeon who performs a craniotomy without a carefully considered constructive hypothesis places himself on a level with the practitioner of the stone age."

Electrocortical stimulation was performed as a necessary adjunct to surgery, to confirm the epileptogenic nature of the tissue to be resected, and to assure that the resection would not encroach upon areas subserving sensation, motility, or language. Thus, as Penfield noted, "surgical procedures are never primarily experimental. Nevertheless, for the clinician who waits hopefully, chance often fulfills the most exacting requirements of physiological observation, and little by little time fills up the gaps in the evidence." This is the method by which Penfield charted the cortex of man. To be successful, such demanding surgery must be based on a relationship of trust between the surgeon and the patient: trust on the part of the patient in the surgeon's skill and judgment, and trust on the part of the surgeon that the patient will accurately report the effects of cortical stimulation.[26] Penfield admired his patients. He admired their courage in embarking upon what must have seemed to them a daunting procedure and their stamina during the long hours necessary to perform the operation.[27]

DATA POINTS – THE BIRTH OF THE HOMUNCULUS

The precentral gyrus is a motor keyboard and useful movement
is its music –Penfield[28]

The Penfield homunculus arose from Edwin Boldrey's master's thesis, published by McGill University in 1936.[29] Boldrey's thesis is in two parts. The first part is entitled "The Architectonic Subdivision of the Mammalian Brain" and is a study of the cytological architecture of the cortex that Penfield had removed at surgery. The second part, "A Report of Electrical Stimulation of One Hundred and Five Human Cerebral Corticies," is of lasting interest. As the title indicates, Boldrey reviewed the operative

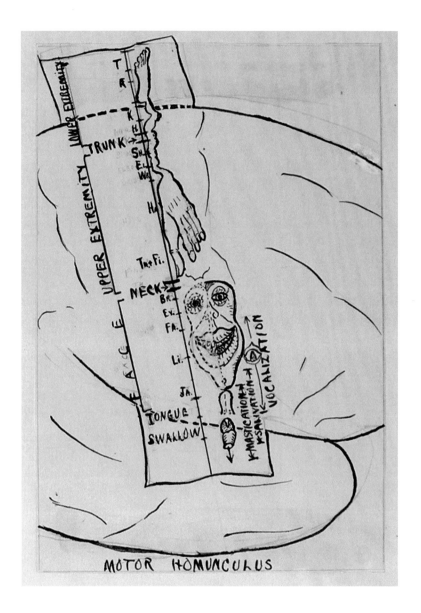

MOTOR HOMUNCULUS

records, brain maps, and operative photographs of 105 patients upon whom Penfield and Cone had operated for the resection of a tumour or of an epileptogenic scar. Each stimulation point was assigned to one of twenty-eight brain maps, each representing a specific function. These included movement and sensation of the tongue, mouth, jaw, face, and throat; swallowing; vocalizing; and sensation and movements of fingers, hand, arm, shoulder, trunk, leg, and foot. Vision and audition were also represented, as were autonomic functions, and head and eye movements. Each stimulation point was placed on the appropriate composite map according to its distance from the Sylvian and Rolandic fissures, thereby creating a cluster diagram of indi-

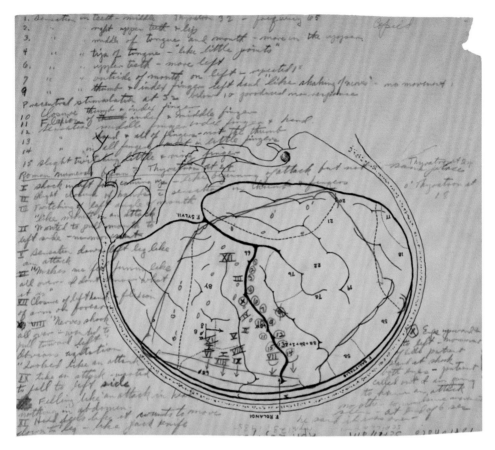

Figure 7.5. *Opposite* The motor strip. Study for the second version of the homunculus. Note the indication of the bilateral motor representation of the face. Hortense Cantile. Osler Library of the History of Medicine.

Figure 7.6. *Above* Penfield's map of the right hemisphere drawn from the surgeon's viewpoint. Stimulation at numbers 1 to 8 produced sensation in the teeth, lips, tongue, and mouth. Stimulation at 9, and at 12 to 15, produced sensation in the hand, thumb, and fingers. Stimulation at III produced twitching of the angle of the mouth. Stimulation at 10 and 11 produced flexion of the index and middle fingers respectively, stimulation at II and VII produced closure of the hand, and stimulation at VII produced flexion of the elbow. Stimulation in the frontal eye field, at I, IV–VI, VIII–XI, and XIII, elicited turning of the head and eyes to the left, and caused the patient to have a seizure. Montreal Neurological Hospital, case F.S., 1935.

vidual data points. Penfield and Boldrey published much of the second part of Boldrey's thesis, augmented by fifteen additional cases, in *Brain* in 1937, under the title "Somatic Motor and Sensory Representation in the Cerebral Cortex of Man as Studied by Electrical Stimulation."[30] It is in this paper that the homunculus first appeared in print – it is absent from Boldrey's thesis – to illustrate the structure–function relationship of the sensorimotor cortex in a single image.[31]

The homunculus appears as an acrobat hanging by his knees from a trapeze, with his head tilted up to look at the audience. The areas devoted to the thumbs, tongue,

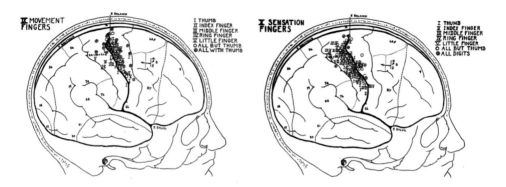

Figure 7.7. Chart IX, "Movement Fingers," and chart X, "Sensations Fingers," from Boldrey's thesis. Each number represents a point where cortical stimulation produced movement or sensation in one or more fingers in the series of 120 patients that Penfield and Cone had operated upon for the resection of a brain tumour or of an epileptic scar. Montreal Neurological Institute, McGill University, Boldrey, "The Architectonic Subdivision of the Mammalian Cerebral Cortex."

and lips are disproportionally large, reflecting their relative importance in the function of the human body, while those devoted to the head, trunk, and legs are small. The homunculus was drawn to illustrate "the invariable consistency of both motor and sensory sequence," and to show that "there are two clearly separable anatomical patterns, one sensory and one motor, and that the sensory and motor elements for each part are closely related to each other."[32] Francis Walshe, his erstwhile friend and the editor of *Brain* from 1937 to 1953, did not share Penfield's view. "I feel," he wrote Penfield, "that your 'homunculus' does indicate graphically your observations, but that it does not indicate any plan of organization in the motor cortex. It represents a partial aspect of the truth, an aspect so fragmentary that no inferences can be drawn from it. I surmise that you will be heartily tired of its horrific appearance – copied uncritically from text to text – before you see the last of it. You may even have to slay it yourself."[33]

Walshe's criticism must have shaken Penfield's confidence in his creation, for he replied, "As far as the homunculus is concerned, it was one of a number of illustrations which we used to try to illustrate the truth. Of course, there is nothing like the homunculus as far as cortical representation is concerned, but it seems to be the only sort of thing that people in general understand. I would kill the damn thing if I could, but that is never possible. It does call attention to certain facts, such as the reversal of the order of representation in the face and neck, as compared with the rest of the body."[34]

The twenty-eight charts on which the homunculus was broadly based are, however, more scientifically rigorous. They do not predict exactly where a specific function will reside in an individual patient, but they do indicate the area where cortical stimulation is likely to find it. Penfield was forceful on this point when he revisited the homunculus in 1950 in *The Cerebral Cortex of Man*: "The relative length of the central cortex devoted to any one structure varies from individual to individual so that it is impossible to locate the arm area, for example, by measuring from the Sylvian or medial longitudinal fissure." However, the sequence in which the functions are represented is accurate. As for the homunculus itself, Penfield was unequivocal, "it is a cartoon … in which scientific accuracy is impossible."[35]

THE CEREBRAL CORTEX OF MAN[36]

Penfield accumulated cortical data points for another decade before committing his findings between to hard covers. *The Cerebral Cortex of Man* is based on some 400 cortical stimulations, most performed by Penfield and Theodore Rasmussen. Penfield and Rasmussen had published sections of the book in scientific journals before *The Cerebral Cortex of Man* came out.[37] This included a detailed description of cortical motor and sensory representations in which the first diagram that would become the new, iconic Penfield homunculus appeared.[38] The book is short, 235 pages of text, and beautifully illustrated with sharp, black line drawings on a stark, white background. It is divided into eleven chapters that address sensory and motor representation, movement of the eyes and head, vision and hearing, vocalization and speech arrest, the second sensory area, the supplementary motor area, and the autonomic nervous system. An additional chapter discusses the effects of ablation of the areas subserving these functions. The remainder of the text is more speculative, addressing consciousness and the elaboration of thought, and the integration of cortical function with that of the upper brain stem. The new homunculus appeared in its pages for the first time and benefited from the criticism of its first incarnation. Where the 1937 homunculus was grotesque and disarticulated, the newly conceived homunculus is elegant and classic. It is a bicephalic creature, cleaved into fraternal twins effortlessly draped across the hemispheres of the brain, one representing the motor function of the cortex, the other the sensory. One is reminded of the figures of *Dawn* and *Dusk* in the Medici Chapel. The new homunculus owes much of its iconic stature to Hortense Douglas Cantlie's ability to render complex ideas simply and to the impact of clear black lines on a white background.[39]

The elusive male genitalia

The case of patient S.K. is an example of the wealth of information that Penfield sometimes recorded on his brain maps. The case is also of interest because a brain map that includes the sensory representation of male genitalia has not previously been published. The patient began having episodic burning sensations of the right

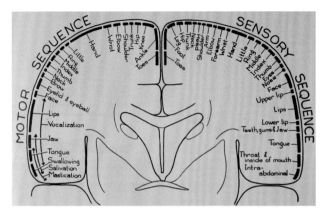

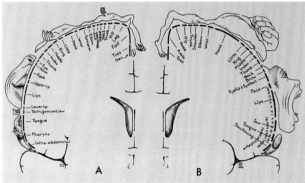

Figure 7.8. *Left*. Diagrammatic representation of motor and sensory responses obtained from cortical stimulation and represented in the plane of the Rolandic fissure. The lengths of the bars indicate the extent of cortical representation of each function. Note that the motor representation for the lips is more extensive than the sensory representation and that the same is true for the hand. The sensory representation of the tongue is more extensive than the motor representation. *Right*. Drawing of the final representation of the sensory (A) and motor functions (B) of the cerebral cortex. Caricatures of each function have been added to the earlier image at left, creating what has become the iconic Penfield homunculus. Penfield and Rasmussen, "Vocalization and Arrest of Speech" and *The Cerebral Cortex of Man*. Osler Library of the History of Medicine.

lower face, neck, and shoulder when he was thirty-one years old. These were sometimes associated with the inability to articulate his thoughts, perseveration (the persistent repetition of a word), and paraphasia (the misuse of words) when he attempted to speak and to write. The attacks progressed to include masticatory movements and salivation, and he was admitted to the MNI when his seizures became generalized. A diffusely infiltrating tumour was suspected in view of the late onset of his seizures and the progressive involvement of different functional areas of the brain. The patient was brought to the operating room a few days after his admission to hospital. Given the detailed brain map and the fifty stimulations that he performed, Penfield's operative note is surprisingly succinct at some 350 words. He

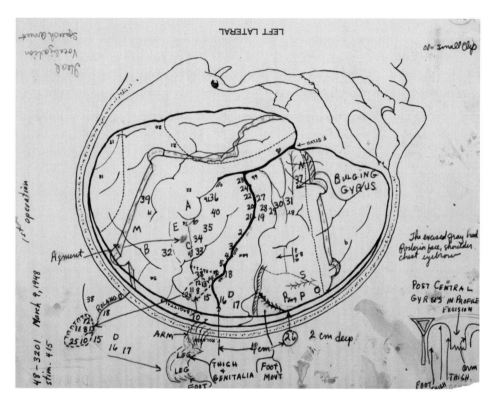

Figure 7.9. Penfield's brain map seen from the surgeon's viewpoint. This is one of the few cases in which responses in the genitalia were produced by cortical stimulation. The central fissure is defined by sensory and motor responses. Stimulation within a narrow segment of the postcentral gyrus, reproduced in the detail at lower left, produced sensations in the right thigh (number 10) and the right gluteus (number 25). This segment was removed just above the sensory arm area, as is illustrated in the mid-lower detail and in the detail at lower right. Resecting this area allowed stimulation of the more medial aspect of the precentral gyrus, which produced sensations in the thigh and genitalia. Montreal Neurological Hospital, case S.K., 1948.

noted that the postcentral gyrus and the posterior aspect of the third frontal convolution (Broca's area) were abnormally splayed over a subcortical mass lesion, confirming his clinical impression of a diffuse neoplastic process.[40] Stimulation of the angular gyrus and of Broca's area generated epileptic activity and resulted in the patient's inability to name objects. The clinico-pathological correlation was obvious: the involvement of Broca's area explained the patient's inability to articulate his thoughts with words and sentences, and that of the angular gyrus was responsible for the patient's inability to express his thoughts in written form.

Penfield then proceeded to identifying the area responsible for triggering the patient's seizures and found that the epileptic focus was in the superior aspect of the postcentral gyrus, in the area representing sensation in the right neck and shoulder. Resecting this area exposed the superior and mesial aspects of the postcentral gyrus to stimulation, which produced a sensation in the patient's genitalia. For whatever reason, Penfield did not note this finding in his operative report. Nonetheless, it is clearly indicated in his brain map, in the vicinity of the representation of the right thigh. This localization is discordant with the localization of male genitalia as published in *The Cerebral Cortex of Man*, where it is represented below the foot area. Penfield, however, was uncertain about this localization, and he undoubtedly had this case in mind when he stated of the male genitalia "its relationship to the foot is not altogether clear."[41] The passage of time has done little to clarify the situation beyond confirming its localization to the medial aspect of the motor strip.

Adrian's cat

One of the most intriguing findings arising from Penfield and Rasmussen's work was the confirmation that there is a second area devoted to sensation within the human cerebral cortex. The existence of a second sensory area in mammals was discovered by Edgar Adrian – later Lord Adrian – who shared the 1932 Nobel Prize for Physiology and Medicine with Sir Charles Sherrington for their work on the physiology of the neuron. Adrian presented a paper to the Physiological Society (London) in 1940, entitled "Double Representation of the Feet in the Sensory Cortex of the Cat."[42] Adrian first delineated the primary sensory cortex of the cat by using sensory evoked responses. This produced a charming feline evocation of Penfield's homunculus. But Adrian also found a second region of the cat's cortex subserving sensation of the forefoot and hindfoot, which was situated below the face area.[43] This site is now referred to as the *secondary somatosensory area* (s-II). Adrian described s-II when he gave the 1942 Hughlings Jackson Lecture at the MNI on the topic of the "Sensory Areas of the Brain,"[44] which no doubt had a great influence on Penfield in his search for the human equivalent of this area. As Adrian found s-II below the inferior aspect of the primary sensory regions in the cat, Penfield looked there for its counterpart in man.

The cases in which Penfield demonstrated s-II were few. One case was reported in Penfield's Ferrier Lecture delivered to the Royal Society (London) in June 1946,[45] and a total of eight cases were reported to the Physiological Society (Bethesda) in 1947.[46] Penfield confirmed the existence of s-II – and the uncertainty of its boundaries – in a report to the American Neurological Association in 1949, in which he stated, "The second sensory area was found to lie in the close vicinity of the upper lip of the fissure of Sylvius. Sometimes it was on the external surface, sometimes within the fissure. It might be placed just anterior or just posterior to the lower end of the Rolandic sensory or motor strip ... The representation of face and mouth separated those second areas from the classical representations of the arm and leg."[47]

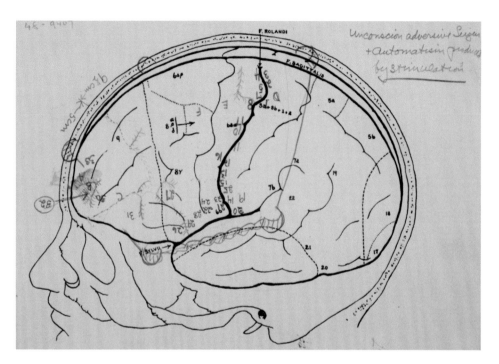

Figure 7.10. Penfield's operative brain map of the left fronto-parietal region shown in the anatomical view to better illustrate the second sensory area (numbers 20 to 24) along the frontal operculum. Stimulation produced sensation in the contralateral arm and shoulder (21), fingers and hand (24), and leg and foot (20, 22, 23). Broca's area is identified by numbers 26 to 29. The arrow indicates the epileptic area. Montreal Neurological Hospital archives, case H.E., 1948.

Two other cases were added in 1954, in Penfield and Jasper's *Epilepsy and the Functional Anatomy of the Human Brain*,[48] including that of patient H.E., which is reported here.

The second sensory area – Cat dream

The patient began having regular episodes of loss of consciousness when he was four years old. The attacks were initially controlled by extracts of the pituitary gland and sedatives, only to recur when he was eight. The attacks changed character after the patient sustained a head injury at the age of twelve, when his head was struck by a swing. His seizures then became nocturnal. They began with turning of the head to the right, which was followed by generalized convulsions. The seizures were accompanied by a recurring nightmare in which a black cat appeared. As Penfield noted, the narrative of the nightmare varied, but the black cat was always present. A tough, yellowed, and atrophic area within the frontal lobe, from which epileptic activity originated, was uncovered at surgery. Stimulation of the upper lip of the Sylvian fis-

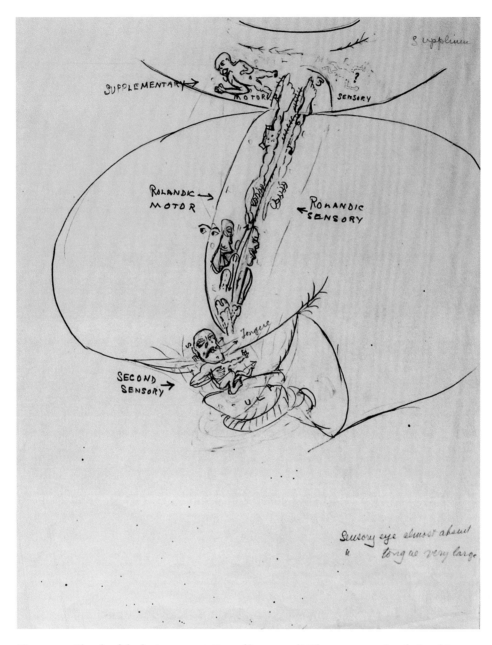

Figure 7.11. Sketch of the last representation of homunculi. The somatotopic relationships within the supplementary motor area and the second sensory area are fanciful, and that of the supplementary sensory area is purely conjectural. The professionally rendered image was published in Penfield and Jasper's *Epilepsy and the Functional Anatomy of the Human Brain* (1954). Osler Library of the History of Medicine.

sure in front of the motor strip produced sensations in the shoulder, arm, hand, fingers, hip, and leg, thus confirming the existence of s-ɪɪ in in the human cortex. An extensive frontal resection was performed, including the scarred, epileptogenic area. The postresection cortical EEG was quiescent and Jasper concluded, "prognosis should be good." And it was: the patient remained free of epileptic attacks –and dreams of cats – following surgery.

The second sensory area is depicted in Penfield and Jasper's *Epilepsy and the Functional Anatomy of the Human Brain*. The sketches on which it is based show faces that don't seem happy to be there. It has all the appearance of an afterthought. Penfield would be more certain of his depiction of the supplementary motor area.

CHAPTER 8

The Supplementary Motor Area

The discovery of the supplementary motor area is one of the most important events of twentieth-century neurobiology. It established that the sensorimotor homunculus has a sibling in the mesial aspects of the frontal lobes, which is poor in localizing the sensations that reach it and synergistic in the movements with which it responds. And yet, it is capable of the most evolved of human activity, speech. Although characterized by Wilder Penfield and Keasley Welch in 1949 as a distinct functional unit, its ancestry harkens back to the late nineteenth century, with the work of Herman Munk, of Victor Horsley and Edward Albert Schafer, and of Cécile and Oskar Vogt.

THE MARGINAL GYRUS

The marginal gyrus of the monkey occupies the mesial aspect of the frontal lobe from the frontal pole to the marginal sulcus, which separates the frontal from the parietal lobe. The posterior aspect of the marginal gyrus in front of the motor strip corresponds to the supplementary motor area (SMA) in man.

Herman Munk, while professor of physiology at the veterinary college in Berlin, observed in 1881 that electrocortical stimulation of the marginal gyrus anterior to the motor leg region in the monkey caused movement of the contralateral arm.[1] Victor Horsley, working in collaboration with the distinguished physiologist Edward Albert Schafer,[2] reported similar responses in greater detail two years later.[3] Horsley and Schafer studied the responses of the marginal gyrus to electrical stimulation in 1883, as part of a larger work on the "Functions of the cerebral cortex."[4] They observed that stimulation of the marginal gyrus extending posteriorly from the level of the genu of the corpus callosum

> gave rise to the contraction of perfectly definite groups of muscles … producing more or less *co-ordinated movements* [emphasis added] of the trunk and limbs … When the stimulus was applied anteriorly the resulting movements affected the upper limbs … when applied near the middle of the excitable part of the convolution, the muscles chiefly or primarily affected were those of the trunk

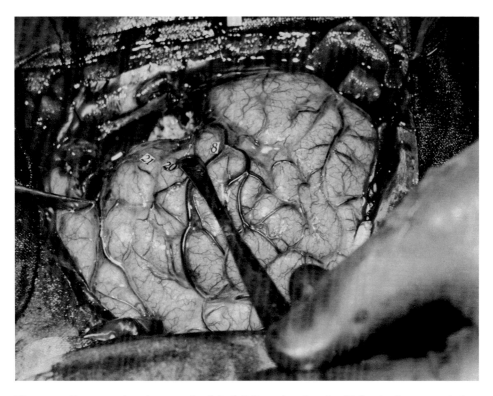

Figure 8.1. Postoperative photograph of the left frontal and parietal lobes in the anatomical view. The resected supplementary motor area is delineated between the two instruments. Montreal Neurological Hospital, case M.C., 1951.

… whilst, when applied posteriorly, muscles of the lower limb alone were called into action.[5]

Horsley and Schafer also observed that the paralysis produced by ablation of the marginal gyrus was limited in severity and duration. Clearly, they had stumbled upon what Penfield would later name the supplementary motor area.

Cécile and Oskar Vogt, working at the Kaiser Wilhelm Institute in Berlin, reported in 1919 that stimulation of the anterior aspect of the marginal gyrus, which they identified as *area 6ab* on their architectonic map of the monkey, produced *coordinated movements* of the upper limb and fingers. They termed this area the *secondary motor field*.[6] The Vogts collaborated with Otfrid Foerster in Breslau, who was the first to identify the sma in man by electrocortical stimulation and ablation. Their collaboration resulted in the first human brain map based on the correlation of cortical function with cyto-architectonic areas. (See figure 3.4.)

Foerster gave the Hughlings Jackson Lecture of the Royal Society of Medicine (London) in 1935, during the Second International Congress of Neurology.[7] Penfield also attended the congress and spoke on the surgical treatment of epilepsy.[8] During his lecture, "Motor Cortex in Man in the Light of Hughlings Jackson's Doctrines," Foerster related his experience with the stimulation and ablation of the Vogts' area 6*ab* transposed to the human brain.[9] (See figure 3.4.) This area lies within the medial aspect of the intermediate frontal lobe, directly in front of the motor leg and foot area. With stimulation of this area, Foerster reported,

> a complex mass-movement of all parts of the contralateral half of the body is obtained. Head, eyes and trunk are turned to the contralateral side and the contralateral arm and leg execute combined movements. As a rule the arm is raised and abducted, the forearm is flexed, the hand is pronated and the fist is closed or opened. I call this compound movement the flexor *synergy* of the arm [emphasis added] … The leg is simultaneously flexed at the hip and knee with dorsal flexion of the foot and toes, constituting a flexor synergy of the leg; or there may be extension of hip and knee and plantar flexion of the foot, an extensor-synergy of the leg.[10]

Ablation of area 6*ab*, Foerster observed, "either gives rise to no detectable symptoms, or, if there are symptoms at first, they disappear very soon,"[11] as Horsley and Schafer had noted five decades earlier. Foerster thus conceived that the role of area 6*ab* was to compensate for damage to the primary motor area within the precentral gyrus.

Epileptic seizures arising from area 6*ab*, Foerster continued, were stereotypical and dramatic:

> all the muscles of the contralateral half of the body are thrown into spasm almost at once; the head, eyes and trunk are turned to the side opposite to the discharging lesion and the arm and leg are involved in tonic-clonic mass-convulsions; in the arm the flexor synergy generally predominates, while in the leg the extensor synergists prevail. Towards the end of the discharge the flexor and extensor synergies alternate with each other by typical clonic spasms.[12]

These features of epileptic seizures arising from area 6*ab* are clearly indicated in Foerster's brain map. (See figure 3.4.)

Area X

The medial aspect of area 6*ab* was revisited in 1939 by Richard Brickner, a psychiatrist at Columbia University, who prevailed upon Clement Mason, a neurosurgeon at the same institution, to operate upon an epileptic young woman "according to the technique of Penfield."[13] Thus, the exposed left frontal lobe was submitted to electrocortical stimulation in an effort to identify an epileptic focus, with little effect, until "the brain was very gently retracted laterally, so the electrode point could be placed upon its medial surface." As stimulation of the mesial frontal lobe reached a point "a little less than 1 cm. in diameter … low down in area 6, probably just above its junction with the posterior tip of area 32[14] … the patient uttered syllables resembling, 'err, err, err,' in what seemed a stereotyped manner." Brickner referred to the small surface eliciting this response as "area X."[15] Although Brickner concluded that stimulation of area X had produced perseveration of speech, he did not consider that it might be involved in the elaboration of language, since, as he noted, "no known part of the speech zone lies near area X."[16] Rather, he thought that there was spread of the electrical current from area X to Broca's area, 10 centimetres away.

PENFIELD AND THE SUPPLEMENTARY MOTOR AREA

Penfield's discovery of the SMA came about through his attempts to treat cerebral tumours and epileptic seizures that originated in the superior and medial aspect of the frontal lobes, a few centimetres in front of the precentral convolution and above the cingulate gyrus. There, "just in front of the motor area of the cerebral cortex of man," he wrote, "is a supplementary representation of movements."[17] Stimulating this area was facilitated by the use of an electrode, some four inches in length, which protruded from a pencil-like hand piece connected to a generator by an electrical wire. The electrode was insulated for the whole of its length except for the very tip, which was the size of a match head. The electrode was pliable and could be bent into a gentle curve, inserted under the superior sagittal sinus, and directed downwards and parallel to the falx to make contact with the cortex of the mesial aspects of the frontal lobe without contusing it.

Penfield and Welch, June 1949

We have few clues as to why Penfield became interested in the mesial intermediate frontal area as a functional unit. His main collaborator Keasley Welch did not study this area in furtherance of a graduate degree – his thesis was on gliobastoma multiforme – but it is obvious that he was assigned the task of studying the effects of stimulation of this area in the monkey, and the effects that Penfield had observed in his patients in whom this area had been submitted to electrocortical stimulation. Penfield and Welch described their results in a paper entitled "The Supplementary Motor Area in the Cerebral Cortex of Man," at the annual meeting of the American Neurological Association in Atlantic City, New Jersey, in June 1949, when the term *supplementary motor area* was used for the first time outside of the MNI.[18]

It appears very likely that Penfield's discovery of the second *sensory* area in man influenced his search for an equivalent area of secondary importance subserving *motor* function. This is clearly stated, not by Penfield but by his friend Clinton Woolsey, a farsighted and imaginative neurophysiologist, who commented on Penfield and Welch's presentation in Atlantic City, by stating,

> We were struck recently when we were demonstrating the [sensory] pattern in the rat, how if you merely did the maneuver of turning over the sensory map and superimposing on the motor, the second sensory area fell in the region where [the supplementary motor area] might be expected to be … It struck us that this area which we call the motor field, area 6, or supplementary as Dr Penfield has called it, may be analogue of the second somatic.[19]

The notion that Penfield was inspired to seek a second area dedicated to movement as an analogue to the second sensory area is strengthened as Penfield and Welch's address on the SMA was immediately followed by an address by Penfield entitled "A Secondary Somatic Sensory Area in the Cerebral Cortex of Man."[20]

Penfield and Welch's address on the SMA was similar to Foerster's 1935 Hughlings Jackson Lecture in which he describes the function of area 6*ab*.[21] Their paper is short, some 1,000 words, but in these few words they eloquently described the effects of stimulation and excision of the SMA and the semiology of epileptic seizures that arise from it.

Foerster did not mention vocalization as a response to stimulation of area 6*ab*, but Penfield had produced vocalization by cortical stimulation in this region, without realizing its significance, as reported in Boldrey's thesis[22] and in Penfield and Boldrey's 1937 paper in *Brain*.[23] Penfield and Theodore Rasmussen reported a larger series of patients in 1949, in which stimulation of the precentral gyrus below the face area and overlapping the area representing the mouth and lips had produced vocalization expressed as vowel sounds.[24] Penfield and Welch now reported vocalization of a different nature in response to stimulation of the SMA. These responses were complex and varied, and consisted of sounds and of exclamations, of the continuous, rhythmic pronunciation of a vowel, and of the repetition of words. *Bilateral* movements of the face and jaw often accompanied these responses. The complexity and rhythmicity of the sounds, and the change in pitch and volume produced by prolonged stimulation, led Penfield to suggest that the SMA "may be of importance in the production of sounds utilized in motor speech."[25] In this context, Penfield noted that in a few cases, true aphasic responses, characterized by the inability to name objects correctly, were obtained when the *posterior* aspect of the left SMA was stimulated.

Stimulation of the SMA often produced complex, synergistic movements of the extremities, trunk, and eyes – much as Foerster had found – in contrast to the more limited movement of single muscles produced by stimulation of the precentral

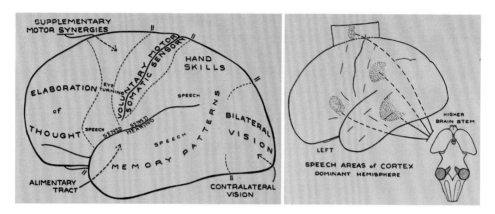

Figure 8.2. *Left*. The first published drawing of the supplementary motor area, indicated by the dashed-line arrow at the top of the drawing. Penfield used the term "synergies" that Foerster had used in 1935 when describing the motor effects produced by stimulation in this area. *Right*. The first illustration to suggest that the supplementary motor area plays a role in the elaboration of language. Note that Penfield excludes the first temporal convolution and the angular gyrus in this caricature. The language areas are integrated as a functional unit by the upper brain stem. Penfield would later elaborate greatly on the relationship of cortical function and the upper brain stem through the centrencephalic integrating system. Penfield, "A Secondary Somatic Sensory Area in the Cerebral Cortex of Man" and "Observations on Cerebral Localization of Function." Osler Library of the History of Medicine.

gyrus. Sensations were felt either throughout the body or in one or both legs. Autonomic responses, such as dilatation of the pupils, also resulted from stimulation, as did cardiovascular responses. Penfield and Welch's description of the resection of the SMA was terse – seventeen words – but to the point: "There has been no permanent deficit in posture or movement following excision of the supplementary motor area."[26]

Stimulation of the SMA also produced auras and epileptic seizures. These often began as a sensation in the epigastrium, abdomen, chest, and head. The common, overt manifestations of an epileptic seizure were arrest of speech, vocalization after an initial silence, and arm movement. Deviation of the head and eyes to the opposite side, pupillary changes, and movements of the extremities appeared as the seizure progressed.[27]

Penfield 1949, 1950

September 1949 found Penfield in Paris at the Congrès Neurologique International to deliver two noteworthy lectures,[28] in which the SMA is illustrated for the first time. Interestingly, echoing Foerster, Penfield refers to the SMA as the area of "supplementary motor synergies."

Most significantly, however, Penfield, for the first time, proposed that the SMA has a role in the elaboration of language, as he states, "it is now evident that speech has three and perhaps four areas of representation in the cortex of man,"[29] these being Broca's area, Wernicke's area within the temporal lobe, the inferior parietal lobule, and the SMA.

Penfield's two sparsely circulated papers from the Paris congress are of great importance as they indicate Penfield's thinking on the site and function of the SMA as it evolved. Penfield's thinking on the SMA continued to evolve into the spring of 1950, as reflected in a lecture that he gave in Germany in April of that year[30] in which he was more explicit in delineating the localization of its language function, in expressing its autonomy from the pre- and postcentral gyri, and in his description of the effects of its excision:

> In the dominant hemisphere there is a narrow zone between the supplementary motor area and the motor representation of the foot, the stimulation of which produces *aphasia*. When stimulation is thus employed, it serves to inactivate, for voluntary use, the cortex adjacent to the electrode. While the electrode is kept in place, the patient is typically aphasic just as he is during stimulation of Broca's area. He can speak, but after the manner of aphasics. The supplementary motor area continues to give its typical electrical response when directly stimulated even after ablation of the Rolandic motor and sensory gyri. Thus it moves the opposite limbs, which are paralyzed on voluntary effort. Excision of the supplementary motor area alone, on one side, produces no detectable deficit in patients after the first postoperative weeks have passed.[31]

Gilles Bertrand[32] elaborated on the motor function of the SMA in his master's thesis, "Studies on Cortical Localization in the Monkey 'Supplementary Motor Area.'"[33] Bertrand found that the SMA functions independently of the motor strip, since movement of the contralateral limb can still be elicited by electrical stimulation after the motor strip has been excised. Nonetheless Bertrand found that the SMA projects into the pyramidal tract in a manner similar to the precentral motor area but independently of it. Furthermore, he also found that it has a much more important ipsilateral projection to the spinal cord than the precentral gyrus does.[34] Bertrand concluded from his observations that "the large ipsilateral as well as contralateral projections to the cord leave no doubt as to the important role [the SMA] must play in the integration of normal coordinated movements, [and that] its role is one of regulation of muscle tone in smoothing down movements and preventing over-shoot, rather than initiation of movement."[35] Bertrand's findings thus provided an explanation of the bilateral and synergistic functions of the SMA that were observed by Foesrter and Penfield.

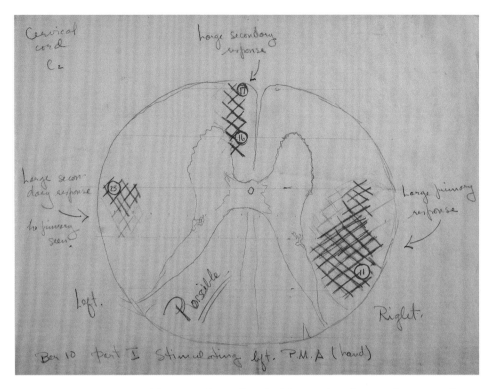

Figure 8.3. Cross-section of the cervical spinal cord of the monkey showing the extent of responses to electrical stimulation of the left supplementary motor area (crosshatching). The crosshatched area on the right of the image shows that the SMA projects primarily to the contralateral pyramidal (motor) tract. There is also a vigorous response to the ipsilateral pyramidal tract, which would account for the role of the SMA in the coordination of movements. A response is also indicated in the ipsilateral sensory dorsal column. Montreal Neurological Institute, McGill University, Bertrand, "Studies on Cortical Localization in the Monkey."

Penfield and Welch, 1951

Penfield's definitive statement on the SMA appeared in a paper entitled "The Supplementary Motor Area of the Cerebral Cortex: A Clinical and Experimental Study," published with Welch in 1951.[36] Since they had given their address to the American Neurological Association two years previously, the number of patients in whom the supplementary motor area had been stimulated had increased from twenty-one to twenty-four, but their conclusions were the same: "Electrical excitation of the mesial and superior surfaces of the cortex anterior to the precentral gyrus in man produced an unexpected variety of responses – vocalization, movements of the head, face, arms, trunk, and legs, inhibition of voluntary activity, aphasia, eye movements, pupillary effects, cardiac acceleration, and arrest of breathing."[37] Seizures arising from the SMA were described in Jacksonian terms, as inhibitory, such as the inability to reply or arrest of speech at the onset of a seizure, and, conversely, as the activation of different muscle groups acting synergistically and bilaterally, which followed.[38] Patient John B. was a victim of such attacks.

Somatotopy

The patient's history was very succinctly put during the Clinical EEG Conference of 28 October 1952:

> At the age of 20 when the patient was serving on a Corvette[39] he was thrown against a bulkhead and was unconscious for an unstated period ... Eight months after he had a major generalized seizure and was unconscious for eight or ten hours. Following this attack he had major seizures at night. Beginning a year ago he has had minor seizures of the following type. He cries out, turns his head to the left and draws his arms together, bending over to the left.

Penfield, who had witnessed one of these seizures while making his rounds, described it in these words:

> He made a low cry and turned rather suddenly to the left, his right arm being extended, his left arm somewhat flexed. His face was in a tonic posture. He was flushed, his mouth was puckered and saliva poured out of his mouth. After about ten seconds he turned back to the right, his eyes well over to the right, his right arm came up and his right knee, which was bent, was raised. This stage lasted only a few seconds. When the tonic posture disappeared he seemed confused for a little time, then he stood up, still a little confused, and then said "I am all right."

The EEG recordings revealed a left frontal para-sagittal epileptic focus, and the patient was operated upon on 31 October 1952:

> The undersurface of the dura was rather yellow, indicating that there had been a subdural haemmorhage as there were a few adhesions toward the midline. There was some atrophy next to the midline in the intermediate frontal region. The cortex within the midline was extremely tough and yellow. This zone of abnormality corresponded pretty well with the supplementary motor area. It is difficult to visualize what could have happened, I suppose that at the time of the blow there may have been tearing of a vein which could have caused the subdural bleeding, but it is rather surprising that that should have produced such a discrete abnormality. The electrographic abnormality corresponded very well with his area.

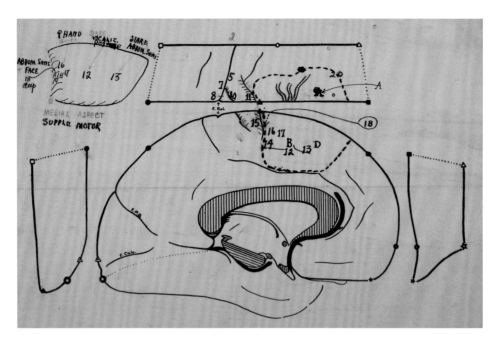

Figure 8.4. Operative brain map attempting to show a somatotopic organization within the supplementary motor area. Penfield was ultimately unsuccessful in showing a consistent somatotopic relationship within the supplementary motor area, and the topic remains unsettled. Montreal Neurological Hospital.

A very epileptogenic focus was found in the mid-aspect of the SMA, marked No. 12 and "B" on the accompanying brain map. Electrocortical stimulation at this point caused the patient to emit a low, continuous sound, stiffen and move his right arm, and extend his left leg. As the movements abated, the patient told Penfield, "I had an attack." Stimulation of the posterior-most aspect of the SMA (No. 14) rendered the patient unresponsive and caused fluttering of the eyelids and clenching of the right fist. Stimulation just above this point (No. 16) produced movements of the right arm as if reaching for the head, and the patient reported a "feeling" in his stomach. Stimulation just anterior to this area (No. 17) produced dramatic results, as described in Penfield's operative note:

There was silence, then fluttering of the eyelid and closure of the lips and opening of the jaw. There was then a rhythmic movement of the whole body with extension of the leg. Stretching movement that came and went twice … Stimulation well down toward [the] cingulate fissure caused patient to say he was having an attack and he spoke during the stimulus. There was flexion of right and left arm in a purposeful way toward his mouth. Patient added that he brought the left arm up for protection.

Stimulation at the anterior aspect of the SMA (No.13) caused the patient to stare and to feel an abnormal sensation in his abdomen. Penfield proceeded with resection of the SMA "down to the cingulate fissure and considerably anterior into the frontal region along the midline … After the removal the electrocorticography suggested a little further removal laterally and this was carried out … This is a complete supplementary motor area removal … His speaking and his movement were quite normal at the close of the excision."

Inspection of the inset in Penfield's brain map reveals his interest in establishing a somatotopic representation of the SMA, with little success. Stimulation of the anterior aspect of the SMA produced staring and abdominal sensation; stimulation of the mid-SMA produced staring, vocalization, and posturing; stimulation of the posterior aspect of the SMA on its crown produced posturing of the hand; and stimulation of its posterior bank produced sensation of the face and of the abdominal area. Similar responses were obtained in other cases, but in noncongruent areas. As it was, Penfield was never able to demonstrate a somatotopic organization in the SMA. He was, however, able to confirm its function in the elaboration of speech.

CHAPTER 9

Speech and Brain Mechanisms

Language is proper to man –Descartes[1]

None of the homuncular figures depicted the language areas, but language was very much on Penfield's mind in the early 1950s. While Keasley Welch was studying the SMA, Lamar Roberts, another research fellow at the MNI, was embarked on a decade-long research project that would culminate in the publication of Penfield and Roberts's landmark *Speech and Brain Mechanism* in 1959. But as Penfield wrote, "in order to set the stage for a study of aphasia,"[2] he and Theodore Rasmussen first published their observations of vocalization.[3]

VOCALIZATION

Pulling the voice out of me
Penfield's earliest addition to the function of the precentral gyrus was his discovery of its role in vocalization, something that had escaped even Foerster's notice. This first occurred, to Penfield's immense surprise, in 1935, as he was mapping the motor strip of patient H.My. Penfield's exuberance is palpable through his operative report and the results of cortical stimulation that produced a phenomenon that had not previously been heard.

The patient was thirty-three years old in 1933, when he was admitted to the MNI with a diagnosis of "epileptic fits." He had suffered four such attacks in the preceding two years, and all were identical. He experienced a feeling of weariness, which was quickly followed by turning of the head and body to the left. He then fell to the floor where he lay, stiff and unconscious, for five to ten minutes. He had an unusual episode during his first admission to the MNI, when he felt as if he were about to have a seizure and stated that there was something wrong with his ability to speak. This was not obvious to the physician who examined him, and the patient's diagnosis was changed from "epileptic fits" to "epileptiform attacks with probably a considerable functional element" – shorthand for hysterical spell – and he was discharged from hospital with a prescription for phenobarbital. The seizures persisted despite this medication and he was readmitted to the institute. The patient

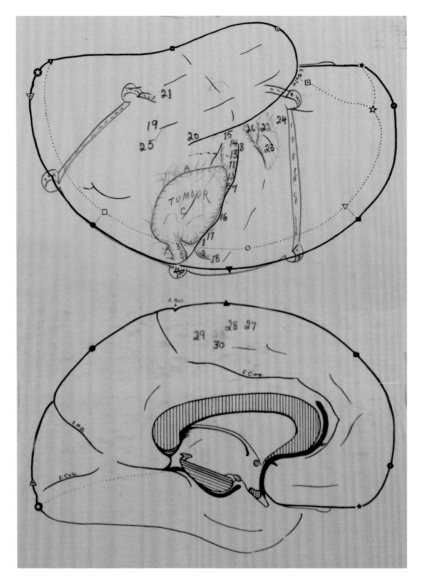

Figure 9.1. Penfield's operative sketches of the case of a patient with a brain tumour originating in the postcentral convolution, in which all three speech areas were stimulated.
The numbers 22–24 and 26 are within Broca's area. When these points were stimulated, the patient pronounced "pardon" when she wanted to say "bed," "wait a minute … moth" when she wanted to say "butterfly." She was unable to say "cow" until the stimulus was withdrawn and said "that is a bird fish" when shown a drawing of a fish. The patient was aware of her mistakes and laughed when she made one. The numbers 19, 20, 21, and 25 are within the posterior speech region. The patient was unable to speak when stimulation was applied at these points, or her speech was hesitant and paraphasic, such as identifying the drawing of a house as "a home, drum," or identifying a flag by saying "that is a Union Jack." Numbers 18 and 27–30 identify the supplementary motor area. The patient said "da, da, da" during stimulation at numbers 27 and 28, remained quiet after the stimulus was withdrawn, and then silently opened and closed her lips until after a time she correctly identified the image shown to her. Involuntary closing of the hand, movement of the foot, posturing of the hand, and turning of the eyes were produced by stimulation at numbers 18, 29, and 30. Montreal Neurological Hospital.

OPERATION REPORT

Montreal Neurological Institute No. 439.

35 years.

Operator: Dr. Penfield.

Operation Date: 4-6-35.   Anaes. Local.

Provisional Diagnosis: Cerebral cicatrix. Jacksonian epilepsy.

Final Diagnosis: Infiltrating tumor of the brain. Jack-
                                 sonian epilepsy.

Operation: Right osteoplastic craniotomy and re-
                                 moval of tumor.

Objective findings: The brain appeared normal. The pressure
was not unduly increased excepting for the fact that one gyrus in the
region of the frontal adversive field was wider than the other gyrii
and was a somewhat lighter red. There did not seem to be an increase
in the number of vessels, but the vascularity produced an increased
redness of the convolutions.

Procedure: A large osteoplastic flap was turned down.
Electrical exploration carried out as described below and a hollow
needle was passed into the gyrus which looked questionable for biopsy.
The needle was introduced at a depth of 3 cm. When the tissue was blown
out of the needle, instead of being 3 cm. in length it was 6. Tissue
also followed out of the tract; in other words apparently there was
a considerable amount of pressure within the convolution itself. The
convolution was then removed with a certain amount of normal tissue
about it. The removal thus was carried up to the pre-central gyrus
but not including the pre-central gyrus. The removal passed to the
midline, exposing the falx. The bone flap was replaced. The decompression was left beneath the temporal lobe, the dura being left
open. The bone flap was fastened with steel wire, the aponeurosis
and scalp were closed by Dr.Erickson in separate layers with silk and
dermal sutures as usual.

Electrical Stimulation: The fissure of Rolando was outlined by
stimulation. When area 5 (marked 5 on the drawing) was stimulated the
patient called out "Oh" in a somewhat groaning tone. This was definitely involuntary vocalization. The location of this point was slightly
less than 1½" above the fissure of Sylvius in the pre-central convolution. A special note is made on some of the observations during this
stimulation. In all, the area was stimulated thirty-one times, each
time producing vocalization. At no other point could any sound be
produced. At a point below this marked 12 vocalization was obtained
of a definitely lower pitch. It is rather difficult to be certain
that this was not simply due to less intensity of vocalization; nevertheless on each occasion when it was repeated stimulation at 5 was higher
than stimulation at 12. The patient was unable to stop the cry or
influence it in any way. At a distance of about 1 mm. from the area
no vocalization would be produced; coming 1 mm. closer the vocalization
would occur in typical fashion. No movements of the arm or face were
obtained at this point and with this intensity of stimulation no motor

Figure 9.2. The first page of Penfield's operative report of the first case in which electrocortical stimulation of the precentral gyrus produced vocalization. Montreal Neurological Hospital, case H.My., 1935.

(continued)

movements were obtained at all anywhere. A stronger stimulation had
to be used to produce flexion of the hand on the same convolution above
this point, and below the point with the same strong stimulation, violent swallowing was produced. Even this strong stimulation, however,
did not produce motor movements of the extremities but only vocalization. So far as I know this is the first example of true vocalization
as the result of electrical stimulation of the human brain. There was
nothing at any time to suggest the formation of words. The patient
was conscious throughout and co-operative. There was no pain associated with the vocalization but at times he complained of pain in the
head which may have been due to the effect of the indifferent electrode
upon his temporal muscle.

Pre-operative mental condition: Clear.

Post-operative condition: Clear.

Pain Localization: Pain was felt in the right temple when
the lateral aspect of the longitudinal sinus was stimulated.

Figure 9.3. Second page of Penfield's operative report. Montreal Neurological Hospital, case H.My., 1935.

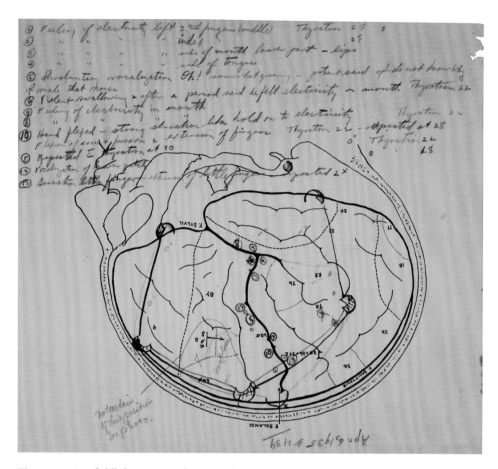

Figure 9.4. Penfield's brain map shown in the surgical viewpoint. The results of cortical stimulation are handwritten, probably by his assistant, Theodor Erickson. Stimulation at points 5 and 12 produced vocalization. See text for details. Montreal Neurological Hospital, case H.My., 1935.

was brought to the operating room on 6 April 1935, due largely to Penfield's clinical acumen in diagnosing a right frontal epileptic focus based on the patient's seizure pattern. A right osteoplastic craniotomy was elevated and a widened, pale gyrus was seen in the midfrontal region, which is referred to as the frontal eye field.

Before he could biopsy what was obviously a subcortical mass lesion, Penfield proceeded with stimulation, which first produced a sensation of electricity in the left side of the mouth and lower lip, and on the side of the tongue. The postcentral gyrus thus identified, Penfield moved the stimulating electrode a centimetre ante-riorly, in front of the sensory representation of the mouth and lips. The effect of stimulation was a shock to both the surgeon and to the patient:

When area marked as 5 on the drawing was stimulated the patient called out "oh" in a somewhat groaning tone. This was definitely involuntary vocalization. The location of this point was slightly less than one and a half inches above the fissure of Sylvius in the pre-central convolution … In all, the area was stimulated thirty-one times each time producing vocalization. At no other point could any sound be produced. At a point below this, marked 12, vocalization was obtained of a definitely lower pitch. It is rather difficult to be certain that this was not simply due to less intensity of vocalization; nevertheless, on each occasion when it was repeated, stimulation at 5 was higher than stimulation at 12. The patient was unable to stop the cry or influence it in any way. At a distance of about one millimeter from the area no vocalization would be produced. No movements of the arm or face were obtained at this point, and with this intensity of stimulation no motor movements were obtained at all anywhere. A stronger stimulation had to be used to produce flexion of the hand on the same convolution above this point [No. 10], and below the point [No. 6], with the same strong stimulation, violent swallowing was produced. Even this strong stimulation, however, did not produce motor movements of the extremities, but only vocalization. *So far as I know this is the first example of true vocalization as the result of electrical stimulation of the human brain* [emphasis added]. There was nothing at any time to suggest the formation of words. The patient was conscious throughout and co-operative. There was no pain associated with the vocalization but at times he complained of pain, which may have been due to the effect of the indifferent electrode upon his temporal muscle.

Penfield elaborated on the results of the thirty-one stimulations performed a points "5" and "12" in a single-spaced, two-page addendum to his operative report. The pertinent comments are reproduced here, as Penfield recorded them.

Stimulation at point #5 the patient cried out in a sort of groan like "oh" or "ah." This was repeated four times with the same result … Patient when asked why he made this noise said "I don't know." The next time it was tested he said, "You have made me do that." The same strength of stimulus produced numerous sensory results in other areas but no motor responses. When #5 was stimulated a fifth time the patient cried out "Oh-h." When asked what he felt he said "Something made me speak."

Penfield obviously realized the significance of the patient's responses: a new cortical function had been discovered, but he needed confirmation and called Colin Russel, the professor of neurology at McGill University and neurologist-in-chief at the MNI, to the operating room to observe the patient as he responded to Penfield's electrode. As point number 5 was stimulated for the seventh time, the patient's mouth "opened widely without any expression of fear or emotion while crying [vocalizing]. The longer the stimulation was continued the louder the tone became and the higher the pitch." As Penfield persisted with cortical stimulation one gets the impression that the patient was a little put off by it all: "When asked whether he felt anything he said, 'felt anything, sure – it felt as though you were puling the voice out of me.'"

One has an increasing sense of discomfort as one continues to read Penfield's report: "Vocalization continued (until his breath probably gave out) for a period of six seconds and ended in a tremolo. He then said 'That hurts, doctor,' – the stimulation was still being continued. When asked about where it hurt he said 'Where the instrument is, and it is continuing to hurt.'" Undeterred, Penfield punctured the cortex for the fifteenth stimulation at number 5 and noted, "At a depth of two millimeters produced vocalization – no latent period." As the stimulations wore on, the patient seemed to regain his spirits, and Penfield and he shared a light moment:

Twenty-second stimulation: Patient was informed that he was to try not to call out when I stimulated and he said he would try. I told him when I was going to stimulate and phonation began almost immediately after stimulation and continued until stimulating was withdrawn. I told the patient "I win" and he replied, "You did" and laughed. He then said, "I guess I would have won if I had been on that side of my head!"

With the pre- and postcentral convolutions and the area from which electrical stimulation had produced vocalization now identified, Penfield proceeded with what had been the initial point of the operation:

A hollow needle was inserted into the gyrus which looked questionable, for biopsy. The needle was introduced to a depth of three centimeters. When the tissue was blown out of the needle, instead of being three centimeters in length, it was six. Tissue also followed out the tract; in other words apparently there was considerable amount of pressure within the convolution itself. The convolution was then removed with a certain amount of normal tissue about it. The removal thus was carried up to the pre-central gyrus, but not including the post-central gyrus. The removal passed to the midline exposing the falx. The bone flap was replaced. The decompression was left beneath the temporal lobe, the dura being left open. The bone flap was fastened with steel wire, the aponeurosis and scalp closed by Dr Erickson in separate layers with silk and dermal sutures as usual.

Thus ended what was intended to be a routine operation.

The patient weathered surgery well, and his recovery was uneventful. The lesion proved to be an oligodendroglioma, and a complete resection was achieved. He had the occasional attack in the first few years after surgery but remained seizure-free thereafter. He died at home of unknown cause at the age of fifty-seven, twenty-three years after his admission to the MNI. Reflecting upon this case, Penfield wrote,

In general, the patient was unable to stop the cry or to influence it in any way. He was as surprised at the first sound of his own voice as we were, and he dissociated himself from this artificial employment of his cortex at once. He knew he had not willed it … At ward rounds, nine days later, the following note was made on the patient's record: When I discussed with the patient his sensation at the time that vocalization was produced on the operating table, he stated that it sounded not as though he was saying anything he wanted to say but as though his voice came with a rush, as something beyond his control. There was no sensation of the mouth, tongue or face at the time of vocalization. He said he felt no sensation anywhere, but "just as though something drawed [sic] it out" of his mouth.[4]

By the time Penfield published "The Cerebral Cortex of Man" in *Brain* in 1937, he had accumulated five more cases in which stimulation of the precentral gyrus had produced vocalization.[5] All the responsive sites were below the hand region. Penfield's final publication on the subject of vocalization appeared in 1949 in a paper entitled "Vocalization and Arrest of Speech."[6] By then, he had accumulated thirty-five cases in which vocalization had been produced by cortical stimulation. Roughly half of the cases were on the right and half were on the left, and Penfield concluded, "there is a zone in the sensorimotor convolutions of each hemisphere in which vocalization, lip movement and tongue movement are represented bilaterally. These areas may be called the word articulation zones," which he clearly distinguished from the areas of the brain that were "essential to the mental processes involved in speaking."[7] It is these areas to which he next turned his attention.

LANGUAGE

During the great debate on the lateralization of articulate language to the left hemisphere that took place at the Imperial Academy of Medicine of Paris in the spring of 1865, Jean-Baptiste Bouillaud, at one time dean of the Faculty of Medicine of the University of Paris, stated that the movement towards localization of function to specific areas of the brain was irrevocable.[8] He was proven correct in 1870 when Gustav Fritsch and Eduard Hitzig, in Berlin, demonstrated motor responses elicited by the electrical stimulation of the precentral gyrus in the dog.[9] Of course, animal studies were unsuitable for the investigation of language, a problem that had de-layed the acceptance of localization of language in Broca's time. However, the Napoleonic wars and the vicissitudes of nineteenth-century life sometimes created the equivalent of human experiments. This is the point that Ernest Auburtin, a prominent Parisian physician, made during a meeting of the Academy of Anthro-pology of Paris in 1863 when he commented on the localization of language: "when a bullet traverses the anterior lobes and abolishes speech without altering intelli-gence in any way, is this not for the physiologist the same as if the wound had been made with the goal of scientific observation?" He made his point by recounting the case of an unfortunate soul who had shot himself in the head after losing heav-ily at the gambling tables:

> Among these cases of trauma, which I consider to be as demonstrative as vivi-sections, there is one that is noteworthy: … A wounded man who had just shot himself point blank in the forehead in an attempt at suicide was brought to l'Hopital Saint-Louis. The anterior lobes of the brain were exposed but were undamaged. Intelligence was intact, as was speech. This unfortunate survived many hours, and the following experiment was performed on him. As he was questioned, the flat of a large spatula was applied to the anterior lobes. Speech was suddenly suspended as light compression was applied; the word that was begun was cut in two. The faculty of language reappeared as soon as the com-pression ceased.[10]

On the basis of such evidence and the accumulation of clinical cases, Broca, Meynert and Wernicke, and Jules Dejerine identified the anterior and posterior speech regions. The clinico-pathological method, on which these observations re-lied, was limited in that aphasia was often accompanied by other neurological deficits, and the damage that the brain exhibited at autopsy was often diffuse. De-spite these difficulties, Broca was able to accurately localize articulate language to the *pars opercularis* and *pars triangularis* of the left frontal lobe, Wernicke localized the aphasia that bears his name to the posterior aspect of the first and second tem-poral convolutions, and Dejerine localized agraphia and alexia to the angular gyrus. Although Fedor Krause in Berlin,[11] Harvey Cushing in Boston,[12] Victor Horsley in London,[13] and Otfrid Foerster in Breslau[14] pioneered in the localization of sensory and motor function to the pre- and postcentral gyri, it was not until Penfield took up the stimulating electrode that the localization of language was confirmed by direct observation in awake patients. Language-competent areas could now be more precisely delineated, their function determined, and their rel-ative importance established.

Preston Robb

Preston Robb graduated from McGill Medical School in 1939. He trained in neurology at the MNI, and at Johns Hopkins and Harvard Universities. Robb returned to the MNI after his training, where he was appointed neurologist-in-chief in 1968.[15] Penfield had assigned Robb to study the effects on language of resections within the language dominant hemisphere while he was a resident at the MNI, in furtherance of his master's degree.[16]

Robb's research came at a turning point in Penfield's interest in language. Between 1930 and 1946, Penfield had depended on a patient's ability to count during cortical stimulation in order to delineate the speech areas. By the time Robb arrived at the MNI Penfield had begun to stimulate the cortex while the patient named small objects that could be held in the hand or depicted on index cards. If patients were unable to name the object or its image, they were asked to describe its use verbally or by pantomime.[17] On some occasions, the patients were also asked to read. Electrocortical stimulation was not, however, the first method used by Penfield in his attempt to identify the language areas by disrupting a patient's ability to speak. Prior to this he had tried injecting the local anaesthetic nupercaine into the cortex in a putative language area.[18] This failed to interfere with speech, and worse, it created small cysts within the cortex. Harkening back to Auburtin, Penfield then attempted to generate an aphasic response by applying pressure to the cortex with the ball of his thumb. This also proved ineffectual. Finally, he used electrical stimulation, which did interfere with the ability to speak as long as the stimulus was applied.[19]

Robb's study included the first patient in whom the more extensive and refined language tasks were used. That patient, P.M., also has the distinction of being the first individual in whom the role of the angular gyrus in the comprehension of written language was demonstrated by cortical stimulation.[20] This case was previously unknown as it had only appeared in Robb's thesis and is reported here along with the patient's brain map.

The patient had an unspecified illness that caused him to be unconscious for two weeks in 1936, when he was twenty-five years old. Five years later he sustained a head injury with loss of consciousness, after which he began to have epileptic seizures. These persisted despite a prolonged trial of medication, and he was admitted to the MNI in March 1946. A PEG showed that the temporal horn of the left lateral ventricle was enlarged, indicating atrophy of the anterior temporal lobe. A large, left-sided craniotomy was elevated and

the temporal lobe was found to be thinned out, yellow, and tough. There were a number of small gyri and a good deal of tissue that could have been giving rise to epileptic activity. The abnormality extended back to a point about 2 cm. behind the central [Rolandic] fissure. The rest of the brain appeared normal … When

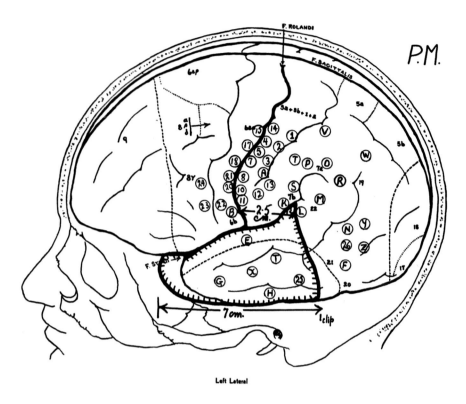

Figure 9.5. The first brain map of language areas based on electrocortical stimulation. Only positive responses related to language are described. "Electrical stimulation of the cortex produced vocalization at point 17. Stimulation at 20 and 22 stopped counting. Stimulation at points 23 and 24 (Broca's area) caused counting to slow and stop. The patient was unable to name objects correctly during stimulation of point 26. He eventually called a key a 'lock for key.' The patient was then shown a pen and as point 26 was restimulated, he said 'That is a …' then he yawned. After withdrawal of the stimulation he said, 'That is a …' and made motions of writing with his hand. Two minutes later he was able to name the pen correctly. The patient was unable to name objects when point 'N' was stimulated and this persisted for one to two minutes after stimulation was withdraw. He could not name a pen nib when point 'O' was stimulated. Rather, he called it part of a pen. At point 'P' he called a key a fountain pen, then named a pencil correctly. At point 'R,' after some deliberation, he named a match correctly during stimulation. At point 'S' he could not name objects during stimulation and all he could say was 'ka-ka.' At point 'T' he was able to read aloud during stimulation. At point 'S,' after stimulation, he was able to continue for a few words, then said 'ga-ga.' Stimulation at 'Y' did not stop reading the first time, then, when repeated twice he would say two words correctly and then the words would be inaccurately used and pronounced. Stimulation at 'M' interfered with reading. Stimulation at 'K' interfered with reading numbers. He tried to read the numbers but got them wrong. Stimulation at point 'J' prevented him from naming objects. Stimulation at point 'X' prevented him from naming objects correctly, for example, when presented with a pair of scissors he said, 'That is a rink' … 'that is a pair …' Then he signified with his hands that he knew what it was. Stimulation at 'R' caused him to slow down gradually and he said 'kur-kur.' Stimulation at 'P' failed to stop counting. Stimulation at 'L' caused him to slow down. When repeated, he continued counting without interruption. Stimulation at 'J' stopped counting slowly. When repeated he was able to continue counting. Stimulation at 'K' caused him to skip when counting." Montreal Neurological Institute, McGill University. Robb, "A Study of the Effects of Cortical Excision on Speech in Patients with Previous Cerebral Injuries."

the supramarginal gyrus was stimulated he was able to say syllables like "Ka-Ka" when trying to name an object. He said numbers but neither the pronunciation or the order was accurate. During stimulation of the posterior temporal region, in the vicinity of the angular gyrus, he was unable to name objects. He could say, "That is a …" but could not complete the sentence with the key word. *Stimulation in the vicinity of the angular gyrus arrested reading* [emphasis added]. At one point he was able to name an object after some deliberation but was unable to read. There were other points further away from the angular gyrus in which reading, naming objects and counting were not affected by stimulation.[21]

The pre-and postcentral gyri identified and the posterior language areas delineated, resection of the abnormal temporal lobe proceeded apace: "The temporal lobe was removed to a point exactly 7 cm. from the anterior end of the middle fossa. The line of removal was 2.5 cm. posterior to the central fissure."[22] The resected tissue thus included point "X," 4.5 centimetre from the temporal tip, where stimulation had "prevented [the patient] from naming objects correctly. For example, when presented with a pair of scissors he said, 'That is a rink' … 'that is a pair …' Then he signified with his hands that he knew what it was … In the postoperative period [the patient] developed an amnesic type of aphasia which increased to complete aphasia."[23]

P.M. was one of fifty-one patients that Penfield had operated upon in whom Robb was able to correlate the site and extent of resection with postoperative aphasia. This led him to conclude, "when 4 cm. from the tip [of the temporal lobe] were excised the postoperative aphasia was only very transient. When 7 cm. were excised the postoperative aphasia was more persistent and consisted mostly of an amnesic aphasia and an auditory agnosia,"[24] Since that time, it is only under the most unusual circumstances that a dominant temporal resection for epilepsy performed at the MNI extends beyond four centimetres from the temporal tip.

The first language map

Robb continued to work with Penfield on the localization of language after the publication of his thesis, examining newly admitted patients pre- and postoperatively and assisting Penfield in the operating room as he stimulated the cortex in Broca and Wernicke's areas. By 1947, Robb had collated thirty-three cases in which cortical stimulation had interfered with speech during the performance of the new, more refined language tasks. Robb presented his results to the Association for Research in Nervous and Mental Disease in 1947, in an address entitled on the "Effects of Cortical Excision and Stimulation of the Frontal Lobe on Speech."[25] It was at this meeting that Penfield and Robb presented the first composite brain map based on interference with language resulting from cortical stimulation.

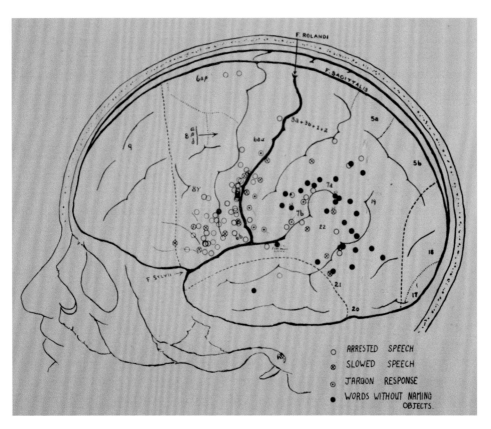

Figure 9.6. The first composite language map to be published. It is based on stimulation of the dominant hemisphere in 33 patients on whom Penfield operated. Robb, "Effects of Cortical Excision and Stimulation of the Frontal Lobe on Speech."

Robb observed that stimulation of the posterior aspect of the third left frontal convolution produced "a pure motor deficit, while the ability to speak but the inability to name objects occurred with stimulation of the posterior temporal or parietal lobes." These effects could not be elicited by stimulation of the homologous areas in the right hemisphere. Robb also expressed the opinion that

> All of the lateral aspect of the left frontal lobe with the exception of the third frontal convolution may be removed and, at most, there will be only transient aphasia. The posterior part of the third left frontal convolution may be removed and recovery will be possible: however, the postoperative aphasia will be much more prolonged as compared to that seen following excision of other areas.[26]

Lamar Roberts would take up the study of language localization where Robb left off and largely contradict Robb's opinion on the resectability of the language areas.

Penfield and Roberts

Undoubtedly heartened by the early results of cortical stimulation observed by Robb, Penfield saw the opportunity to more accurately delineate the language areas by cortical stimulation using a wider variety of tasks. Lamar Roberts, who had recently taken up a fellowship at the institute, devoted a decade to the study of the structure–function relationship of language. Roberts had obtained his medical degree from Duke University and came to the MNI for his neurosurgical training in 1947, as Robb was finishing his study of language localization. Roberts would later be appointed the founding director of the Department of Neurosurgery at the University of Florida, Gainesville.

Roberts identified seven types of language-related responses to cortical stimulation. Arrest of speech and slowing of naming and counting were considered nonaphasic responses, and they could be obtained from stimulation of either hemisphere. There were five types of responses that Roberts classified as aphasic: (1) distortion, mispronunciation, and repetition of words and syllables; (2) confusion of numbers while counting; (3) the inability to name [anomia] while retaining the ability to use words; (4) misnaming using inappropriate words with evidence of perseveration; and (5) misnaming without perseveration.[27] Of note, Roberts found that the first four types of aphasic responses could be obtained from Broca's area, the inferior parietal lobule, the first and second temporal convolutions, and the intermediate precentral region at the midline (the SMA). The fifth type of aphasic response, misnaming without perseveration, was obtained only with stimulation of the first two temporal convolutions and in the peri-Sylvian aspect of the parietal lobe.[28]

Roberts initially identified three areas where cortical stimulation produced aphasic responses. These he localized to the *pars opercularis* and *pars triangularis* of the left frontal lobe, as Broca had discovered; to the posterior aspect of the first and second temporal convolutions behind the level of Heschl's gyrus, as first described by Meynert and Wernicke; and to the supramarginal and angular gyri, as described by Jules Dejerine. Despite having identified a few aphasic responses obtained with stimulation of the left SMA, Roberts was not prepared to state unequivocally that it was a fourth language area, although he and Penfield did entertain that possibility. Roberts published these observations in his master's thesis, "A Study of Certain Alterations in Speech during Stimulation of Specific Cortical Regions," in 1949.[29] Roberts's doctoral dissertation, "Alterations in Speech Produced by Cerebral Stimulation and Excision," followed in 1952.[30] "The only additions" to his thesis, Roberts stated in the introduction to his dissertation, "are the production of misnaming without perseveration in the left Broca's and supplementary motor areas and an increased number of 'aphasic types of responses' in the supplementary motor

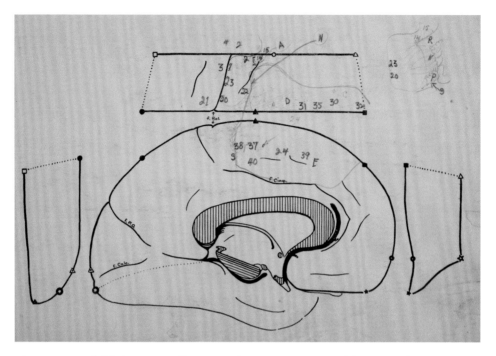

Figure 9.7. Penfield's brain map illustrating the responses obtained from stimulation in the dominant supplementary motor area. With stimulation at number 30, the patient hesitated but continued naming objects. At 31, 32, 35, 36, and 37 she stopped naming objects, but was able to do so correctly when stimulation was withdrawn. She also had difficulty naming at 33, responding, "that is a bull, that is a cla, that is a cow." The patient was initially silent when number 39 was stimulated, then said "that is a –" very slowly. Eventually she said, "I don't know what it is for." The continuous line indicates the extent of the resection. Postresection stimulation at letters N, P, and R produced posturing of the upper and lower extremities, and this area was also resected. Montreal Neurological Hospital, case E.G.

area during electrical arrest."[31] Thus, Roberts's dissertation established the SMA as a fourth area subserving the faculty of language.

Broca's area – I could not think of the words

Patient C.St-D. was twenty-six years old when he began to have seizures. These were of two types, one focal, and the other generalized. The focal seizures consisted of trembling of the right hand, which he was unable to move voluntarily and with which he was unable to grasp. The generalized seizures were heralded by stiffening of the right side of the body and uncontrolled jerking of the right arm. This was followed by the inability to speak properly, and tonic-clonic convulsions. A flurry of seizures occurring over several days left the young man with difficulty speaking and permanent weakness of the right arm and hand. He was admitted to the MNI in May 1953. Radiological and electrophysiological examinations shed no light on the source of the seizures. Nevertheless, Penfield concluded the Clinical EEG Conference by stating, "In spite of the lack of evidence of superficial lateralization of an epileptogenic focus, the clinical story is clear enough to justify exploration, and a suspicion of a focal lesion above the fissure of Sylvius, and just posterior to Broca's area … Exploration will be carried out."

Accordingly, a left-sided craniotomy was elevated. Penfield found that an underlying lesion had widened the posterior aspect of the inferior frontal convolution – Broca's area. Gentle palpation revealed a softened area bounded circumferentially by firmer tissue. The lesion breached the cortical surface just behind Broca's area, and Penfield diagnosed a tumour whose size he estimated at "about that of a robin's egg." Cortical stimulation directly in front of the tumour resulted in the patient's inability to speak because, as he told Penfield when the stimulus was removed, "I could not think of the word." Stimulation just below that point caused the patient to identify the image on a card as the image that had preceded it, a phenomenon referred to as perseveration and an integral part of the aphasic syndrome. Penfield proceeded with resection of the posterior aspect of the lesion, which exposed the posterior bank of the *pars orbicularis*. He took advantage of this unusual access to Broca's area and proceeded to stimulate it. This caused the patient to be silent when he was asked to identify a comb and to snap his fingers, as if he was trying to remember its name. When the stimulus was removed the patient answered "it's for your hair," and then correctly said a "comb." The patient's speech was slurred after the resection of the tumour had been completed, but Penfield noted, "there was no evidence of aphasia." Pathological examination of the resected tissue revealed a benign piloid astrocytoma, a type of brain tumour that is cured by resection.

The significance of this case lies in Penfield's stimulation of the posterior bank of the *pars opercularis*, which proved that language is not restricted to the crown of the gyrus, as some had suggested.

Penfield received a letter from the patient's wife four years after surgery, in which she was pleased to report that her husband had been in excellent health since the operation. He was not taking any medication, and they lived a very happy and active life.

Wernicke's area – Gradenigo's syndrome
Patient T.M. was nine years old when he developed an infection of the left middle ear. The infection spread to the mastoid bone and the subdural space, and he developed double vision. He underwent an uneventful mastoidectomy and drainage of the subdural empyema. He developed generalized seizures at the age of twenty-two, which were presaged by epigastric discomfort and difficulty finding his words. These episodes caused him to be admitted to the MNI two years later, in 1949. The

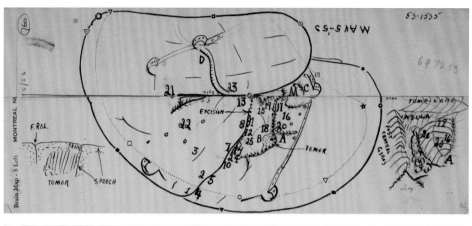

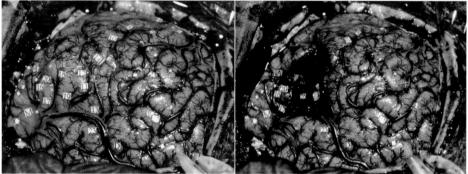

Figure 9.8. *Top* Penfield's operative sketch outlining Broca's area and its relationship to the mostly subcortical tumour, which is seen pointing through the cortex (arrow). Stimulation at 16 and 20 caused inability to speak, the patient stating after stimulation, "I could not think of the word." Upon stimulation at 17, the patient named the image he had seen immediately before. The detail at left illustrates the relationship of the tumour to the precentral gyrus in cross section. The detail at right illustrates Broca's area after the resection of the tumour and the effect of stimulation of the postero-lateral bank of the *pars opercularis*. Aphasic responses were obtained with stimulation at 26. Montreal Neurological Hospital, case C.St-D., 1953.

Figure 9.9. *Bottom Left*. Intraoperative photograph (anatomical viewpoint) of case C.St-D. before the resection of the tumour. *Right*. Photograph taken after the resection of the tumour, exposing the lateral bank of the *pars opercularis* of Broca's area. Stimulation at point number 26 produced aphasic responses. Montreal Neurological Hospital, case C.St-D., 1953.

patient's case was discussed at the Clinical EEG Conference. The diagnosis was obvious: the seizures began in the language-dominant temporal lobe because of the epigastric sensation and the word finding difficulties. The cause of the seizures would have been obvious to anyone who had practised neurology in the preantibiotic era: Gradenigo's syndrome.[32] First described in 1904, the syndrome begins with infection of the middle ear that spreads to the mastoid bone. When the infection

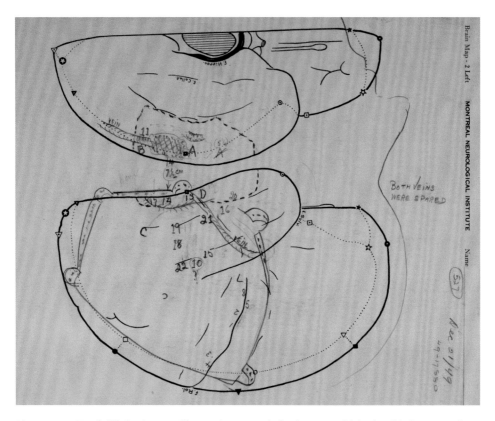

Figure 9.10. Penfield's brain map illustrating a postinfective scar within the third temporal convolution. The dashed line indicates the extent of the resection. Stimulation at number 15 caused the patient to misname scissors as "squashers" and "squasher ware." At 18 he misnamed a butterfly as "water" and at 22 he responded "that is a woman's habnet" when shown a picture of a woman's hat. He was unable to name what was shown to him when the stimulating electrode was applied at 19. These aphasic responses were all within the posterior aspects of the second and third temporal convolutions. There was no interference with speech at numbers 16 and 21. Montreal Neurological Hospital, case T.M., 1949.

reaches the apex of the mastoid it interferes with the function of the sixth cranial nerve, which produces double vision. Often, the seventh cranial nerve is also affected and the patients develop a Bell's palsy. If left untreated the infection spreads to the inferior aspect of the temporal lobe. The end result is a cerebral scar that matures over time to produce temporal lobe epilepsy. All of this would have been evident to the attendees of the EEG conference and would have been sufficient to justify surgical exploration. But the patient had a seizure while undergoing an EEG examination. The seizure originated from the left inferior temporal region and quickly spread to the lateral surface in the left temporal lobe, before evolving into a major convulsive attack. The clinical and EEG findings were therefore concordant, and Penfield brought the patient to the operating room, where a large bone flap was elevated.

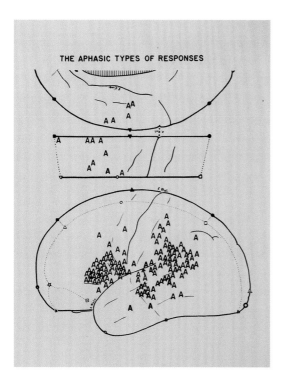

THE APHASIC TYPES OF RESPONSES

Figure 9.11. Composite brain map in which each letter "A" indicates a point where electrical stimulation produced an aphasic response. Montreal Neurological Institute, McGill University, Roberts, "Alterations in Speech Produced by Cerebral Stimulation and Excision."

This uncovered thick adhesions between the undersurface of the dura and the inferior aspect of the left temporal lobe. The cortex was markedly scarred and highly epileptogenic. Penfield proceeded with cortical stimulation and, as he noted in his operative report, "the speech area in the temporal lobe was outlined rather carefully." Stimulation of the posterior aspect of the first and second temporal convolutions above the cicatrix caused the patient to misname scissors as "squashers" and "squasher ware," and a butterfly as "water." When shown a picture of a woman's hat he responded "that is a woman's habnet." Penfield's resection was limited to the scarred third temporal convolution, avoiding the areas where stimulation had interfered with speech. The patient had one major seizure during the first year following surgery but then remained seizure-free for the next thirty-six years.

The language zone

Roberts's doctoral dissertation constituted his contribution to *Speech and Brain Mechanisms*, published by Penfield and Roberts in 1959.[33] Beyond identifying the areas subserving language, Penfield and Roberts made the following observations:

> So far as can be determined, there is no difference between the effects of the electrical current when applied to the dominant Broca's area, supplementary motor area, or parieto-temporal region as regards the various alterations of speech. The

reason for this lack of difference could be that these three areas are connected by transcortical and subcortical pathways in a single system. An electrical disturbance set up in any part of the system might disrupt the function of the whole system[34] …

The closer the lesion is to Broca's area … and the adjacent precentral face area, the more the motor components of speech are involved. The nearer the lesion is to the vicinity of the junction of the parietal, temporal and occipital lobes, the more reading and writing are affected; and the more the posterior superior temporal region is involved, the greater the difficulty in the comprehension of spoken words.[35]

Jules Dejerine and his wife, Augusta Dejerine-Klumpke, had expressed a similar opinion in 1905 in their monumental and exquisitely illustrated *Anatomie des centres nerveux* (Anatomy of the Neural Centers).[36] Referring to the posterior third frontal convolution, the inferior parietal lobule, and the posterior temporal gyri as the *language zone*, and having described the transcortical fibre system linking them, the Dejerines wrote,

any alteration of the language zone at any point in the surface that it occupies does not result in difficulties limited to this or that modality of language, but an alteration in all modalities of language, with pre-dominance of those difficulties corresponding to the … centre directly affected by the lesion. Motor aphasia predominates if the lesion is centred on Broca's area, word deafness predominates if the lesion destroys the posterior part of the first temporal convolution and word blindness predominates when there is a [lesion in the] angular gyrus.[37]

This brilliant insight had been achieved purely by reason and the clinico-pathological method, without need of electricity.

Handedness, speech, and cerebral dominance
Jean-Baptiste Bouillaud first suggested that right-handedness and left-hemisphere dominance for speech are associated, in an address to the Imperial Academy of Medicine in the spring of 1865.[38] Broca made Bouillaud's concept his own when he spoke before the Society of Anthropology of Paris a few months later. Based on the association of right-handedness and the lateralization of speech to the left hemisphere it was quickly but erroneously assumed at the time that left-handers were right-hemisphere dominant for speech.[39] Preston Robb was one of the first to challenge this assumption as he stressed "the importance of not assuming speech to be opposite the dominant hand" in his thesis.[40] Roberts was more emphatic than Robb, stating, "the left cerebral hemisphere is dominant in practically all individuals re-

gardless of handedness, except those who have gross lesions of the left hemisphere within the first few years of life."[41] Although Roberts was unaware of it, Broca had recognized that the right hemisphere can subserve speech in individuals who have sustained an injury to the left hemisphere in infancy or early childhood, as he informed the Anthropological Society of Paris in 1865: "a subject in whom the third *left* frontal convolution, the usual seat of articulate language, is atrophied since birth would learn to speak … with the third *right* frontal convolution, as the child born without the right hand becomes as skilful with the left hand as one normally is with the other."[42]

Charles Branch, Theodore Rasmussen, and Brenda Milner at the MNI confirmed Roberts's observation on the prevalence of left-hemisphere dominance for speech using the Wada test.[43] This test consists of injecting the short-acting barbiturate amytal into one carotid artery. The hemisphere supplied by the carotid artery is thus inactivated and produces a contralateral paralysis. The opposite carotid artery is injected a few days later. The patient becomes temporarily aphasic when the hemisphere responsible for language is perfused with the barbiturate. The hemispheric dominance for language was thus established and correlated to a patient's handedness. Branch and his coworkers found that most individuals are left-hemisphere dominant for speech regardless of handedness.

Rasmussen and Milner also recognized that children who had sustained damage to the language zone had a high probability of being right hemisphere dominant for speech, as Broca had surmised.[44]

Functional integration

The Dejerines were not the first to conceive of language as a functional unit integrated by fibre systems. This concept was first formulated by Jean-Baptiste-Maximien Parchappe de Vinay, a respected and influential neuropsychiatrist whose major interest was in cerebral syphilis. Parchappe conceived of language as a holistic function involving multiple regions on both sides of the brain, which were connected by white matter fibres.[45] For Parchappe, the integration of language as a functional unit – a faculty – was made possible through short "U" fibres connecting a gyrus to the one adjacent to it, through longer intrahemispheric fibres connecting one cortical area to another, and by the massive fibre bundle of the corpus callosum connecting homologous areas of both hemispheres. Surprisingly, Penfield did not believe that intracortical fibres or the corpus callosum played a significant role in the integration of language or in the recovery from aphasia. Rather, he conceived that this was achieved through reciprocal connections between the language-competent cortex, the thalamus, and the upper brain stem, as part of what he referred to as the *centencephalic integrating system*. This mechanism of integrating language was first proposed by Penfield in his 1949 address to the Congrès Neurologique International in Paris. It was restated by Roberts in 1952, and by Penfield and Roberts in 1959 when they wrote, "It is proposed that comprehension of speech occurs after impulses have been received in the higher brain stem and both cortical auditory areas, and during interaction between the higher brain stem and the left hemisphere. Following interaction between the higher brain stem and the left hemisphere, impulses pass to both cortical motor areas and hence to the final common pathway to those muscles used in speech – spontaneous speech occurs during these transactions."[46]

Penfield first published an illustration of the subcortical system for integration of speech in the Paris address of 1949, in which he included the SMA. It was reproduced with minor modifications in Roberts's 1952 dissertation and in *Speech and Brain Mechanisms* in 1959.

The recognition of different areas devoted to language did not imply that all had equal importance in its elaboration, as Penfield and Roberts realized:

> We believe that the most important area for speech is the posterior temporo-parietal region, including the posterior parts of the first, second, and third temporal convolutions behind the vein of Labbé, the supramarginal gyrus, and the angular gyrus. The next important area for speech is that of Broca … The supplementary motor area on the medial, and a little on the superior aspect the hemisphere in front of the precentral foot area is dispensable; lesions here can produce prolonged dysphasia, and it probably is very important if the other araea of speech are destroyed.[47]

This statement requires clarification. The role of the third temporal convolution in language is subtle. Brenda Milner had never noted a speech deficit resulting from resection of the third temporal convolution (personal communication), although it appears to have a role in recognizing the shape of letters. The vein of Labbé is no longer considered to be a reliable indicator of the anterior limit of the temporal language area. The anterior limit of the temporal language area is considered to be at the level of Heschl's gyrus[48] or at the junction of the Rolandic and Sylvian fissures.[49] These usually correspond to a length of four centimetres from the temporal tip, as Robb had first realized. Further, despite the apparent casualness with which they regarded resection of Broca's area, Penfield and Roberts do interject a word of caution, stating, "Despite the *suspicion* [emphasis added] of dispensability of the anterior speech area of Broca, we still advise that this area, which can be outlined so clearly by stimulation, should be clearly avoided during surgery."[50]

Penfield and Roberts had established this hierarchy based on the differences in the severity and the duration of the deficits that followed a lesion in each of the speech areas. Once again, and unbeknownst to them, Jules and Augusta Dejerine had preceded them in this realization:

We should not believe however that lesions of the language zone alter the different modes of language equally. In fact, there exists a veritable hierarchy presiding over the modalities of language resulting from education and the acquisition of images. Thus, images are that more fixed, that more resistant the earlier they are acquired. Auditory images are first acquired and most deeply etched by the process of education, and govern the process of inner language. The motor images of articulation rapidly follow, and their union with the preceding ones is intimate, precocious, and constitutes the ever-present basis of inner language. Only much later does the child learn to associate the visual image of words and the auditory and motor images of speech as they are transcribed or printed. As for writing, it is but the reproduction on paper of the visual images of letters and words and the last mode of language that is learned.[51]

Plasticity and speech

Lamar Roberts alluded to *plasticity* in relation to recovery from aphasia in his dissertation and used the term in a paper entitled "Functional Plasticity in Cortical Speech Areas and Integration of Speech" in 1956.[52] Roberts's concept of plasticity held that transient aphasia occurs when a part of the dominant hemisphere for language is damaged and the remaining healthy brain compensates for the lost tissue through its interaction with the upper brain stem. If there is greater tissue loss the aphasia may be permanent, and whatever improvement is experienced by the patient will result from the transfer of language to the opposite hemisphere, through the action of the bilateral interconnections of the centrencephalic integration system with the temporal and frontal lobes. Roberts's concept of plasticity assumed that the right cerebral hemisphere has the potential to subserve speech throughout life.

As is the case with much that was written on language in the twentieth century, Broca had already addressed it in the nineteenth.[53] For Broca, both cerebral hemispheres were equally able to subserve speech. That this task fell to the left one, Broca believed, was due to the earlier intra-uterine development of the left hemisphere.[54] Thus, for Broca, both hemispheres had the same potential for speech but the left frontal lobe was primed at birth to take on this function. The right hemisphere also had this capacity, but it remained dormant as long as the left frontal lobe was intact. It could be called into service even in adulthood but would be successful in restoring speech to the aphasic patient only if she had the drive and determination to relearn to speak as she did as a child, and a teacher as dedicated as a parent willing to help her.[55]

Current opinion favours a multifactorial process in the recovery from aphasia in left hemisphere language-dominant individuals, which includes, as Roberts suggested, recruitment of residual, functional left hemisphere tissue and activation of homologous areas within the right hemisphere.[56]

The Surgical Treatment of Temporal Lobe Epilepsy

A most encouraging field of therapy –Penfield[1]

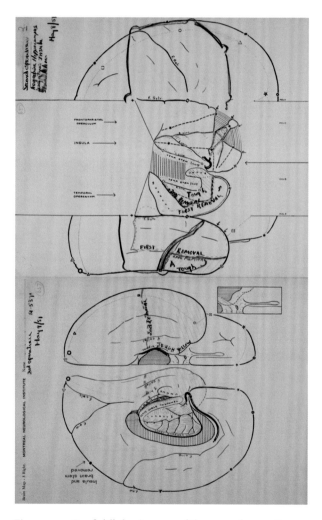

Figure 10.1. Penfield's brain map of the second operation performed upon a patient who had undergone the ineffectual resection of the first two temporal convolutions. A second procedure resected the third convolution, the uncus, the amygdala, and the hippocampus, and alleviated the patient's seizures. Montreal Neurological Hospital, case T.S., 1951.

CHAPTER 10

The Importance of Scars

PENFIELD'S FIRST OPERATION FOR TEMPORAL LOBE EPILEPSY

Penfield operated upon his first epileptic patient soon after he arrived at the Royal Victoria Hospital. The patient's clinical history is sparse, the original admission note having been lost. I have reconstructed it from Penfield's operative note and William Cone's report of his examination of the resected specimen, which have been preserved.[1] Penfield's operative report of patient R.M. is typical of the format that he used throughout his career. The findings observed at surgery, the results of cortical stimulation, the pathological findings, the technical details of the operation, and a note on prognosis were recorded. After Herbert Jasper's arrival at the MNI, Penfield also included a summary of the EEG findings, and Jasper's separate, detailed report was added to the patient's chart. The pathology reports remained unchanged well into the twenty-first century. They contain a summary of the patient's history and physical examination, and a copy of Penfield's operative note. The gross appearance of the resected specimens is described, and the results of microscopic examination are reported in great detail. William Cone, who was both neurosurgeon-in-chief and head of neuropathology at the MNI until his death in 1959, signed the pathological reports, as did the fellow training with him in neuropathology at the time. Penfield's operative report and Cone's pathology report on Penfield's first epilepsy case are reproduced here as they appear in the MNI archives.

R.M. sustained a fracture to the right side of his skull when he was thrown from a horse as a child in 1918. He was operated upon then, and a frontal contusion was uncovered and a subdural hematoma was evacuated. The injury left him weak and numb on the right side, and with intractable focal motor seizures that recurred up to twenty times a day. These led him to consult Penfield shortly after his arrival in Montreal, in November 1928. The patient's examination revealed a left homonymous hemianopia and left facial weakness, a spastic left upper extremity, and spastic contracture of the neck muscles, which caused his head to tilt to the left. There was diminished two-point discrimination of the left hand, and the left deep tendon reflexes

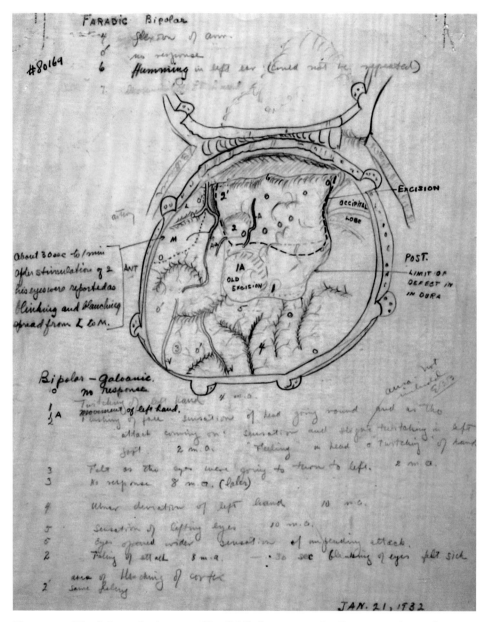

Figure 10.2. Hand-drawn brain map of Penfield's first temporal epilepsy case, drawn from the surgeon's viewpoint. The bold "1A" enclosed by a circular dashed line indicates the site where Penfield performed a first resection in 1928. The area marked "Excision" was resected during the patient's third operation, on 21 January 1932. The text at left enclosed by a square bracket refers to the area delineated by dots and labeled "L" and "M," which blanched after stimulation at point number 2 and in which an artery is shown to end abruptly. Blanching of the cortex was also observed with stimulation at point 2. Montreal Neurological Hospital, case M.R., 1934.

were hyperactive. The patient's history and physical findings indicated a right hemi-spheric lesion involving the sensorimotor region.

Stanley Cobb and the highly influential epileptologist William Lennox came from Boston to consult on the case and undoubtedly to observe Penfield operate using the techniques that he had recently learned from Foerster. Penfield performed a small right fronto-parietal craniotomy and resected a small cortical area anterior to the motor hand region, which he had identified by cortical stimulation. This procedure, however, was ineffective in controlling the patient's seizures. Nonetheless, a slight change was noticed in the patient's seizure pattern in that the *right* side of the body was now also involved early on in the attack. Undoubtedly thinking that the original lesion may have been bifrontal, Penfield performed a second operation, a left frontal craniotomy, in May 1929. No abnormality was found, no resection was performed, and the procedure was ineffectual. A third surgical exploration was undertaken on the right hemisphere, on 21 January 1932. The original right-sided craniotomy was extended to expose the temporal lobe, which was found to be scarred and atrophic. Cortical stimulation identified the motor strip, and stimulation of the mid-temporal lobe caused the patient's eyes to blink and the frontal and temporal operculum to blanch. The vascular reaction undoubtedly influenced Penfield's decision to resect the posterior aspect of the right temporal cortex to its junction with the occipital lobe. This operation was successful in greatly reducing the frequency of the patient's seizures. Penfield's operative report and Cone's pathological report are reproduced here, in their original format:

OPERATIVE REPORT

M., Robert.	Royal Victoria Hospital No. 80169.
<u>Operator:</u>	Dr Penfield.
<u>Operation Date:</u>	1-21-32.
Anaes. local.	
<u>Provisional Diagnosis:</u>	Cerebral cicatrix. Jacksonian epilepsy.
<u>Final Diagnosis:</u>	The same.
<u>Operation:</u>	Right, temporal frontal osteoplastic craniotomy. Excision of cerebral cicatrix. Transplantation of fascia from thigh.

<u>Objective findings:</u>   The same area of honey-combed bone was encountered in the bone flap coextensive with the defect in the dura over the temporal lobe. The dura was not under increased pressure except for the pathological areas to be described. The brain appeared quite normal, the convolutions of good consistency. The area of previous excision in the motor area was not in any way adherent but it must be borne in mind that this lay directly beneath the bone. On turning the bone flap there was no evidence of attachment of the brain to the

bone. There was no connective tissue scar in the area of excision and stimulation at the bottom produced a normal physiological response without any sensation of an attack. The inferior horn of the lateral ventricle came almost to the surface because of the extreme thinness of the temporal lobe over it. When the fluid escaped the whole temporal lobe collapsed. There was a zone of brain as thin as a membrane over the lateral aspect of this inferior horn. This became thicker on the undersurface of the temporal lobe. An area of the brain was bounded sharply by a definite line posteriorly, less definitely in other directions. There was a small cup-shaped area just posterior to the fissure of Sylvius marked 2 in the illustration, stimulation of which invariably produced the premonitory signs of an attack. This consisted of a feeling of the head turning. The patient states that his head seems to go around regularly before an attack. Between this cup-shaped area and the area of old excision was a strip of cortex covered with pia arachnoid about 1½ cms. in width. It is interesting that there has been no regrowth of the denuded pia over the denuded areas of brain at least grossly. The inside of the ventricle appeared normal. The [choroid] plexus passed well down into the inferior horn. After removal of the pathological tissue a plexus of arteries was encountered over a dome-shaped structure which was taken to be the Island of Reil.

Stimulation: During the progress of the stimulation the brain became more resistant to response. The fact that we did not produce a generalized seizure is probably due to the small attacks which were induced and which developed resistance. Stimulation just above the old excisions gave twitching of the left hand and stimulation in the old excision gave movement of the hand. Stimulation at 2 in the small area just posterior to the fissure of Sylvius with 2 m.a. [milliamperes] gave face sensation of head going around and approach of an attack. With this sensation was a twitching of the left hand. Stimulation below this over the temporal lobe at the nearest point but [sic] the fissure of Sylvius gave a similar result as far as feeling of an attack is concerned. It is of great interest that stimulation of zone 3 which must correspond with the frontal adversive field made the patient feel as though "his eyes were going to turn to the left," and stimulation just above the area of the old excision gave him on the first occasion a sensation of lifting his eyes upward and on the second occasion with longer stimulation his eyes were seen to open wide and had the sensation of an impending attack. This area was not removed and did not appear pathological. On one occasion stimulation at this lower portion of the temporal lobe was reported by the patient as humming in the left ear. This could not be repeated. Following stimulation at 2 prime nearly one minute the pallor which was present on one gyrus L spread upward to an adjacent gyrus and during that time his eyes were reported as blinking convulsively.

<u>Procedure:</u> The pathological tissue was removed with sutures around the full extent indicated in the drawing, that is, just below the old excision and extending backward to the occipital lobe. In front the brain was dissected slowly so as not to injure the middle cerebral artery and the plexus of arteries over the isthmus of Riel was left in place. The ventricle was left widely open. Fascia was removed by Dr Cone from the thigh and the defect in the dura was closed completely. A considerable area of decompression was left in the bone this time. The bone flap was closed with silver wire and a drain inserted into the ventricle. The aponeurosis and scalp were closed as usual. The patient's condition was excellent throughout. On the way to his room, however, just as he reached the elevator he became suddenly pulseless. On reaching his room there was no arterial pressure what-ever in the arm but the pulse returned quickly with intravenous glucose.

PATHOLOGICAL REPORT

3-1338. M., Mr Robert. Royal Victoria Hospital No. 80169.

Age: 24 years.

<u>Operation:</u> Right, temporal, frontal, osteoplastic craniotomy.
Excision of cerebral cicatrix.
Transplantation of fascia from the thigh.

<u>Operator:</u> Dr Penfield.

<u>Date of Operation:</u> 1-21-32.

<u>Clinical Data:</u><u>Subjective</u>—

1. Fracture of skull, 1918 followed by exploratory operation and disclosure of contused brain in the left hemisphere.
2. Left-sided Jacksonian convulsions and left-sided weakness since the accident.
3. Re-exploration of hemisphere, November, 1928 with removal of scar left [sic] temporal parietal region.
4. Continuance of seizures following this operation with alteration in pattern, the right side of the body being involved early in the seizure.
5. Left craniotomy in May 1929 with negative exploration of left hemisphere.
6. Continuation of seizures up to present time; pattern indefinite but predominantly left-sided.

<u>Objective</u>—

1. Abnormal posture with deviation of head to the left and flexion of left arm.
2. Left homonymous field defect.
3. Unequal pupils; right larger than left.

4.   Left facial weakness.

5.   Relative weakness of left arm.

6.   Diminished two-point sensibility and slight astereognosis of the left hand.

7.   Ataxia in finger-nose-finger test, left hand.

8.   Hyperactivity of all tendon reflexes.

REPORT – LABORATORY OF NEUROPATHOLOGY

Gross: Specimen consists of a portion of brain weighing ten grams and containing a cerebral cicatrix to which thickened arachnoid is attached firmly for an area of 4 by 3 centimeters. Several artery clips mark the situation of the larger pial vessels which are fairly numerous. A second portion weighing four grams is of similar appearance but beneath the thickest meningeal covering is a cyst or space which measures about 1 by 1 by 2 centimeters. The denser cicatricial layer just beneath the arachnoid is about one-half of a centimeter thick and grossly appears as a dense layer of fibrous connective tissue. Numerous portions of bone with a fat [sic] dura most of which are circular shaped, as from burr openings, are preserved in 10% formalin. One piece to which is attached a dense portion of dura is being decalcified. Material has been placed in 10% formalin, formalin ammonium Bromide and Zenker's.

Microscopic: The main portion of this specimen has been handed over for special study upon vascular innervation of brain scar. The Gold Stains simply show gliosis.

Diagnosis: Cerebral cicatrix, right temporal.

This was the first of many patients on whom Penfield would operate for the treatment of temporal lobe epilepsy, but it was not yet recognized as a specific clinical entity with a distinct pathological substrate. Thus, the results of surgery for temporal lobe epilepsy were not analyzed separately from all operation performed for focal epilepsy arising from a cerebral scar.

THE ROLE OF EEG

Penfield's 1935 review of the effects of cortical resection on epilepsy, "Epilepsy and Surgical Therapy," was marred by an overly subjective assessment of outcome and by an unrealistically short follow-up period. Penfield attempted to correct these deficiencies when he updated his outcome analysis for inclusion in *Epilepsy and Cerebral Localization*, which he published with Theodore Erickson in 1941.[2] For this new analysis the effects of surgery were segregated into five groups, depending on the percentage by which a patient's seizure had decreased in frequency. This way of

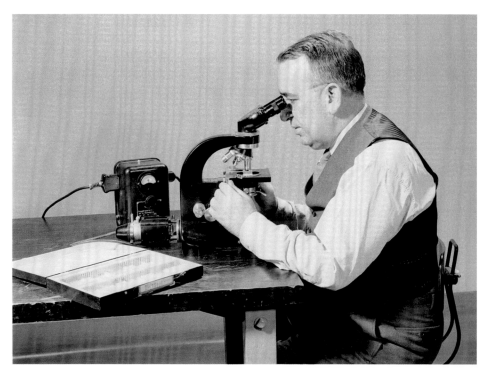

Figure 10.3. William Cone examining a specimen removed at surgery. Montreal Neurological Institute, McGill University.

classifying postoperative results had been devised by Penfield's mentor, Allan Whipple, at the Presbyterian Hospital in New York City.[3] In this classification, group *four* was comprised of patients who were completely free of seizures following surgery. Group *three* patients had a 75% decrease in seizure frequency. Patients in these two groups were considered as having had a "satisfactory" result. Group *two* patients had a decreased seizure-frequency of 50%, and their outcome was considered "fair."[4] Group *one* patients had a 25% decrease in attacks, and patients whose operation did not result in a decrease in seizure frequency fell into group *zero*.

Penfield and Erickson analyzed the outcome of 115 patients who had been operated upon between 1929 and 1939 and for whom at least one year had elapsed since surgery. In the majority of patients the follow-up period ranged from three to five years. As Herbert Jasper arrived at the MNI in 1938, the role of EEG was not a factor in the analysis. The results of surgery were not as impressive as those that Penfield had reported in 1935: 43% of patients whose craniotomy resulted in the resection of a cortical scar had a satisfactory outcome according to Penfield's new grading scale, and in 35% the outcome was "fair." Surprisingly, one quarter of patients who had only an exploratory craniotomy and no cortical resection also had a "fair" outcome.

Table 10.1
Results of surgery, 1929–39

Procedure	No. of cases	Outcome (%)					
		4	3	2	1	0	Worse
Resection of a meningocerebral cicatrix	62	22.5	22.5	32	10	11	2
Resection of a cortical cicatrix	53	19	21	19	9	30	2
Exploration	35	2.5	2.5	20	0	69	6

Note: Five patients underwent ligation or excision of a cortical artery, and seven patients died as a result of surgery. Modified from Penfield and Erickson, Epilepsy and Cerebral Localization.

One is hard pressed to explain a "fair" outcome resulting from exposure of the cortex to operating room air. Penfield offers no explanation, and none is forthcoming.

One of the most significant conclusions that Penfield drew from this early surgical experience was the realization "that the best results from radical surgical therapy occur in those cases in which a removable localized lesion is found in an otherwise comparatively normal brain."[5] In the presence of such a lesion the resection was limited and tailored to incorporate the scarred area and the epileptogenic zone surrounding it. If there was no obvious lesion, there was no resection. Penfield continued to apply this approach to the treatment of temporal lobe epilepsy for the next twenty-five years, until his discovery of medial temporal sclerosis.

World War II had a great impact on the MNI's staff as their activities were directed to the war effort.[6] Nonetheless, patients were still treated for epilepsy during the war years, and all now underwent preoperative EEG as an aid to preoperative localization. But what was the value of this new technology? Was it reliable, and how was it to be integrated into Penfield's approach to the diagnosis and treatment of epileptic patients? These questions could only be assessed clinically in patients such as T.E.

The patient was five years old when he came down with a severe headache and a febrile illness of such severity that he was not expected to survive. He nonetheless recovered, but he was dysphasic, with a tendency to substitute one word for another.

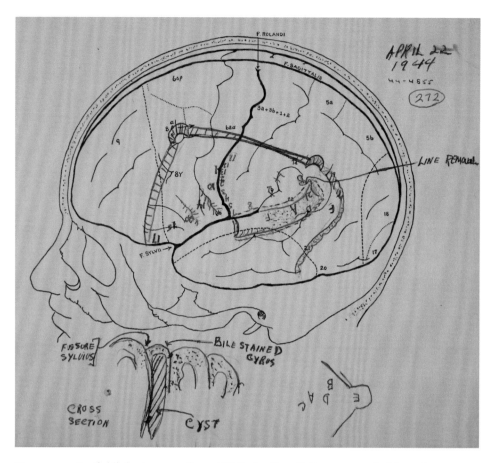

Figure 10.4. Penfield's brain map of case T.E. Epileptic activity was recorded from the areas represented by letters A–E, which are clustered about the discoloured portion of the first temporal convolution. The discoloured area overlay a cystic cavity, as indicated in the detailed drawing, which depicts a cross-section of the parietal and temporal lobes at the level of the lesion. The Sylvian fissure separates the parietal operculum from the cystic cavity within the first temporal convolution. The cortex overlying the cystic cavity and the posterior-most aspect of the temporal lobe were injected with nupercaine to assess their language competency. Montreal Neurological Hospital, case T.E., 1954.

His seizures began eleven years later when he was sixteen years old. These were characterized by lip smacking and swallowing movements, during which he stared blankly and had a tendency to drop things from his right hand. The diagnosis was apparent to Penfield, who observed, "the story suggests the possibility of a localized meningitis or brain abscess which occurred at the age of five, followed by aphasia. The attacks now suggest an origin in the temporal region. He will have an electrogram [*sic*] and x-rays of his skull." The EEG revealed evidence of a focal epileptogenic lesion in the left temporal lobe. Thus, there was concordance of the history, clinical findings, and electrophysiology. A left-sided craniotomy was elevated:

> The posterior part of the temporal convolution was somewhat narrow and was stained as though by bile, being brownish in color. The electrocorticographic activity had been localized quite clearly over it. This discolored gyrus was the outer covering of [a] cyst, the gyrus being thinned out to a thickness of 2 to 3 mm. as it covered the cyst wall. The cyst itself extended downward along the fissure of Sylvius being a measured depth of 3 cms from the surface to the bottom of the cyst … [It] opened easily and its surface was everywhere shining and smooth. It seems most likely that it was the remnant of a former intracerebral hemorrhage, and that the cyst contained yellow fluid for a considerable period of time, and that it is the original blood pigment, which stained the walls of the cyst and the covering gyrus … The first temporal gyrus was then removed as far forward as the lower end of the postcentral gyrus. This was extended back so as to include the angular gyrus. The removal of the gyrus opened the cyst widely. It is possible that the excision should have been carried out farther posterior, and the continuation of *this gyrus posteriorly was injected with nupercaine[7] at the time the rest of the gyrus was injected. There was no interference with speech following this nupercaine injection* [emphasis added]. If there is further trouble I would expect it to be posterior rather than anterior and further removal could be carried out easily.

This case is a remarkable example of the correlation of clinical and electrographic findings with the site of a structural lesion. The posterior aspect of the first temporal convolution – Wernicke's area – was atrophic, discoloured, and soft to the touch, indicating a remote cerebral haemorrhage and cystic degeneration of the underlying white matter. These impressions were confirmed when Penfield incised the atrophic cortex and entered into a mature cyst whose inner walls were smooth, shiny, and xanthochromic. Electrocorticographic recordings showed that the cortex about the cyst was highly epileptogenic. The abnormal area of cortex was far enough posteriorly on the first left temporal convolution that identifying the posterior speech region was warranted. Stunningly, Penfield injected the gyrus with nupercaine, a local anaesthetic, as described in the preceding chapter. Confident in a procedure that he would later judge as damaging and ineffectual, Penfield resected the first temporal gyrus as far back as its junction with the angular gyrus. That the patient's illness occurred when he was a young child probably resulted in a shift of the posterior speech region to the opposite hemisphere.[8] This explains why he did not experience postoperative aphasia, as would be expected with such a posterior excision in the dominant hemisphere. Penfield need not have been concerned about another operation.

Table 10.2
Results of surgery, 1939–44

Procedure	No. of cases	Outcome (%)				
		4	3	2	1	0
Resection	59	25	31	14	12	19
Exploration	16	0	0	32	14	54

Note: There was one postoperative death. The percentages have been rounded up. Modified from Penfield and Steelman, "The Treatment of Focal Epilepsy by Cortical Excision."

This one sufficed. T.E. remained free of epileptic attacks until his last follow-up in 1991, forty-six years after his operation.

THE ABSENCE OF SCARS

The concordance of pre- and intraoperative EEG localization with a structural lesion led Penfield to review the role of EEG in epilepsy surgery over the five-year period 1939–44. These data were reported at the March 1947 meeting of the American Surgical Association.[9] There were seventy-five patients in the study, of which fifty-nine had undergone the resection of a traumatic cortical scar, of a brain abscess, or of a cortical area damaged *in utero* or during the birth process. Included among the latter were patients with microgyria, a cortical malformation that Penfield was the first to describe, and which is now recognized as one of the commonest causes of focal epilepsy.[10]

Sixteen patients had an exploratory craniotomy without resection. Thus, the advent of EEG does not appear to have diminished the proportion of patients operated upon unnecessarily. Nonetheless, the study of these patients allowed Herbert Jasper to discover that localized "sharp waves" recorded from the preoperative EEGs and "spikes" recorded from the ECOG were associated with a structural, epileptogenic lesion. This would be useful in the diagnosis of temporal lobe epilepsy once mesial temporal sclerosis was recognized as its cause, but this had yet to be achieved. Another significant observation was that hyperventilation, over-hydration, and metrazol were all useful in generating epileptic sharp waves in patients with focal epilepsy whose EEG was initially normal. Metrazol, a stimulant, was also used in the operating room following the resection of an epileptic area to uncover any residual

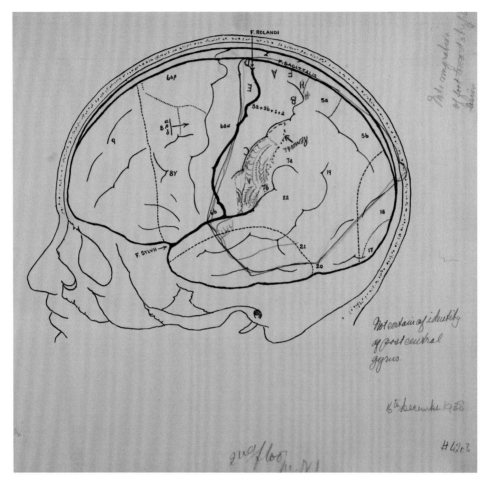

Figure 10.5. Penfield's brain map of a patient who had focal sensory seizures with secondary generalization, illustrating an area of focal microgyria. Montreal Neurological Hospital, case M.B., 1938.

epileptic activity. Nonetheless, Penfield reported an overall rate of satisfactory outcomes, 56%, that was not significantly different from what he and Erickson had reported in 1941. Nevertheless, Penfield recognized that "the simpler the electrographic record is and the better it is localized, the better the prognosis of a successful excision."[11] But he remained dubious of the role of EEG without corroborating evidence because, as he explained, "a well localized, simple electroencephalogram, not supported by … evidence of a lesion, has sometimes led us to a useless exploration, i.e., a craniotomy without excision."[12]

Despite the lack of improvement in surgical outcome, Penfield's 1947 analysis is significant in that for the first time, he analyzed the effects of surgery based on the site of the lesion, and discrepancies were observed. Thus, a satisfactory outcome was

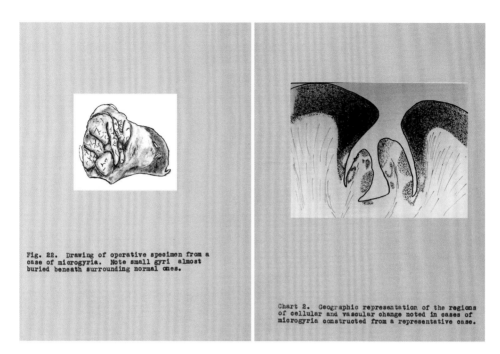

Fig. 22. Drawing of operative specimen from a case of microgyria. Note small gyri almost buried beneath surrounding normal ones.

Chart 2. Geographic representation of the regions of cellular and vascular change noted in cases of microgyria constructed from a representative case.

Figure 10.6. *Left.* Drawing of microgyric cortex removed by Penfield. The uniform tissue to the right of the image is subcortical white matter to which two small vascular clips are attached. *Right.* Cartoon of a cross-section of the image at left depicting the area of microgyria between two normal gyri. The cortex of the microgyria is markedly thinned, and there are islands of subcortical gliosis and white matter strands projecting toward the surface. Montreal Neurological Institute, McGill University, Humphreys, "Study of the Vascular and Cytological Changes in the Cerebral Cicatrix."

obtained in 70% of patients whose seizures originated in the frontal lobe exclusive of the precentral gyrus, but a satisfactory outcome was achieved in only 50% of the patients who were operated for temporal lobe seizures.[13]

In retrospect, this was undoubtedly due to the more extensive resections of epileptogenic tissue achievable in the frontal lobes, compared to the limited resections that Penfield performed in temporal cases. The relatively poor results of surgery for temporal lobe epilepsy were due to ignorance, at the time, of the importance of the mesial structures in its etiology and to the fear of encroaching upon them, which might produce the Klüver-Bucy syndrome. Nonetheless, Penfield correctly concluded from his analysis that "radical excision seems to offer a reasonable possibility of cure"[14] but that "craniotomy which does not include removal of abnormally functioning cortex has no chance of success."[15] In temporal epilepsy, however, the lesion was hidden from the surgeon's view within the mesial temporal structures.

CHAPTER 11

The Dreamy State

Psychomotor epilepsy usually goes unrecognized[1]

John Hughlings Jackson described psychomotor epilepsy in a case report that he published in 1888, in a paper entitled "On a Particular Variety of Epilepsy."[2] The case was that of a physician whose epileptic attacks were characterized by what Jackson called a "dreamy state."[3] While in this state the patient, to whom Jackson referred as patient 5, attended to mundane tasks and professional activities, all the while unaware that he was doing so, and for which he had no memory. This behaviour would later be referred to as "automatism." Patient 5 described one of these episodes in the diary that he kept of his illness:

> I was attending a young patient whom his mother had brought me with some history of lung symptoms. I wished to examine the chest, and asked him to undress on a couch … Whilst he was undressing I felt the onset of *a petit mal*[4] … The next thing I recollect is that I was sitting at a writing-table in the same room, speaking to another person, and as my consciousness became more complete, recollected my patient, but saw he was not in the room. I was interested to ascertain what had happened, and had an opportunity an hour later of seeing him in bed, with the note of a diagnosis I had made of "pneumonia of the left base." I gathered indirectly from conversation that I had made a physical examination, written these words, and advised him to take to bed at once. I re-examined him with some curiosity, and found that my conscious diagnosis was the same as my unconscious, – or perhaps I should say, unremembered diagnosis had been.[5]

The onset of the dreamy state, Jackson wrote, was often preceded by a sensory warning, which was most characteristically an unrecognizable smell or taste, or a rising epigastric sensation. In patient 5's case, however, the warning was a feeling of recollection, a feeling of *déjà-entendu*, the sense that he had previously heard what he was currently hearing. Chewing movements or lip smacking heralded the onset of patient 5's seizures, during which he performed acts of which he was unaware and for which he was amnesic, as he described in his diary. Jackson also recognized that patients with this particular variety of epilepsy could visualize complicated scenes arising from past experience – complex episodes of *déjà vu* – yet remain aware of their illusory nature. Jackson referred to this phenomenon as "mental diplopia," by which he meant that a patient was conscious of two events at the same time, one being the illusion, the other the awareness that it was an illusion. Penfield would evoke this concept, to which he referred as "double consciousness," when he needed to explain how patients whose temporal lobes were stimulated could relive a past experience, yet remain conscious of events occurring in the operating room. To Jackson, the onset of the seizures – epigastric sensations, lip smacking – indicated "an epileptic discharge beginning in some part of the gustatory centers"[6] of the brain, which David Ferrier, in his animal studies, had erroneously localized to the uncus of the temporal lobe. Thus, Jackson accurately localized psychomotor seizures to the uncinate process but for the wrong reason, and the term "uncinate fits" entered the medical vocabulary to denote psychomotor seizures.

Jackson returned to patient 5 – to whom he now referred as "Z" – in 1898, after he had died from an overdose of chloral hydrate.[7] A small, cystic, smooth-walled cavity within the left uncus was found at autopsy, confirming Jackson's earlier suspicion. Unfortunately, the brain was inadequately preserved and the cause of the lesion could not be ascertained. The prevailing opinion at the time was that an arterial thrombosis had occurred, although an occluded artery could not be identified in the vicinity of the cyst.[8] Patient 5 – Z – was later identified as Arthur Thomas Myers, a physician at the Belgrave Hospital for Children. He lived next door to Jackson, in Manchester Square, London.[9]

The next major advance in our understanding of temporal lobe epilepsy came in 1938, in a paper entitled "Psychomotor Epilepsy," authored by Erna and Frederic Gibbs and Bartolome Fuster, from the Illinois Psychiatric Institute. The authors reviewed the EEGs of 300 patients suffering from psychomotor seizures and found that they originated from the anterior aspect of the temporal lobe.[10] They concluded their highly influential paper by stating, "Patients with psychomotor epilepsy are rarely benefited by treatment with any or all of the antiepileptic substances at present available … In severe cases surgical removal of the discharging region should be attempted."[11] Worthy comment, but still, one had to know where to operate in the absence of an obvious lesion, and it was known that some regions of the temporal lobe were dangerous to approach.

THE KLÜVER-BUCY SYNDROME

Aurora

Heinrich Klüver was a highly innovative and influential neurophysiologist who performed seminal work on the occipital and temporal lobes. After immigrating to the United States from Germany, Klüver obtained a doctorate in psychology from Stanford University for his studies on visual imagery in children. From Stanford he went to the University of Minnesota, where he met Karl Lashey, with whom he enjoyed a lifelong friendship and professional collaboration. Klüver took dual appointments in the Departments of Psychiatry and of Biological Sciences at the University of Chicago, where, according to Paul Bucy, he was a brilliant star.[12]

Klüver became interested in the effects of mescaline on the visual system after he had personally experimented with the ingestion of mescal buttons.[13] Klüver got the opportunity to study the effects of mescaline on a primate when a female rhesus monkey named Aurora was assigned to his laboratory. Aurora had undergone ablation of the uterus and ovaries as a prelude to experimentation in the department of endocrinology, but she became unmanageably aggressive following surgery. She was reassigned to Klüver because of his affinity for monkeys. Klüver injected Aurora with mescaline in December 1936 as part of an experiment to assess its effect on visual function. The injection, however, caused Aurora to exhibit chewing and licking movements and to fall into a convulsion. Recalling Jackson's paper on uncinate fits, Klüver prevailed upon Paul Bucy, a neurosurgeon, to remove both of Aurora's uncinate processes. To do this Bucy had to remove the amygdala and hippocampus, the parahippocampal and fusiform gyri, and the lateral temporal convolutions. The effects of this procedure were as dramatic as they were unexpected. Klüver and Bucy published the results of their experiments in 1937 under the heading "Psychic Blindness and Other Symptoms."[14] They elaborated upon their findings in subsequent papers[15] – the last one was published in 1955[16] – but the initial publication was enough to strike fear in the heart of any neurosurgeon contemplating approaching the mesial temporal structures.

What Klüver and Bucy describe as *psychic blindness* is now referred to as visual agnosia, the inability to recognize objects by their appearance, although vision is not impaired. The "other symptoms" referred to in the title of their paper were a tendency to explore objects orally by licking, biting, and chewing them; obsessive, repetitive exploration of anything placed in her visual field; tameness; and hypersexuality. The lateral temporal neocortex was not felt to be responsible for this behaviour, because neurosurgeons had resected it, at least unilaterally, with no such effects. Clearly then, the cause lay in the medial structures of the temporal lobes, and neurosurgeons approached them with the greatest reluctance.

Aurora was killed – Klüver and Bucy's word – in December 1938, two years to the day after she had entered Klüver's laboratory.[17] As for Klüver, he spent the last years of his life as a recluse in his laboratory, caring for his monkeys.

THE UNCUS

Despite concerns with the Klüver-Bucy syndrome, Penfield followed where the pathology led him, and gradually, gingerly, his resections began to encroach upon the uncus, a knuckle-like structure containing the amygdala and the *pes hippocampi*, if it was discoloured, atrophic, or hardened. One such case was that of patient S.L., a thirty-five-year-old New Zealander referred to Penfield in October 1950 by Mr Murray Falconer, a neurosurgeon. The patient had sustained numerous concussions with loss of consciousness while playing rugby, football (soccer), and boxing. He had his first seizure at the age of twenty-one, following a surgical procedure to set a broken nose. The seizures were preceded by an aura consisting of a progressively louder buzzing sound heard in both ears and ending in a loud bang. On other occasions, the aura consisted "of a sudden illusion of great silence," when "even the breeze rustling in the trees are hushed." This aura, unlike the other, was always followed by a generalized, tonic-clonic seizure, as was a third aura, which consisted of an olfactory hallucination characterized as a peculiar smell. A PEG showed that the left lateral ventricle was slightly enlarged, which suggested atrophy of the left temporal lobe. Penfield elevated a left-sided bone flap and observed that the first temporal convolution was yellowed and tough as it curved along the temporal pole and well into the uncus.

Stimulation from an electrode inserted to a depth of 1.5 centimetres in the first temporal convolution caused the patient to respond, "yes I am going to, I am going to." When asked what he had experienced, the patient stated, "all the noise was jumbled, upside down, like a crossword puzzle." Cortical stimulation within the second and third temporal convolutions produced aphasic responses. The resection was therefore limited to the first temporal convolution and extended down to the uncus and medially to the point where stimulation had produced the patient's aura. Summarizing his thinking, Penfield concluded his operative report by stating, "The excision was carried out on the basis of reproduction of the patient's aura and from the objective changes in the first temporal convolution. It is likely that the tendency for attacks will be reduced but prognosis for complete cessation must be very guarded."

Penfield's prognosis proved to be overly pessimistic. After a short period of intermittent attacks, the patient became seizure-free and remained so until his death from lung cancer, twenty-eight years after surgery. His referring surgeon, Murray Falconer, relocated from New Zealand, where he had been recognized for his expertise as a lumbar spine surgeon, to Guy's-Maudsley Hospital, London, where he, and MNI fellow Peter Schurr, founded an epilepsy surgery program.[18] The gliotic changes that Penfield noted extending along the first temporal convolution into the uncus would later be recognized as an integral constituent of mesial temporal sclerosis.

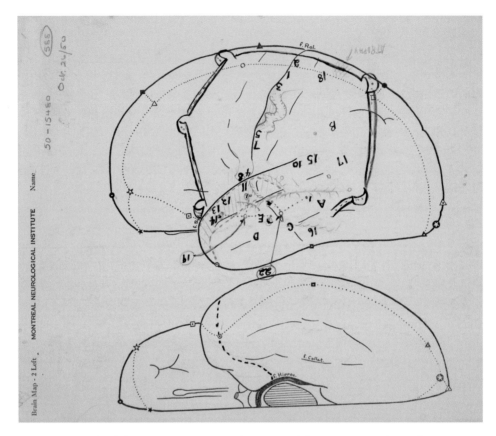

Figure 11.1. Penfield's brain map illustrating the extent of the resection performed in patient S.L., which included the first temporal convolution and the uncus. The postcentral gyrus was atrophic, which is represented by its wavy appearance. Montreal Neurological Hospital, case S.L.

THE NEGLECTED SPIKE

S.L.'s case was included in the analysis of a series of patients operated upon for temporal lobe epilepsy that Penfield and his fellow, Herman Flanigin, reported to the American Neurological Association in Atlantic City in 1950.[19] Their study included fifty-one patients operated upon between 1939 and 1949. The follow-up period extended from one to eleven years. Most of the patients were found at surgery to have a scar from penetrating or nonpenetrating trauma, or from an injury sustained during birth – what Penfield referred to as "birth compression," squeezing of the head through a narrow birth canal. The extent of resection varied from the temporal pole alone to the anterior half of the temporal lobe. The uncus had been included in the resection in only ten cases and the hippocampus in only two. Penfield and

Flanigin found that 50% of the patients had a satisfactory outcome by the criteria that Penfield had previously established. Of note, the incidence of satisfactory outcomes reached 60% when birth compression had caused the epileptic scar. Penfield would soon recognize a difficult passage through the birth canal as *the* major cause of psychomotor epilepsy, but not yet.

Although preoperatives and cortical EEGs had been used routinely to help localize the epileptic focus, the results of surgery were little better than they had been before clinical electrophysiology had come to the MNI. This, however, was not for lack of insight on the part of Herbert Jasper and his brilliant colleague, John Kershman. Jasper and Kershman suspected that the epileptiform activity recorded from the lateral temporal cortex originated from the medial structures.[20] This explained why the cortical EEG recorded epileptic activity from the lateral cortex in the absence of a visible structural lesion there and the relatively poor results obtained from lateral temporal resections. Penfield, however, was reluctant to venture into the mesial temporal lobe because he feared producing some elements of the Klüver-Bucy syndrome. Further, he had expressed the opinion that "the electrogram [the ECoG] without objective change in the cortex … is not yet to be trusted as the final guide to excision."[21]

However, not everyone agreed with Penfield. Herbert Jasper, Henri Pertuiset, and Herman Flanigin published their own analysis of the temporal lobe series in 1951, in a paper entitled "EEG and Cortical Electrogram in Patients with Temporal Lobe Seizures."[22] Significantly, Jasper and his collaborators found that "with strictly unilateral electrographic abnormalities in the preoperative tracing, sixty-seven percent of the patients showed good results" following surgery. Jasper, Pertuiset, and Flanigin also described how the role of ECoG had evolved in the intraoperative investigation of temporal lobe epilepsy:

Electrographic recording was first carried out on the exposed surfaces of the temporal lobe; then, with electrodes insulated except for their tips, records were taken from the inferior surface, including the temporal tip, the uncus and the hippocampal gyrus. After removal of the tip of the temporal lobe, it was possible to record directly from the insula and, in a few instances, from the *pes hippocampi* through the opened ventricle.[23]

Could the EEG and ECoG activity recorded from the lateral cortex in which there was no lesion have originated from the mesial strictures hidden from the surgeon's view? A positive answer was suggested almost as an afterthought, as Penfield and Flanigin noted at the end of their paper, "One patient has been operated on a second time since the termination of this analysis. It was found that there was *induration of the cortex* [emphasis added] in the remaining uncus and hippocampal gyrus. This

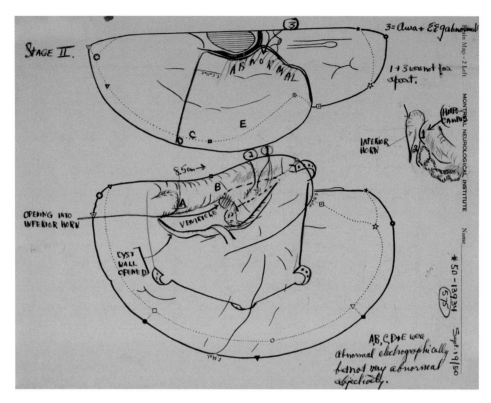

Figure 11.2. Brain map of a patient following a left lateral temporal resection and in whom the temporal horn of the left lateral ventricle was entered. The hippocampus is visible at the floor of the ventricle, as illustrated in the detail at right. Stimulation at number 1, near the insula, produced nausea. Stimulation at number 3, over the amygdala, and at number 2, on the hippocampus, produced the patient's aura and epileptic spikes. Penfield wrote at bottom right, "A, B, C, D, +E were abnormal electrographically but not very abnormal objectively." The third temporal convolution was nonetheless resected to 8.5 centimetres from the temporal tip. Montreal Neurological Hospital, case D.H., 1950.

was excised, and he has had no further seizures during the few months that have followed operation."[24] That patient was J.O.

A singular case

There are instances when a single observation alters the course of neurology. Such was the case of patient J.O., which led to the discovery of mesial temporal sclerosis as the substrate of temporal lobe epilepsy. It is a measure of the importance that Penfield ascribed to this case that fragments of it were published on three occasions. It was first mentioned in Penfield and Flanigin's review of temporal lobe cases as one of ten in which the uncus was resected. It was then included in Jasper's follow-up paper on the role of EEG in selecting patients for temporal resection. It was last

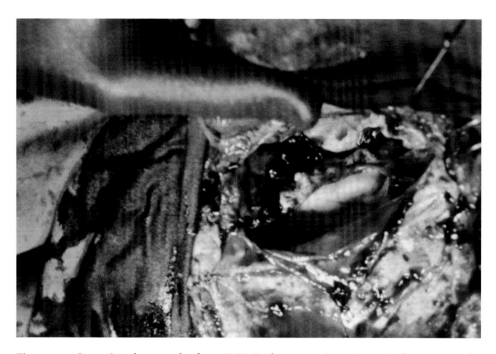

Figure 11.3. Operative photograph of case D.H., in the same orientation as in the corresponding brain map. The dura has been opened over the anterior–inferior aspect of the temporal lobe. A moist, green drape covers the unopened dura. The inferior aspect of the temporal lobe has been resected, and the temporal horn of the lateral ventricle has been opened. Penfield's thumb is retracting the inferior-most aspect of the operative site to expose the hippocampus, which appears as the cylindrical structure at the bottom of the exposure. This is the best intraoperative photograph of the hippocampus taken by Penfield. Montreal Neurological Hospital, case D.H., 1950.

referred to in Penfield and Jasper, *Epilepsy and the Functional Anatomy of the Human Brain*. However, the patient's detailed history and brain maps are published here for the first time.

The patient's birth and early childhood gave no indication that he would become epileptic at the age of fourteen. There was no history of epilepsy in his family. He had not had a febrile seizure or an infection of the nervous system, and he had not sustained a head injury. Yet, one night in 1942 he had his first temporal lobe seizure. Penfield described the attacks when the patient, now twenty, was admitted to the MNI:

It is quite clear that he was automatic in the first attack and that this was followed by status [epilepticus] and difficulty speaking for about three days. His attacks since then have been ushered in by an "olfactory" hallucination consisting of a smell like burning oil. After this, he becomes automatic for a considerable period (raises right arm) and is said to make a gesture with his right hand approximating thumb to finger. In attacks seen here in X-ray department, he spoke unintelligible words in the beginning but the attack was followed by sleep and he spoke normally on awakening.

Radiological examinations revealed that the temporal horn of the left lateral ventricle was larger than the right – a finding that is now universally recognized as an indicator of mesial temporal sclerosis. Herbert Jasper concluded that EEG recordings were characteristic of "a deep left temporal focus," and Penfield ended the Clinical EEG Conference, where the patient's case had been discussed, by stating that operation seemed justified. Accordingly, the patient was brought to the operating room on 24 February 1948:

> The dura was opened … the middle fossa[25] of the skull seemed to be quite small from before backwards … The temporal lobe appeared normal … The central fissure was located. It seemed to lie farther forward than we expected. Electrocorticography was carried out and abnormality found in the second temporal convolution. Electrodes placed underneath the temporal lobe also showed some abnormality. Stimulation was then carried out to determine where speech arrest was produced, and it was concluded that it would be dangerous to speech if the usual 5 cm. of the anterior end of the temporal lobe was removed; consequently … a removal back as far as 4 cm. from the anterior limit of the middle fossa was carried out … There seemed to be a fairly definite toughness of the uncinate gyrus itself … Stimulation of the uncus definitely reproduced the olfactory aura and produced a seizure. The uncus was removed by suction … After that, an electrogram was taken and spike discharges were still found to be present in the second temporal convolution. A little further removal was carried out, but it was decided that it would be dangerous to speech to make any further removal. This area will have to be watched in the future.

The brain map that accompanies Penfield's operative report is one of the most detailed that he drew, which reflects Penfield's burgeoning interest in the mesial temporal structures. Surprisingly, the map is drawn on an older template than the one that was in use at the time. The later map had a section illustrating the undersurface of the temporal lobe, which was absent in the older one. Thus, Penfield had to sketch in the temporal undersurface by hand in order to illustrate the sites where recording of epileptic activity was obtained and where stimulation produced the patient's attacks. This appears as an inset at the top of the brain map. The results of stimulation of the uncus and of the parahippocampal gyrus (Nos 11, 24, and 25)

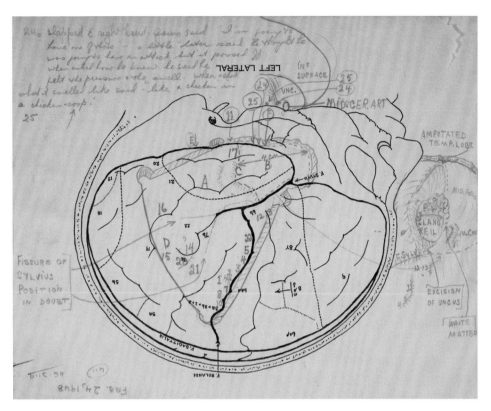

Figure 11.4. Penfield's brain map of the first operation performed on patient J.O. The under-surface of the temporal lobe is sketched in at the top of the illustration, where the uncus is labelled "unc." The small circle next to the uncus represents the middle cerebral artery. Epileptic activity was recorded, and epileptic attacks were generated, from the uncus and hippocampus at numbers 11, 24, 25, and at letters E and F. Epileptic activity spread from the undersurface to the lateral surface of the temporal lobe and to the angular gyrus, as represented by the letters A–D. The resection did not extend to the body of the hippocampus and left the epileptic areas indicated by 11 and E intact. Number 17 indicates an area from which aphasic responses were obtained, which limited the extent of the lateral resection. The detail at right illustrates the cavity created by the resection of the anterior temporal lobe. The operation did not alleviate the patient's seizures. Montreal Neurological Hospital, case J.O., 1948.

were dramatic, and the breathless tone of the dictated report suggests that they were as much of a surprise to Penfield as to the patient:

[The] patient said "I feel a what-you-may-call-it coming on." Head turned, then he began to swallow and make motions to his face. Right hand is twitching; left hand towards his face. His thumb and second finger of the left hand are gripped together in his usual manner. His toes are spread apart. Brain becoming cyanosed. Patient swallowing. He is moving his right arm and his left arm around and around over each other. This act obviously was produced by stimulation on the uncus or uncinate gyrus, I think. Duration – two minutes, 30 seconds.

When the area was restimulated,

[He] slapped with [his] right hand, [and] said, "I'm going to have one of those." A little later [he] said he thought he was going to have an attack but it passed off. When asked how he knew, [he said that] he felt the pressure and the smell. When asked what it smelled like, [he] said, "like a chicken in a chicken coop."

A third stimulation, a little more posteriorly, was just as startling:

[The] patient said, "Oh brother," and seemed to go into an attack. [His] eyes stared and he moved his hands as he had before and began to masticate. After about a minute or two, [he] spoke and said "I rang the bell. I wanted to speak to Bill." He explained that Bill was working for the mayor, and corrected this to the "King." [He was] unable to tell us whether he had the smell this time.

The array of EEG electrodes was repositioned on four occasions, so as to cover the whole of the lateral temporal lobe, its undersurface, and the uncus. This underscores the significance that Jasper assigned to this case. Jasper's report detailing the results of the cortical EEG takes up two pages of small, single-spaced type, with corrections and marginal notes. The reason for this unusually lengthy report was the unequivocal spread of epileptic activity from the uncus to the lateral temporal neocortex, which was one of the few times when this was recorded from the exposed brain. As Jasper noted in his report,

With stimulation … on the uncinate gyrus anteriorly, the patient had a seizure. In the [EEG] this attack was marked by some rapid discharges … from the electrode nearest the stimulation point on the uncus, and after fifteen seconds interval there appeared suddenly a burst of rhythmic, high voltage … sharp waves recorded from all electrodes, both on the under surface and on lateral surface of the temporal lobe.

For Jasper, then, the most striking feature of the cortical EEG was "the setting off of a rhythmic system," characterized by "a sudden explosive discharge involving all electrodes and was obviously triggered from stimulation of the uncinate gyrus." This was vindication of what he and Kershman had proposed a few years earlier from their studies of scalp EEGs.

Penfield's resection was limited to the lateral neocortex, and uncus, which included the *pes hippocampi*, but left the body of the hippocampus intact. Penfield concluded his operative report on a cautionary note, stating that the extent of the removal that he had performed had been limited by the proximity of speech representation and that further removal might be necessary in the future. He was correct in his prognosis but not because epileptic tissue had been left near the speech region. Rather, Penfield had to reoperate because he had failed to resect the body of the hippocampus.

The patient was free of seizures for a short time after surgery, but they recurred with increasing frequency and severity. There had also been a change in the patient's seizure pattern, the seizures being now of two kinds. One was characterized by a rising sensation in the throat, the presence of a strong smell, grunting sounds, and swallowing motions. The other began with a ringing sound "like a tuning fork that a singer uses," which appeared to come closer and closer to him. This was followed by the inability to speak, with the patient explaining that he knew what he wanted to say but could not find the words with which to say it. He was readmitted to the MNI in 1951. As his case was reviewed, Jasper recalled that after the final resection at the original operation, "there remained a fairly active spike focus on the inferior surface of the left temporal lobe … this being located on the stump of the uncinate or fusiform gyrus" as well as at the lateral resection margin, where excision had been limited by the presence of language function. The locations of the residual sites of epileptic activity were concordant with the patient's new seizure pattern and Penfield and Jasper concluded, "The electrocorticogram argued quite strongly at the last operation for further removal and subsequent developments indicate that this was valid evidence. Further excision seems justifiable in the light of our experience in the last four years with regard to excisions of the temporal lobe." By this was meant that the operation should be directed primarily at the residual hippocampus.

The patient was returned to the operating room on 3 October 1951, and Penfield observed, "The anterior part of the middle fossa was filled with fluid caught in a web of the most delicate tissue, this tissue vanished when it was sponged and then left almost nothing to pick up. This allowed unimpeded inspection and electrographic recording from the insula and the stump of the hippocampus."

Stimulation of the hippocampus "reproduced what seemed to be the patient's aura in the form of feeling in the epigastrium and a taste sensation." Accordingly, "the hippocampus and hippocampal gyrus were removed back a little bit." The operative sketch however indicates that more than "a little bit" of the hippocampus

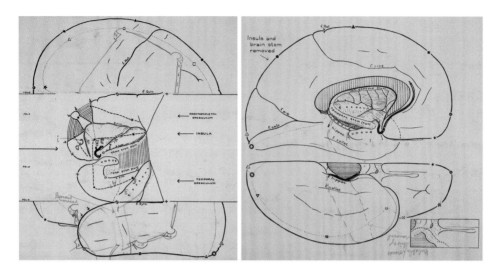

Figure 11.5. Operative drawings showing the extent of the mesial temporal resection performed at the patient's second operation. Resection of the hippocampus cured the patient of epilepsy. Montreal Neurological Hospital, case J.O., 1951.

was removed. The patient only had the occasional minor attack over the next twenty-five years.

This case reinforced Penfield's recent experience, that mesial structures – the uncus, amygdala, and hippocampus – could be resected, at least unilaterally, without incurring cognitive or behavioural deficits and resulted in better seizure control than if they were left behind at operation. As Jasper later pointed out, "the persistence of the neurosurgeon in exploring deeper structures"[26] led to one of the most important findings of twentieth-century epileptology, that the cause of psychomotor epilepsy lay in the mesial temporal structures.

CHAPTER 12

Incisural Sclerosis

He has shown us where the lesion lies[1]

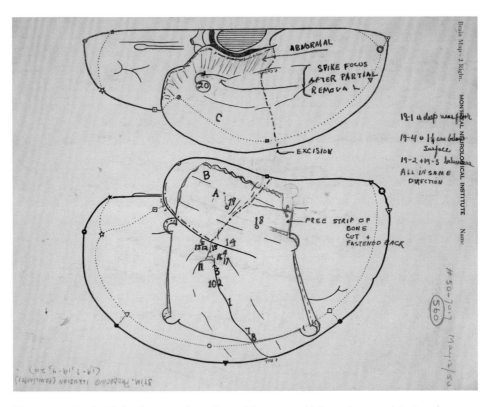

Figure 12.1. Penfield's brain map of a patient with temporal lobe epilepsy and incisural sclerosis involving the anterior part of the first temporal convolution, the uncus and the hippocampal gyrus. Epileptic spikes were recorded from the hippocampus once the lateral temporal lobe had been resected. Montreal Neurological Hospital, 1950.

The discovery that the resection of the mesial structures of the temporal lobe could convert an unsuccessful operation into one in which seizures were abolished was momentous: the role of the mesial structures in psychomotor epilepsy was revealed, and the unilateral resection of these structures was found to be innocuous – at least for the time being. The mesial temporal structures clearly required more study, and

Penfield assigned the task to three exceptional residents then at the institute: Maitland Baldwin,[2] Kenneth Earle,[3] and William Feindel.[4] The importance with which Penfield viewed research into the mesial temporal structures is reflected by his choice of these individuals to carry it out: Baldwin became the first director of neurosurgery at the National Institutes of Health, Bethesda, Maryland; Earle was appointed chief of neuropathology at the Armed Forces Institute of Pathology, Washington, DC; and Feindel succeeded Penfield and Rasmussen as director of the Montreal Neurological Institute.

THE AMYGDALA

Although Jackson's patient "Z" harboured a small lesion within the uncus, Jackson realized that the manifestations of uncinate fits were too complicated to originate from the uncus alone, and he wrote in 1899,[5] "the discharge lesions [*sic*] in these cases are made up of some cells, not of the uncinated gyrus alone, but of some cells of different parts of a region of which this gyrus is a part – a very vague circumscription, the uncinated region."[6] Jackson was correct. The uncus is a knuckle-like projection of the parahippocampal gyrus situated anteriorly and medially on the undersurface of the temporal lobe. (See figure Ana.2.) It is reached surgically by resecting the anterior aspect of the first temporal convolution and following it downward as it curves around the temporal pole. The uncus contains a cluster of cells gathered into a small nucleus referred to as the amygdala because of its shape, which is reminiscent of an almond. The uncus also contains the *pes hippocampi*, the anterior-most projection of the hippocampus. Thus, the amygdala became a legitimate target in the investigation of temporal lobe epilepsy, and a depth electrode was developed at the MNI to record from it and its immediately vicinity. This electrode allowed the recording of epileptic spikes originating from the amygdala and the peri-amygdaloid region and to investigate the role that these structures played in initiating psychomotor seizures. This was performed in the following way, as described by Wilder Penfield

Figure 12.2. *Opposite top* Penfield's brain map. The "X" between letters A and B indicates the point at which a depth electrode was inserted in the second temporal convolution to reach the amygdala. The detail at the left shows the tip of the electrode within the amygdala. Stimulation of the amygdala produced the patient's aura. Montreal Neurological Hospital, case H.M., 1952.

Figure 12.3. *Opposite bottom* Operative photograph of the right hemisphere seen in the anatomical orientation, corresponding to the view in the previous illustration. The posterior frontal lobe is at right, where the precentral gyrus is identified by numbers 5, 7, and 8. The parietal lobe is at the left, where numbers 1–4 identify the postcentral gyrus. The depth electrode has been inserted through the temporal cortex, so that its tip lies in the amygdala. Montreal Neurological Hospital, case X.B, 1952.

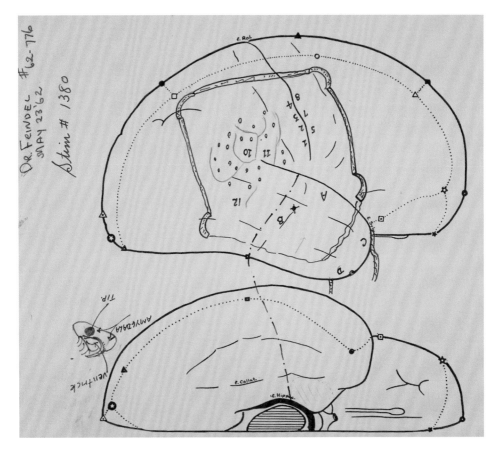

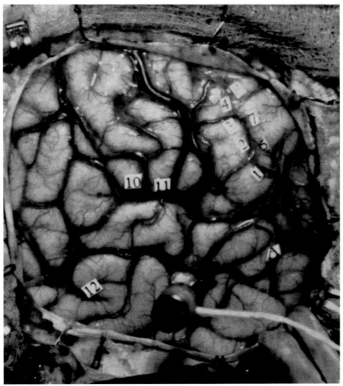

and Maitland Baldwin in their influential paper "Temporal Lobe Seizures and the Technique of Subtotal Temporal Lobectomy"[7] and using coordinates that Baldwin had determined in his master's thesis:[8]

> It is possible to pass an electrode, coated except at the tip, into the temporal lobe and stimulate the uncus, amygdaloid nucleus or various portions of the superior temporal surface before deciding on excision. The electrode is introduced and then the current is switched on and off. An electrode, for example, passed directly inward in a plane 4 cm. from the temporal tip will enter the amygdaloid nucleus at a depth of 4 to 5 cm.[9]

Using this technique, William Feindel, Wilder Penfield, and Herbert Jasper discovered the role of the amygdala in psychomotor epilepsy, as they reported in a paper entitled "Localization of Epileptic Discharge in Temporal Lobe Automatism," which Feindel read before the American Neurological Association in 1952,[10] and which Feindel and Penfield published in a greatly expanded paper in 1954.[11] Feindel and his coauthors observed that the habitual aura and typical features of temporal lobe epilepsy could be reproduced by stimulation within and around the amygdala. The auras produced were emotional, such as a feeling of fear; visceral, such as a rising epigastric sensation; and alterations of consciousness, such as feelings of *déjà vu*. Epileptic seizures, characterized by brief periods of automatism and amnesia, were also produced, during which epileptic spikes originating in the amygdala spread to the lateral temporal cortex.

William Feindel wrote of the discovery of the role of the amygdala in the semiology of psychomotor epilepsy for the MNI house journal *Neuroimage* in 1998, to mark the centennial of Hughlings Jackson's paper.[12]

Amygdaloid Seizures with Automatism and Amnesia

In 1951, Dr Penfield encouraged me to study the 155 patients with temporal lobe epilepsy, especially those with automatism and amnesia who had undergone operation, mostly temporal corticectomy, in the preceding ten years. Analysis of the seizure patterns in 50 of these patients showed that a variety of features preceded automatism, the most common being sensation, conscious confusion, motor features, and some type of head sensation. Of note especially was the dreamy, faraway feeling (emphasized by Hughlings Jackson) as well as a sense of fear, flushing or pallor of the face and auditory or visual hallucinations.[13] Armed with this detailed information we then observed in the operating room in patients under local anaesthesia during surgical treatment, the responses to cortical and deep temporal stimulation. During that year, in 16 patients, we were able to produce the typical features of temporal automatism with sometimes striking cortico-graphic ictal changes. The anatomical sites for the stimulation clustered in and about the amygdala. The functional implications of our findings in the operating room were most intriguing: that the amygdala could serve as the generator of temporal lobe seizures, the hallmarks of which were automatism and amnesia. A search of the literature and especially the writings of Hughlings Jackson turned up this case of "Dr V." [*sic*] who resembled our first reported case. The results were all the more exciting to me, having just returned to the MNI from three years at Oxford in the Department of Human Anatomy with Le Gros Clark. He had investigated in the monkey the anatomical connections of the temporal lobe and was studying with Margaret Meyer, the central connections of the olfactory system.[14] Also in the Department was Alf Brodal as a visiting professor, completing his extensive review on the function of the hippocampus and the amygdaloid nucleus.[15] So a substantial part of our final paper became devoted to the anatomy of the amygdala and its powerful connections. The electrographic findings at operation included the important demonstration of low voltage fast activity and suppression of cortical spiking during the induced ictus. In the laboratory, Pierre Gloor and I were able to reproduce this circumstance by amygdala stimulation in cats.[16] Subsequent experimental studies of the amygdala amply confirmed in detail the important physiological role of this structure.[17] The immediate logical conclusion from our study in 1951 was that surgical excision must include the amygdala to secure satisfactory relief of seizures. Whether the hippocampus should also be included with that removal is a controversial point that still demands scientific clarification. When Brenda Milner, with Penfield and Scoville, emphasized the risks to memory function of hippocampal removal, it appeared even more advantageous to focus on excision of the amygdala, but to keep the hippocampal section to a minimum, based on its electrographic abnormality recorded at the time of operation.

CHASLIN'S GLIOSIS

Jasper and Kershman had suggested, more than a decade before Penfield turned his attention to the amygdala and hippocampus, that the "electrographic localization" of the clinical manifestations of psychomotor epilepsy "frequently seems to be deep to the temporal lobes (e.g., the hippocampus) near the midline."[18] The failure to recognize the importance of the mesial temporal lobe, Jasper and Kershman conceded, was due to "lack of knowledge regarding the function of these deeper-lying structures and of their relation to general cortical function."[19] This was about to change as Penfield assigned Maitland Baldwin and Kenneth Earle to review the role of the mesial structures in temporal lobe epilepsy.

Philippe Chaslin, a psychiatrist at the hospice at Bicêtre, in Paris, described the pathological appearance of the hippocampi in epileptic patients in 1889, in a paper entitled "Note on the Pathological Anatomy of Essential Epilepsy."[20] Chaslin found the hippocampi of epileptics to be hard, shrunken, and their outer surface to be smooth or slightly roughened. Microscopic examination revealed a proliferation of glial cells interspersed within glial fibrils and glial fibre bundles. Chaslin described these pathological changes as *Sclérose névroglique* – neuroglial fibrosis, which is referred to as Chaslin's gliosis in the French-speaking world. Chaslin's paper was largely forgotten until Spielmeyer reported similar changes in 1929,[21] which he ascribed to ischemia secondary to vasoconstriction. Earle, Baldwin, and Penfield refocused interest in the hippocampus in a paper that they read at the 1952 meeting of the American Association of Neuropathologists in Atlantic City, New Jersey.[22] Their paper is short, less than 500 words, but in it they describe the lesion at the origin of temporal lobe epilepsy and suggest a mechanism for its occurrence.

Earle and Baldwin reviewed the cases of 120 patients upon whom Penfield had operated for temporal lobe epilepsy. They found that seventy-eight patients had a history of a difficult birth, of perinatal anoxia, and of early postnatal head injury, from which Penfield concluded that a prolonged or difficult birth could be invoked as the "etiological mechanism" in psychomotor seizures. His conclusion was supported by the radiological findings, which showed that the middle fossa in these patients was smaller on the affected side, indicating a pathological process operant within the first two years of life. The PEG findings were also concordant with Penfield's hypothesis, as they revealed that the temporal horn of the lateral ventricle in affected patients was larger on the affected side, which indicated loss of tissue of the medial aspect of the anterior and mesial temporal lobe.

The epidemiological and radiological findings led to a fresh look at the histopathology of the tissue that Penfield had resected. The macroscopic appearance was much as Chaslin had described: "The uncus, hippocampal gyrus and part of the first temporal convolution [were] shrunken, yellow and avascular."[23] The microscopic findings were also reminiscent of Chaslin's: "Histological study of the excised areas usually revealed a diffuse increase in fibrous astrocytes in the atrophic cortex. In some, there was definite loss of neurons with cystic degeneration in a few cases. In others, the loss of neurons was not apparent, but fibrous astrocytes were increased in the grey matter."[24] These histological findings involved "the uncus, hippocampal gyrus, and part of the first temporal gyrus."[25] Thus, Earle, Baldwin, and Penfield recognized that neuronal loss and gliosis are the defining characteristics of what Penfield referred to as *incisural sclerosis*.[26] Penfield preferred this term to Chaslin's descriptive term, *neuroglial fibrosis*, because, as Penfield emphasised, "the sclerosis is of that portion of the brain that lies on the incisura of the tentorium. It is that portion of the brain which, if the head is squeezed, must herniate through."[27] Thus, *incisural sclerosis* implied an etiological mechanism, which revived the vascular hypothesis.

The tentorium cerebelli is a thickened membrane that lies between the inferior surface of the temporal lobes and the upper surface of the cerebellum. It has a scythe-like opening toward the midline called the *incisura* through which the brain stem passes as it joins the cerebral hemispheres to the spinal cord. The medial structures of the temporal lobe, and most notably the uncus, lie immediately above the incisural opening. Pressure inside the cranium causes the uncus and other mesial temporal structures to herniate through the incisura, wedging them between the brain stem and the edge of the tentorium. This is a common occurrence in patients with a mass lesion in a cerebral hemisphere, and it is often a terminal event.

Penfield proposed that herniation of the mesial structures might occur during prolonged and difficult labour as excessive pressure is applied to the head due to a narrow birth canal or from the vigorous application of forceps. The herniated tissue would then interfere with the blood supply to the mesial temporal lobe by compressing the anterior choroidal artery.[28] The resultant ischemia of the amygdala and hippocampus, however temporary, would then initiate a pathological process that evolved into incisural sclerosis and eventually caused temporal lobe epilepsy. Penfield supported his hypothesis by invoking the well-recognized susceptibility of the hippocampus to anoxia and by observing that experimental compression of the head of stillborn infants resulted in incisural herniation.[29]

Sometimes, Penfield wrote to illustrate his point, "the history suggested the actual cause," and he related the cases of a patient in whom

> there was a history of difficult, instrumental birth. On x-ray examination the right half of the skull appeared slightly smaller than the left … His seizures were characterized by a psychical hallucination, a cephalic aura, and automatism, accompanied by movements of mastication. Electroencephalograms indicated that the seizures originated in the right temporal lobe … There were marked atrophy, toughness, and avascularity of the first temporal convolution, and this abnormality extended into the uncus and hippocampal gyrus. Close to the tip of the inferior horn [of the lateral ventricle] the tissue was gelatinoid, grey, and tough. Histologically, this gelatinoid tissue contained numerous fibrous astrocytes and some giant astrocytes. The uncus and hippocampus showed pronounced increase in fibrous astrocytes.[30]

Although its etiology is still debated, incisural sclerosis, which is now referred to as *mesial temporal sclerosis* so as not to imply a specific pathophysiological mechanism, is universally recognized as the commonest cause of temporal lobe epilepsy.

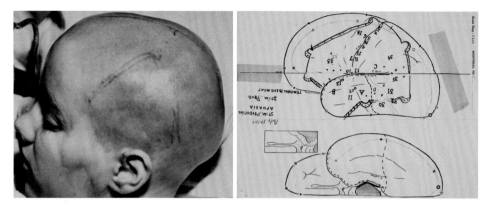

Figure 12.4. *Left*. Operative photograph illustrating the diamond-shaped incision line, favoured by Penfield, in a patient prepared for a left temporal craniotomy. *Right*. Brain map of the same patient. Numbers 1 to 18 identify the pre- and postcentral gyri. Number 33 indicates Broca's area. Numbers 31, 32, 34, and 35 indicate the posterior speech region. Montreal Neurological Hospital, case O.L.

Jason Mixter, the distinguished neurosurgeon, recognized the importance of Penfield's discovery by stating, "he has shown us where the lesion lies."[31]

THE MONTREAL PROCEDURE

The discovery of a structural lesion within the mesial temporal structures from which epileptic spikes were generated and spread to the lateral neocortex led Penfield and Baldwin to modify the tailored temporal resections that Penfield previously performed into a standardized procedure that included resection of the mesial structures. Initially referred to as "the Montreal procedure," this standardized and highly successful operation is widely known as an "anterior temporal lobectomy and amygdalo-hippocampectomy." Penfield and Baldwin described this new operation to the American Surgical Association in May 1952 in an address entitled "Temporal Lobe Seizures and the Technic of Subtotal Temporal Lobectomy."[32] The procedure is described here as Theodore Rasmussen and William Feindel performed it, with the author assisting. After sterilization of the scalp and infiltration of the incision line, a large craniotomy was elevated, designed to expose the frontal lobe and frontal operculum beyond Broca's area, the parietal lobe beyond the inferior parietal lobule, and the first and second temporal convolutions. An array of sixteen recording electrodes was affixed to the edge of the skull and the blunt electrode tips were applied to the cortex in such a way as to cover the whole of the exposed hemisphere in a representative fashion. If necessary, a few electrodes could be replaced about a particularly active area to better define is limits. Electrocortical stimulation

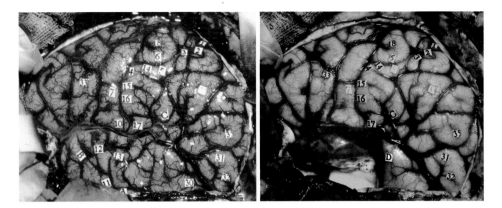

Figure 12.5. *Left*. Operative photograph of the left hemisphere corresponding to the brain map in the preceding illustration. A depth electrode was inserted at number 12. *Right*. Postoperative photograph. The lateral temporal cortex has been resected to approximately four centimetres from the temporal pole in the first stage of the operation, and the uncus, amygdala, and anterior hippocampus were resected under direct vision in the second stage of the operation. The temporal stem is seen as the white, slightly haemorrhagic tissue within the resection cavity, and the insula is just discernable as the structure with a slight sheen above the temporal stem. The letter "D" indicates an area where minor electrographic changes were recorded following the resection, which were not felt to be significant. A uniformly white, thin cottonoid sponge is seen at the bottom of the resection cavity. Montreal Neurological Hospital, case O.L.

was performed with the recording electrodes in place, to identify the sensory and motor strips and the speech areas if amytal testing had identified that the resection would be in the language-dominant hemisphere. Cortical stimulation began in what was supposed to be the postcentral gyrus, which usually responded to a lower current, and then moved to the motor strip, and finally to the presumptive speech areas, if necessary. The results of stimulation and of ECOG recordings were dictated to a secretary. Each contact point that produced a response was identified with a small, numbered ticket, and points where epileptic activity was recorded were marked with a lettered ticket. These were then drawn onto a brain map. The assistant who wielded an atomizer filled with a sterile physiological irrigating solution kept the exposed cortex moist.

On occasion, a seizure was triggered by stimulation. It was the assistant's job to support the patient's head while the recording electrodes were removed from the cortex. The final step before resection was to stimulate and record from the mesial structures. This was performed using two specially constructed electrodes, each with four contact points one centimetre apart. The last contact point was at the tip of the electrode, and the space between the contact points was insulated. The electrodes were inserted at 3.5 centimetres from the temporal tip and at a depth of 3.5–4 centimetres to reach the amygdala, and at 4.5 centimetres along the same convolution and at a similar depth, to reach the *pes hippocampi*. Eight recording electrodes that had been used to record from the cortex were deactivated and were replaced by the eight contact points from the newly inserted depth electrodes. A recording was obtained from these deep contacts and from the electrodes that remained upon the cortex. A satisfactory recording having been obtained, each contact of the depth electrodes was stimulated separately in an attempt to trigger an aura. This usually occurred when the deepest contact of the anterior depth electrode, the one within the amygdala, was stimulated. The proposed incision line was marked with a thin white thread, a photograph was taken, the exposed brain was covered with a thin piece of cellophane to keep it moist and to protect it from inadvertent contact with a sharp instrument, and the resection was begun.

The lateral neocortex was first resected, beginning with the first temporal convolution parallel to the Sylvian fissure and extending posteriorly to the vein of Labbé in the nondominant hemisphere or to four centimetres in the language dominant hemisphere. The incision was then curved inferiorly across the second and third temporal convolutions and into the fusiform gyrus, where the incision was redirected anteriorly. The lateral neocortex was then undermined and amputated as the surgeon cut through the temporal stem of white matter. The tip of the temporal horn of the lateral ventricle was entered, which facilitated the resection of the uncus, the amygdala, and the *pes hippocampi*. The resection included the anterior hippocampus if spikes had been recorded from the hippocampal depth electrode. Electrodes were then applied behind the resection margins of the body of the hippocampus and of the lateral temporal lobe, and a second ECOG was performed. The hippocampal resection was extended posteriorly if spikes were still recorded from its surface. Similarly, further resection of the lateral neocortex was carried out if this could be done without encroaching on the posterior speech region. Initially, the insular cortex was also resected. This part of the procedure was abandoned when it was found that adding an *insulectomy* to the resection could produce contralateral paralysis due to the manipulation of the branches of the middle cerebral artery that supplied the insula.[33]

In later years the skin incision was changed from that of a diamond shape to the shape of a question mark, which allowed greater exposure of the hemisphere. Similarly, the osteoplastic bone flap was abandoned for an unanchored, free bone flap that gave better access to the inferior and medial aspects of the temporal lobe.

The extent of the hippocampal resection raised some concern when the role of the hippocampus in memory was discovered. Thus, two therapeutic approaches evolved at the MNI: limiting the hippocampal resection to the amygdala and *pes hippocampi*, favoured by William Feindel,[34] or letting the intraoperative ECOG dictate the posterior extent of the hippocampal resection, which was favoured by Theodore Rasmussen.[35]

SECTION THREE

The Ghost in the Machine

Where is the place of understanding[1]

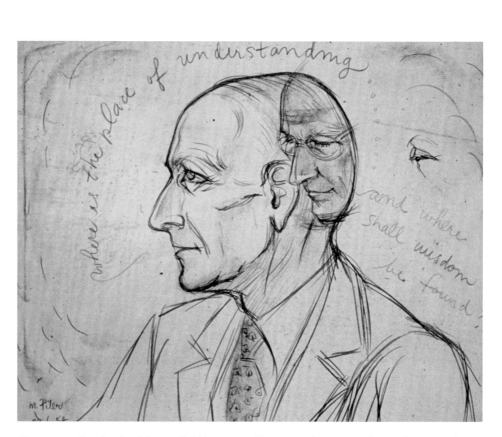

Figure 13.1. Sketch of Wilder Penfield by Mary Filer, 1954. The quote is from Job 28:12 and reads, "Where is the place of understanding and where shall wisdom be found." Montreal Neurological Institute, McGill University.

CHAPTER 13

The Labyrinth of Memory

There are many types of memories that are independent of each other –Broca

The idea that memory is divisible first arose with Franz Gall's proposal that there is a specific site in the orbital region of the brain that is responsible for the memory of words. Gall, who conceived of phrenology, and who wrote in French, referred to this attribute as *la mémoire des mots, la mémoire verbale* – the memory of words, verbal memory – which he distinguished from the general faculty of memory. This conjecture was based on Gall's observation as a child that two of his schoolmates who had a facility for recitation from memory had prominently bulging eyes. Much later, Gall tells us, it came to him in a flash of inspiration that the bulging of his schoolmates' eyes was due to the over-development of the frontal cortex as it rested on the orbit. As Gall imagined it, this cortical hypertrophy reshaped the bone of the orbital roof, causing it to project downward into the orbital cavity and push the eyeball forward. In this fanciful reminiscence from childhood was born the doctrine of phrenology for, if one faculty could deform the skull, so could others.[1] Gall further considered that memory had three other components beside the verbal, each causing its own protrusion on the brain and skull. These were the memory for objects and facts, the memory for locations, and the memory for faces. Gall's localization of an aspect of language – the memory of words – to the frontal lobes of the brain was taken up by Jean-Baptiste Bouillaud, a distinguished and influential figure of nineteenth-century medicine and onetime dean of the Faculty of Medicine of the University of Paris. Bouillaud exerted a great influence on the young Pierre-Paul Broca, which ultimately led to the localization of articulate language to the posterior aspect of the third left frontal convolution.[2] Like Gall, Broca did not believe that memory is a holistic function distributed diffusely throughout the cortical ribbon. Rather, he thought as we do today that there are different aspects of memory, most notably the memory for verbal and nonverbal language, and a memory specific for numbers, for spatial orientation, and for the recognition of faces.[3] Penfield and his new research fellow, Brenda Milner, who were about to discover the multiple facets of memory, were not aware of this historical background.

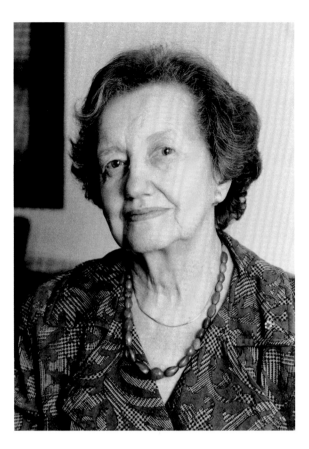

Figure 13.2. Brenda Milner in
midcareer. Montreal Neurological
Institute, McGill University.

THE HIPPOCAMPAL AMNESIC SYNDROME

Penfield's contribution to the study of memory began in August 1946, when he encountered patient P.B.,[4] who had been suffering from psychomotor epilepsy for six years before his admission to the MNI. His attacks began with a feeling of unreality, when all about him seemed silly and absurd. This was followed by a period of unresponsiveness lasting several minutes, during which he performed purposeless movements, such as chewing and fumbling with his fingers. He also performed more complex, purposeful acts, such as making his way to his porch where he kept a barometer, taking a few readings, and recording them in his logbook. He had no memory of having done any of this when he recovered from his spell, but upon verification, he found that his recordings were accurate. The patient's EEGs recorded epileptic activity from the left temporal lobe and he was brought to the operating room on 14 August 1946, where a left craniotomy was raised. The anterior aspect of the first temporal convolution appeared atrophic. "There were electrographic abnormalities anteriorly over the temporal lobe," Penfield noted, "but stimulation did not reproduce the patient's attacks. The lobe was removed in its anterior 4 cm., but, as there were no visible abnormalities, the removal was carried out on electrographic evidence alone."[5] The resection was restricted to the lateral cortex, as this was Penfield's technique at the time. There was transient, postoperative aphasia, but the patient's convalescence was otherwise unremarkable. Forebodingly, however, William Cone was unable to find any significant abnormality in the resected specimen.

The patient's seizures persisted and, as Penfield noted, "he had some distressingly long attacks of epileptic automatisms, which he feared would cost him his employment. He was ready, he said, 'to take a chance on anything.'"[6] Accordingly, he was readmitted to the MNI in September 1951, for reevaluation. Brenda Milner had joined the Department of Psychology at McGill University in 1949 as Donald Hebb's graduate student. Hebb thought that Milner's time would be well spent by examining Penfield's patients for her dissertation.[7] And so it was that she examined P.B. before his second operation and found no indications that his memory was deficient.

The patient underwent three EEG studies during his second admission to hospital. One recorded epileptic activity from the previously operated left temporal lobe, and another recorded epileptic activity from both temporal lobes. The third recording was more ominous, as the epileptic activity arose from the right temporal lobe before spreading to the left one. Despite these new findings, Penfield and Jasper concluded that the patient's seizures were "arising from the medial structures of the left temporal lobe that had been left in place at the time of his first operation."[8] Since Penfield had by now performed a number of operations in which the hippocampus had been resected with impunity, it was decided that the left hippocampus should be removed, to complete the temporal lobectomy begun five years earlier.[9]

The patient was returned to the operating room on Friday, 28 September 1951. The dural opening was limited so as to expose the previously resected area in the anterior aspect of the left temporal lobe. The anterior part of the first temporal convolution that had not been removed in the previous operation was followed as it coursed anteriorly and curved around the temporal pole towards the uncus and to a yellowed hippocampus. The yellowed appearance suggested to Penfield that the hippocampus was damaged and reinforced his conclusion that it was the source of the patient's seizures. Penfield's confidence in having made the correct decision to operate on the left side was undoubtedly buoyed when epileptic spikes were recorded from the hippocampus, and stimulation produced the patient's typical automatism.[10] Penfield removed the uncus and the anterior half of the hippocampus by suction aspiration and so there was no tissue available for pathological examination. Nonetheless, Penfield recorded in his operative report, with an academically detached tone, "the surgeon found marked sclerosis of this area and it is believed that the pathological condition was an example of incisural sclerosis produced by herniation of the inferior mesial temporal cortex through the incisura."[11]

Penfield's apparent equanimity was replaced by consternation as it became obvious that all was not well: "After operation we were stunned to discover that the patient had a severe retrograde amnesia. It included, at first, all the things he should have been able to remember in recent years. By the time he left the hospital, the amnesia for the past had improved until it included only what had happened in recent months. But more important than the retrograde amnesia was that he could no longer remember the new events of each day after he turned his mind to other matters."[12]

Distressed, Penfield sought an explanation for this unique, disastrous outcome, and turned to patient J.O., on whom he had performed the same operation a few days after he had operated upon P.B. but whose outcome had been dramatically different:[13] "If this case is compared to that of J.O., the extent of the resection of the brain tissue seems to be the same. But it was only in Case P.B. that memory loss was a feature. The real difference seems to be that the latter was having progressive memory difficulty before operation and he had severe retrograde amnesia associated with each attack. On the other hand, J.O. had no such difficulty at any time."[14]

This statement, published in 1954 in Penfield and Jasper's *Epilepsy and the Functional Anatomy of the Human Brain*, is at odds with Milner's preoperative evaluation and with Milner and Penfield's 1955 account of P.B.'s case.[15] There was therefore no explanation for the patient's short-term memory loss. Nonetheless, Penfield remained undeterred: "We continued to carry out unilateral temporal lobectomies including medial temporal structures, but with utmost caution. The results in the treatment of this form of epilepsy were, and still are, remarkably successful. We took great care not to do the operation if there was any suspicion of a bilateral lesion."[16] Then, on 21 October 1952, it happened again.

As is often the case in medicine and surgery, a single case raises many questions but provides few answers. A second case, however, is always informative. And so it was that Penfield remained perplexed at P.B.'s outcome until almost a year to the day, when he encountered patient F.C., a twenty-eight-year-old glove cutter who had suffered from psychomotor seizures since the age of twelve. His attacks were characterized by a feeling of depersonalization, automatisms, and amnesia. His automatisms could be quite elaborate, as when he cut a number of gloves perfectly but had no memory of having done so. The EEG localization of his epileptic focus was problematic. Some recordings revealed unilateral activity and others showed bilateral activity. Sometimes the activity arose from the frontal lobes and sometimes from the temporal lobes, but most consistently it arose from the left temporal lobe. So it was to the left temporal lobe that Penfield ascribed the origin of the patient's seizures.[17] The PEG was supportive of this localization, as it showed that the left hemisphere was slightly smaller than the right. As was now routine, the patient underwent preoperative neuropsychological evaluation. The patient described himself as forgetful, especially for what he read. His self-assessment was borne out when Milner found that his scores were low on verbal memory tests, without any evidence of other impairments.[18] The decision was taken to operate upon the left temporal lobe, and Penfield turned a bone flap on 21 October 1952. Epileptic activity was indeed recorded from the undersurface of the temporal lobe, and electrical stimulation of the hippocampus produced the patient's automatisms. Penfield found that the uncus and hippocampus were yellowed and tough, and that the hippocampus was herniated through the incisura. "It is clear," Penfield recorded in his operative note, "that the cause was birth compression," and he resected the lateral temporal lobe, the uncus, and the hippocampus. Pathological examination of the resected tissue revealed incisural sclerosis.

Penfield had no reason to be concerned with his patient's postoperative course. True, he was aphasic, but this was expected as he had undergone a large dominant temporal lobe resection. Transient aphasia was a common occurrence in such cases and was expected to recover gradually, as it did. But, "as the language difficulty lessened," Penfield noted, "it became increasingly apparent that there was a grave disturbance of recent memory."[19] From past experience, and having removed obviously abnormal tissue in this case, Penfield could not have expected any neurological deficit, let alone a cognitive one. Neurocognitive testing was repeated on two successive days, three weeks after surgery. The most striking finding, which stunned his examiners, was that the patient did not recognize them on the second day of testing nor did he remember any of the tests that he had undergone or even that he had been tested at all! His scores on test for verbal memory, on which he had scored poorly preoperatively, were now markedly lower. He was also unable to recall simple geometric forms on a test that was independent of verbal ability. Thus, his loss of immediate recall was now generalized and not specific to the deficiencies that had been observed preoperatively.

Nothing could be done for patient F.C.'s memory deficiencies but to wait and hope that time would heal his wound. He returned to the MNI for reevaluation in 1953, 1954, and in 1955. Unfortunately, his results on tests for recent memory remained unimproved. He could not recall events that had occurred a few hours earlier, or even as little as five minutes before, if he was distracted. And yet, his memory for past events and for skills that he had acquired in the past had returned and it was intact, so that he could continue working as a glove cutter.

An explanation for this unforeseen complication, encountered twice in thirteen months, was required. It came from Herbert Jasper and an EEG recorded during the patient's last visit to the MNI, as Penfield reported:

The electroencephalogram of June 19, 1955 showed a very definite residual epileptogenic process. It was in the *right* anterior temporal region, the side opposite that of operation, and was strictly lateralized, with no recurrence of the abnormality on the left side. Our associate, Dr Herbert Jasper, concluded that this was the continuation of the original contralateral abnormality seen (on the right side) in preoperative studies.[20]

Thus, ongoing EEG activity from the mesial aspect of the right temporal lobe indicated that it was damaged, presumably from incisural sclerosis. Penfield and Jasper now surmised that, before surgery, the *right* mesial temporal epileptic activity had been transmitted to the *left* temporal lobe, which had functioned well enough to preserve the patient's memory. This was lost when the left temporal lobe was resected. And, if this was the case for F.C., it must also have been the case for P.B. Milner and Penfield had discovered that memory is divisible, that the hippocampi are responsible for recent memory, and that one well or partially functioning hippocampus is sufficient to preserve it.

Milner and Penfield reported P.B. and F.C.'s cases to the American Neurological Association in Chicago on 13 June 1955, in a paper entitled "The Effect of Hippocampal Lesions on Recent Memory."[21] The clinical syndrome that they described was clearly stated:

> Careful psychological study of our cases indicates that the major defect in these patients is loss of ability to record current experience although past memory may seem to be normal. The conclusion must be that this zone of grey matter plays an essential role in the recording of conscious experience. There is no indication from our evidence as to whether the essential structure in this mechanism is hippocampus (Ammon's horn) or hippocampal gyrus or whether the two act together.[22]

As to why this occurred, Milner and Penfield were unequivocal:

> Our conclusion in regard to these cases is that there was, preoperatively in each, an unsuspected but more or less completely destructive lesion of the right hippocampal zone. The seizure was arising in the left uncal and hippocampal area which, though epileptogenic, was carrying on normal function. The operation would thus deprive the patient of hippocampal function on both sides.[23]

How they arrived at his conclusion is worth noting:

> In each case the surgeon found marked sclerosis of the area and it is believed that the pathological condition was an example of incisural sclerosis produced by herniation of the inferior mesial temporal cortex through the incisura of the

tentorium at the time of birth. Such a mechanism may produce ischaemic injury or destruction, which may be bilateral as well as unilateral. In these two cases the electrographic findings favor a bilateral injury.[24]

Penfield later noted,

To find an explanation for this unexpected memory loss, *I* [emphasis added] turned to the Laboratory of Neuropathology. We were at that time in the midst of a pathological study, which was to be published by Earle, Baldwin & Penfield (1953).[25] In this report, the examination of 157 such cases led to the conclusion that the most frequent cause of temporal lobe epilepsy, even when it made its appearance years after birth, was the sclerotic scar produced by herniation of the hippocampal margin of the temporal lobe through the incisura of the tentorium into the posterior fossa during compression of the infant's head as it passed through the mother's birth canal. Such compression of the infant's head may, of course, produce herniation, with injury, on one side or on both.[26]

It would be another twenty years before Penfield could validate his claim that the right hippocampus was damaged in P.B.'s case.[27] Nonetheless, the hippocampal amnesic syndrome had been described and memory had been demonstrated to be divisible into short- and long-term components.

THE MOST EXTENSIVELY STUDIED PATIENT IN THE HISTORY OF NEUROSCIENCE

Penfield and Milner were not the first to recognize the effect of bilateral hippocampal lesions on memory. That distinction belongs to Glees and Griffith who published a paper entitled "Bilateral Destruction of the Hippocampus (Cornus Ammonis) in a Case of Dementia" in 1952.[28] Paul Glees was a noted neuroanatomist[29] who did postgraduate work with Wilfrid Le Gros Clark at Oxford University when Le Gros Clark was interested in the hippocampus. While at Oxford, Glees examined the brain of a seventy-three-year-old woman who had suffered a stroke, which had resulted in prominent memory loss, confusion, and, eventually, dementia. The most striking feature of her brain, Glees noted, was that the hippocampi were largely destroyed, while the remainder of the brain appeared unaffected. From the patient's clinical history and postmortem findings, Glees wrote, "it seems justifiable to draw the tentative conclusion that the destruction of hippocampus in humans leads to a deranged mental condition in which loss of recent memory and a state of confusion are prominent symptoms … The hippocampal formation of the adult seems essential for recent memory."[30]

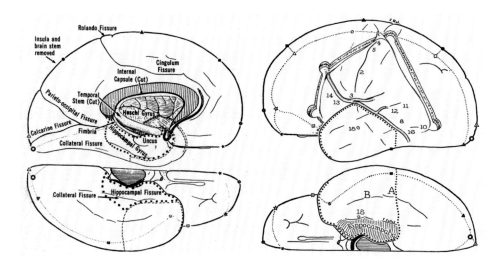

Figure 13.3. *Left*. Drawings of P.B.'s operations. The fine dotted line indicates the resection of the lateral neocortex performed in 1946, and the uninterrupted one represents the resection of the hippocampus performed in 1951. *Right*. Drawing of F.C.'s operation. The dotted line represents the resected area. The hatched area indicates sclerosis of the hippocampal region. Montreal Neurological Institute, McGill University.

Glees and Griffith's paper was published in the April–May 1952 issue of *Monatsschrift für Psychiatrie und Neurologie*, a respected European journal, but this does not appear to have been known to Milner and Penfield when they addressed the American Neurological Association in June 1955. It was, however, Milner and Penfield's presentation of June 1955 that proved seminal in linking the hippocampi to recent memory, for the abstract of their presentation caught the eye of William Beecher Scoville, of Hartford, Connecticut. Scoville recognized that the memory deficits reported by Milner and Penfield were identical to those of a patient that he had operated upon, the patient who would enter scientific literature as H.M. and who Scoville invited Milner to examine.[31]

Scoville was an imaginative neurosurgeon – he designed one of the first spring clips for the treatment of cerebral aneurysms – who was at the time treating schizophrenic patients by frontal lobotomy. He was, however, dissatisfied by this procedure and sought a less destructive method that would achieve the same goal of quieting the demons that afflicted these poor individuals at a time when pharmacology had nothing to offer. Scoville devised a new procedure in which the mesial structures of both temporal lobes were resected, but the frontal lobes remained intact. As most of his patients were severely affected by their psychosis, whatever cognitive deficits might have resulted from this procedure were not obvious to Scoville until he performed what he unabashedly described as a "frankly experimental operation"[32] on a nonschizophrenic patient, H.M., who was disabled by epileptic seizures.[33] It was immediately obvious to Scoville that the bilateral resection of the uncus, amygdala, hippocampus, and para-hippocampal gyrus had a devastating effect of H.M.'s memory. Scoville brought this observation to the attention of the Harvey Cushing Society on 23 April 1953 in a paper entitled "The Limbic Lobe in Man," in which he stated, "bilateral resection of the uncus and amygdala alone, or in conjunction with the entire pyriform amygdaloid hippocampal complex, has resulted in no marked physiologic or behavioral changes with the one exception of a very grave, recent memory loss, so severe as to prevent the patient from remembering the locations of the rooms in which he lives, the names of his close associates, or even the way to toilet and urinal."[34] Scoville mentioned this observation during the discussion that followed Milner and Penfield's 1955 presentation and took the opportunity to acknowledge Penfield's priority in recognizing the effects of bilateral hippocampal lesions on recent memory:

> Dr Penfield was keenly interested in our report [of 23 April 1953] of memory loss in these bilateral cases, inasmuch as it *confirmed his own previous theories and personal observations* [emphasis added.] He invited Dr Milner to review nine of our 35 bilateral, and unilateral medial temporal lobe resections who were sufficiently cooperative to permit quantitative testing. It was refreshing to observe the authoritative manner in which she quantified these results … Briefly, she found that removal of the uncus and probably the amygdala going back up to four centimeters caused no loss, whereas a more extensive removal going back five centimeters or more from the temporal tips produced a measurable deficit on formal tests of recent memory. The two radical removals,[35] which went back eight and nine centimeters to include probably the anterior two-thirds of the hippocampal complex, resulted in a very grave and almost total loss of recent memory, unaccompanied by other changes of intellect or personality.[36]

SCOVILLE AND MILNER 1957

Scoville and Milner published their paper based on her study of H.M., "Loss of Recent Memory after Bilateral Hippocampal Lesions," in 1957.[37] Penfield and Milner published "Memory Deficit Produced by Bilateral Lesions in the Hippocampal Zone," based on the study of P.B. and F.C.'s cases, in 1958.[38] Milner's prior publication with Scoville of what Penfield considered to be his original observation on the role of the hippocampi and memory chilled the burgeoning relationship between them and was still remembered sixty years later.[39] Nonetheless, Penfield supported Milner's ongoing study of H.M., which she did until one of her graduate students, Suzanne Corkin, took a position at the Massachusetts Institute of Technology and followed

H.M. thereafter for the very practical reason that Cambridge was closer to the patient's residence in Connecticut.[40] With regard to the defect produced by bilateral hippocampal resections, Milner, with her usual care with language, described it perfectly when she chaired a symposium on "Disorders of memory after brain lesions in man," in 1968:

> The main features of the amnesic syndrome seen in man after bilateral destruction of the mesial parts of the temporal lobes are now well known. There is no impairment of attention and no loss of preoperatively acquired skills or of intelligence as measured by standard tests. What seems to be selectively impaired is the transition from short-term to long-term memory; these patients can recall events from the remote past; they can also perceive and reason normally, but as soon as their attention is diverted to a new topic they no longer remember what went before. Hence they show a continuous anterograde amnesia for events of daily life, together with some retrograde amnesia for the period immediately preceding the critical brain lesion.[41]

CONFIRMATION

Patient P.B.

Penfield and Milner had correctly deduced the critical role of the hippocampi in recent memory, and their conclusions had been supported by Milner's study of H.M. But the evidence was circumstantial: EEG findings suggestive of right hippocampal dysfunction in a patient whose left hippocampus Penfield had ablated and Scoville's assessment of the structures that he had removed. Enough for a firm presumption but lacking in certainty. Certainty came in 1964 with the death of patient P.B. from a pulmonary embolus. Gordon Mathieson, the head of Neuropathology at the MNI, performed the postmortem examination of P.B.'s brain. Mathieson found that Penfield had excised the anterior part of the *left* parahippocampal gyrus and uncus, the amygdala, and all of the hippocampus except for 2.2 cm of its most posterior extent. The *right* amygdala was intact but the parahippocampal gyrus was gliotic, and the right hippocampus was shrunken, pale, and sclerotic.[42]

Penfield referred briefly to these findings during an address to the Royal Society of Medicine in 1968, and he did not publish them until 1974 and then only at the insistence of Theodore Rasmussen.[43] Despite his initial lack of interest in publishing the results of P.B.'s postmortem examination, Penfield did not minimize their importance:

> This autopsy enables us to confirm the hypothesis put forward in 1958 by Penfield and Milner that the patient had, before operation, a partial destructive lesion of

the contralateral hippocampal zone, and that the second operation deprived him of hippocampal function bilaterally. Furthermore, it enables us to localize this lesion to the pyramidal cell layer, and to a lesser extent, the gyrus dentatus, the parahippocampal, and other temporal lobe gyri being intact on the right side. The 22 mm of the posterior part of the left hippocampus were inadequate to maintain normal memory function. It is probable that some, or perhaps even all, of his seizures arose in the severely damaged right hippocampus. The presence of an intact right amygdaloid nucleus is interesting in that it did not maintain memory function.[44]

Penfield had in the past referred to playback from a tape recorder or from a film-strip to illustrate how memories are revived by electrical stimulation of the temporal neocortex. He also referred to a meeting with "Jones," a hypothetical past acquaintance, to explain the revival of a past experience, and how it might influence the present in life outside the operating room.

Jones first appeared in 1959, in a paper that Penfield published in *Science* on the function of the interpretive cortex.[45] As Penfield described it, as you encounter an individual that you previously knew, "a signal seems to flash upon consciousness to tell you that you have seen that man before. Eventually, you recognize his countenance, his actions, and his voice, and it comes to you that the man is Jones: The sight and sound of the man has given you instant access, through some reflex, to the records of the past in which this man has played some part."[46] But it is not an instantaneous sense of familiarity alone that is revived: "if Jones had been a source of danger to you, you might have felt fear as well as familiarity before you had time to consider the man. Thus, the signal of fear as well as the signal of familiarity may come to one as the result of subconscious comparison of present with similar past experience."[47]

So much for the temporal cortex, but what is the role of the hippocampus in this construct? Penfield addressed this, somewhat summarily, in 1973 as he and Gordon Mathieson were preparing to publish the results of P.B.'s postmortem examination. This revealed, as Penfield had suspected, that the anterior aspect of both hippocampi were damaged but that the posterior aspects were intact. Thus, "the summarizing key of access"[48] to our past experience with Jones lies within the posterior hippocampus and the neuronal circuits joining it to the interpretative cortex. A new experience with him is first temporarily recorded within the anterior hippocampus and, if felt to be significant, it rapidly makes its way to the posterior hippocampus where permanent connections are. Thus, damage to the anterior hippocampi would result in loss of short-term memory, but long-term memories would remain accessible as long as the posterior hippocampus remained intact.

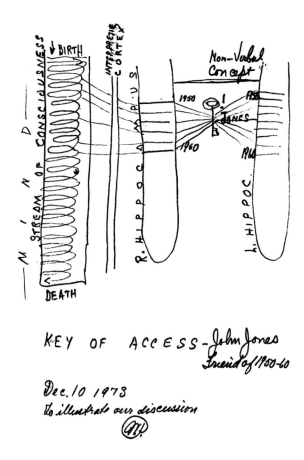

Figure 13.4. Penfield made this drawing to elucidate his idea on the mechanism of memory during a discussion with Brenda Milner. The key to the stream of consciousness is within the upper brain stem. The hippocampi and the interpretive cortex are responsible for scanning and recall of past experiences to assure appropriate responses to new ones. See the text for details. Montreal Neurological Institute archives, Penfield's sketch drawn for Brenda Milner, illustrating the role of the interpretive cortex and hippocampi in memory. Montreal Neurological Institute, McGill University.

Brenda Milner was sceptical of this construct, and Penfield drew a diagram to illustrate his concept, in the hope of convincing her.

As recalled by Milner,[49] the left side of the sketch is meant to represent the stream of consciousness flowing from birth to death, as it is supplied by new rivulets generated within the interpretive cortex. The key to recalling a relationship with John Jones, which lasted from 1950 to 1960, lies within the posterior hippocampi. Milner remained unconvinced. Nonetheless, she recognized that Penfield's sketch was an illustration of his "speculative, inquiring mind" and revealed that even a few short years before his death, "he was wishing right to the end to understand the baffling retrograde and anterograde amnesia in those patients who had taught him and all of us so much."[50]

P.B.'s autopsy was at the time the most detailed and rigorous evidence that bi-hippocampal lesions result in loss of the capacity to form recent memories. Confirmation of the structures resected by Scoville would not come for another thirty-four years.

Patient H.M.

Patient H.M. had a long and by all accounts happy life well into his dotage.[51] As part of his ongoing evaluation, he underwent magnetic resonance scanning at the Brigham and Women's Hospital, Boston, in May 1992 and again in August 1993, the latter when he was sixty-seven years old, forty years after he had been operated upon.[52] The MRI scanner was appropriate for the time, but, at 1.5 Tesla, it did not provide the resolution of current machines. Nonetheless, the MR images revealed that Scoville had over-estimated the longitudinal extent of his hippocampal resections by about one-third. A third MR was performed in 2006, but little more was revealed except changes associated with advancing age and dementia.[53]

H.M. died from complications of arteriosclerotic heart disease on 2 December 2008, at the age of eighty-two. As prearranged, a postmortem MRI scan of his brain was performed at the Massachusetts General Hospital, Boston, and he was autopsied there the following day. The brain was removed, photographed, and deposited in the pathology department, where it hardened for ten weeks in a bath of formaldehyde, before being resubmitted to MR imaging. Little of note was added to the information revealed by previous MR images, except that the extent of the resections, which Scoville had estimated at 8 cm, could now be accurately measured at 6 cm on the left and at 5.5 cm on the right.[54] Thus, the resections that Scoville had performed were similar to those performed by Penfield.

H.M.'s brain was transported to the University of California, San Diego, where it was cut into thin sections, scanned, and reconstructed into 3-dimensional, digital images.[55] However, the images are not those of the twenty-seven-year-old patient studied by Milner but those of an eighty-two-year-old man who had had occasional generalized seizures in the last years of his life and who had become progressively more confused, until, finally, dementia had set in. He had sustained small, recurrent strokes affecting the cortex and white matter, and had suffered from arteriosclerosis, kidney disease, and colon cancer.[56] Thus, the postmortem examination of H.M.'s brain may be informative on the aged brain but adds little to Gordon Mathieson's examination of P.B.'s brain performed at the MNI.

H.M.'s brain unfortunately became a source of contention between the MIT researchers and the San Diego group.[57] The issue was whether a small, newly uncovered lesion in the left frontal lobe of H.M.'s brain had contributed to his memory deficit. The MIT group thought not, while the San Diego group thought it might have. The MIT group was correct, in my opinion. The lesion was present in a part of the brain that is frequently contused without any noticeable consequences to memory, even when the lesion is much larger and more destructive than the one found in H.M.'s brain. Furthermore, there was no such lesion in P.B.'s brain, whose memory deficits were as florid as H.M.'s.

THE WADA TEST

The significance of Penfield and Milner's hypothesis and its confirmation by P.B.'s autopsy cannot be overstated. They demonstrated that memory is not a single function but that it has at least two distinct components, one immediate and the other long-term, and that the former localizes to the hippocampal formations.[58] This realization, however, was not without practical consequences: what was one to do with patients whose epilepsy was refractory to medical management but who showed evidence of bitemporal epileptic activity on their EEG recordings? The obvious answer was simply that they could not be operated upon because the nonresected hippocampal formation could also be dysfunctional and that the operation would lead to amnesia. Thus, patients with intractable temporal lobe epilepsy who might have benefitted from surgery were denied operation. This distressing situation prevailed until Theodore Rasmussen turned to Brenda Milner with what seemed an impossible task: to determine preoperatively whether a patient with bilateral temporal EEG abnormalities could sustain the resection of the hippocampus responsible for the epileptic attacks, without the loss of immediate recall. Rasmussen suggested that Milner devise simple psychometric tasks that the patient could perform while one half of his or her brain was anesthetized to determine if the opposite hippocampus was functioning normally. This, Rasmussen felt, could be accomplished during the performance of the Wada test.

Juhn Wada brought the Wada test to the MNI while on a fellowship there in 1955 and 1956. Wada had devised the procedure while still in Japan. Its purpose was to limit the unpleasant effect of electroconvulsive therapy in the treatment of schizophrenia by anesthetizing the hemisphere submitted to the electric current. It was first used at the MNI to lateralize language in left-handed or ambidextrous patients who were being considered for surgery, to lateralize language function.[59] The Wada test was performed on consecutive days, one day testing one hemisphere, the next day the other. A catheter was placed in one carotid artery into which a short-acting barbiturate, amobarbital, was injected. This resulted in the temporary anesthesia of the injected hemisphere while the other remained alert and was challenged with a number of tasks that tested its ability to remember a word, a rhyme, a sequence of numbers, a drawing, a path through a maze. If the patient correctly recalled what had been said or shown, then the anaesthetized hippocampus could be removed without fear of amnesia. As Milner said in 1977,

> In the surgical treatment of epilepsy it is often necessary to excise the hippocampus radically if the patient's seizures are to be controlled. From the standpoint of memory this can be justified, provided that the medial temporal region of the opposite hemisphere is functioning normally, since material-specific memory deficits consequent upon unilateral lesions interfere little with the patient's life. The situation is, however, quite different whenever there is preoperative evidence of damage to both temporal lobes, for in such cases removal of the hippocampus on the side of the major epileptic focus can produce a global amnesic syndrome that is a more serious handicap than the epilepsy itself. It thus becomes important to be able to determine in advance which patients with suspected bilateral temporal-lobe abnormality can undergo unilateral temporal lobectomy (including the hippocampus) without risk of generalized memory loss. In such cases the carotid-Amytal [amobarbital] technique has proven to be a valid screening procedure, enabling one to assess memory in patients temporarily deprived of the function of most of one hemisphere by the action of the drug.[60]

Rasmussen's faith in Milner was well founded: the amobarbital memory test became a standard part of the MNI's psychometric armamentarium and was adopted the world over.[61] Her studies of P.B., F.C., and of H.M. created the discipline of quantitative neuropsychology and established the separate yet integrated nature of human memory.

MATERIAL-SPECIFIC MEMORY

The term "material-specific memory" was coined by Brenda Milner to mean the ability to recall verbal or nonverbal material presented in a battery of neurocognitive tests. Tests of verbal memory, for example, require an individual to remember a list of words or short prose passages. Nonverbal memory tests require the patient to recall shapes, patterns, faces, and notes and pitches in a short musical excerpt.[62] Milner and her associates found that patients with a left, language-dominant temporal lobe lesion scored poorly on verbal tests, while patients with a right, nondominant temporal lesion scored poorly on nonverbal tests. By 1958, Milner had examined one hundred patients who had undergone a right or a left temporal resection, many with newly devised psychometric tests that she and her research fellows had designed. She presented her results to the Association for Research in Nervous and Mental Disease and reported that patients who had undergone a *right* temporal resection performed poorly in recalling shapes and geometric patterns, and in identifying incongruities in images such as a painting hanging in an animal's cage.[63] The severity of these deficiencies, Milner found, was related to the extent of resection along the inferior aspect of the temporal lobe, which included the hippocampus and parahippocampal gyrus. Milner also found that patients who had undergone a *left* temporal lobectomy did well on visual tasks but performed poorly on verbal ones, such as remembering simple prose passages. As she came to the end of her presentation, she asked, rhetorically,

> What do these findings as a whole tell us of the normal function of the temporal lobes? The data on unilateral lesions show that the left temporal lobe contributes to the rapid understanding and subsequent retention of verbally expressed ideas … The right, minor temporal lobe, on the other hand, appears to be more critically involved in perceptual than in verbal skills. When the right temporal lobe is removed, pictures and representational drawings lose some of their former distinctiveness, and the separate parts are less easily identified … It seems that the right temporal lobe facilitates rapid visual identification, and that in this way it enters into the comprehension of pictorially expressed ideas.[64]

Milner had determined that the hippocampus was the structure within the right temporal lobe that was essential for nonverbal recall.[65] Although she suspected a similar, critical role for the left hippocampus in verbal recall, she was not able to confirm this with the data available to her at the time.[66] Clearly, further study was required on the role of the hippocampi in memory, and this was assigned to her fellow, Philip M. Corsi.

MEMORY AND THE MEDIAL TEMPORAL STRUCTURES

Philip Corsi arrived at the MNI during the academic year 1966–67, with a BA from Dartmouth College and a newly minted MA from McGill University. Corsi's master's thesis[67] had been on auditory discrimination in the presence of contralateral noise. In Milner's assessment, it had "a direct application to problems of hemispheric specialization and cerebral dominance."[68] Thus, Milner recognized in Corsi a talented, creative experimenter who possessed a keen, analytic mind, and she assigned him the study of the role of the mesial temporal structures in material-specific memory. Within a year, he had determined that the severity of verbal memory loss was related to the extent of left hippocampal resection.[69] The following year, he devised a test to assess spatial memory – the Corsi block tapping test – and found that the degree of impairment of spatial memory dependent on the extent of right hippocampal resection,[70] thus expanding on Milner's observations. Corsi published the results of his studies on memory and the hippocampus in his dissertation, "Human Memory and the Mesial Temporal Region of the Brain," published in April 1972.[71]

Corsi compared the effects of right and left temporal resections in seventy-eight patients divided into two groups. Patients in the first group had undergone a right temporal lobectomy, and those in the second group had undergone a left temporal lobectomy. The amygdala had been resected in all patients in both groups. Each group was further divided into four subgroups, depending upon the extent of hippocampal and parahippocampal resections. These structures had been spared in the first subgroup, and resection had been limited to the *pes hippocampi* in the second subgroup. Patients in the third subgroup had undergone the resection of the *pes hippocampi* and approximately one centimetre of the hippocampus and parahippocampal gyrus, and patients in the fourth subgroup had undergone the complete resection of these structures.

All patients were then submitted to a battery of neurocognitive tasks designed to test verbal and nonverbal memory. The results were unequivocal and unassailable: "The severity of verbal memory impairment was found to vary directly with the extent of encroachment upon the hippocampal region in the dominant hemisphere for language." Similarly, patients whose right temporal lobe had been resected "showed a deficit in non-verbal, spatial learning and this deficit varie[d] directly with the extent of medial temporal removal." Simply put, "Whereas the left temporal patients have difficulty in the consolidation of verbal impressions over time, the right temporal patients show a consolidation impairment for non-verbal material."[72]

Corsi's findings were definitive, but they did not answer all questions, as he stated at the end of his thesis: "Although the hippocampus was used as the brainmark [*sic*] for delineating the extent of medial temporal removal, it is not suggested that this is the sole structure associated with the memory disturbances that have been reported. Rather, the entire medial aspect of the temporal region, including hippocampus and parahippocampal gyrus, is taken to be associated with the observed impairments."[73]

The respective roles in memory of the parahippocampal gyrus and of the hippocampus have yet to be fully elucidated.

By 1954, Penfield had published his great works on the structure–function relationship of the cerebral cortex and epilepsy, and he and Brenda Milner had discovered the role of the hippocampus in memory. The remainder of Penfield's life was devoted to conjectures on the creation of experiential phenomena, on the seat of consciousness, on the centrencephalic integrating system, and on what he referred to as the "physiology of the mind."

CHAPTER 14

The Physiology of Mind

Is there a line to be drawn between psychological and physiological phenomena in man? If so, where? –Tolstoy[1]

THE GIRL IN THE MEADOW — MEMORY AND EXPERIENTIAL PHENOMENA

Penfield first described the evocation of a memory by stimulation of the temporal lobes in 1936 when he related the case of a frightened little girl.[2]

Miss. J.V. was seven years old when a stranger accosted her in a meadow and threatened to put her in a rucksack full of snakes. This disturbing encounter caused her to suffer from recurring nightmares in which the scene was reenacted. She began to have epileptic seizures at the age of eleven. These were heralded by a horrifying vision of her experience in the meadow, which was followed by generalized convulsions. She was admitted to the MNI when she was fourteen years old, where a craniotomy uncovered a right parietal-temporal scar.[3] Electrocortical stimulation around that area caused her to say, "Oh, I can see something coming at me! Don't let them come at me! … Don't leave me." She heard accusatory voices and felt a sense of dread. When Penfield asked her to describe what she had experienced in response to cortical stimulation, she answered, "It was like an attack … I saw someone coming toward me as though he was going to hit me." Penfield interpreted her responses to stimulation to indicate that the epileptic discharges began in the visual associative area, which produced her terrifying vision, and then spread to the posterior temporal region close to Heschl's gyri, which caused her to hear voices. Penfield concluded that the visions she saw and the voices she heard were *déjà vu* and *déjà entendu* phenomena of the dreamy state of temporal lobe epilepsy.[4]

At the time that Penfield encountered this patient he was busily preparing his seminal paper on the structure–function relationship of the brain, in which the homunculus made its first appearance, and he was preoccupied with testing the vascular hypothesis of epileptogenesis. Then, as Canada entered the Second World War in September 1939, the MNI directed its activities to the war effort.[5] Penfield thus had little time to devote to the semiology of temporal lobe epilepsy.

Penfield returned to the topic of seizures accompanied by alterations of perceptions in the summer of 1946, in addresses that he delivered at Harvard and Oxford

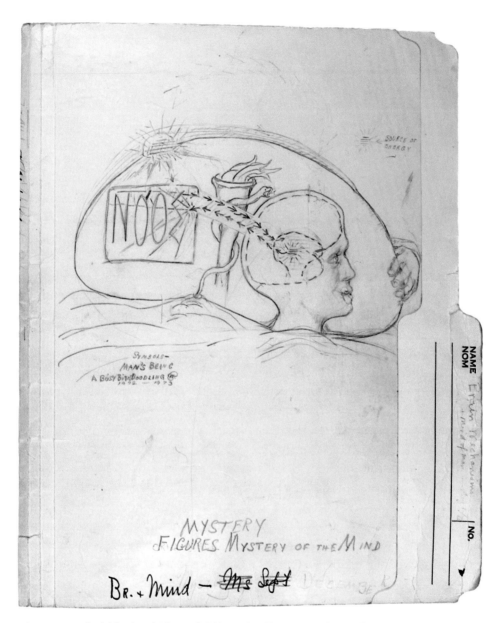

Figure 14.1. File folder in which Penfield kept the illustrations for his "Mystery of the Mind." The drawing represents the brain within the skull, with the centrencephalic system highlighted. The bidirectional arrows represent reciprocal influence of the centrencephalic system and the mind, here labelled as the noos (nous). Osler Library of the History of Medicine, McGill University.

Universities.[6] By then, Penfield no longer considered that phenomena such as those experienced by J.V. were simple *déjà vu* and *déjà entendu*. With the accumulation of cases, Penfield came to realize that what the patients described at surgery – the episode of the young girl in the meadow; a woman who saw herself giving birth to her child – had actually happened and had been brought back to consciousness by stimulation of the cortex. Rather than epileptic "psychical"[7] phenomena, Penfield now considered that what the patients described was "related to the mechanism of memory."[8] Furthermore, it gradually became apparent to him that the revival of memories by the stimulating electrode only occurred in patients with temporal lobe epilepsy, and only when the temporal lobe was stimulated, and no other. Thus, Penfield began to refer to the temporal cortex as "the storehouse of memories."[9] But what his electrode brought forth, Penfield soon realized, were more than simple memories because they included "the emotions which attended the original experience … the reasoning regarding the significance of the event, [and] the individual's own interpretation of the experience … It seems to be the integrated whole that is recorded."[10] Penfield referred to these complex, electrically induced responses as experiential phenomena.

Experiential phenomena – I have lived through it all before (Case M.M.)
As often happened when a case attracted his interest, Penfield sent a talented fellow "back to the charts." In this case, he assigned Maitland Baldwin to review the charts of the 222 patients upon whom he had operated for temporal lobe epilepsy.[11] Baldwin found twenty-five patients in whom Penfield's stimulation of the temporal cortex had produced psychical responses. These were "characterized by various combinations of abnormal experience and unusual behaviour … paroxysms [of] subtle changes in perception, hallucinations and dreams."[12] Baldwin then classified these into two categories: 1. involuntary recollection of past events and 2. unusual interpretations of present experiences. Penfield later referred to the former as *experiential phenomena*,[13] by which he meant the recall of a complete experience – its memory, the emotions that coloured it, and the thoughts that accompanied it – and to the latter as *interpretive illusions*.[14] He would have much to say about illusionary phenomena in the future, but at the time, Penfield's interest lay in experiential phenomena, whose study he considered to be "the beginning of a physiology of the mind."[15]

Penfield conceived of experiential phenomena as distinct units aligned chronologically along the anterior–posterior axis of the first temporal convolution. They also extended vertically downward "through an unending sequence of nerve cells, nerve fibres and synapses"[16] that linked the temporal cortex to the higher brain stem. Transmission of impulses along nerve cells and synapses was akin to a loop and travelled both ways, from cortex to the brain stem and back.

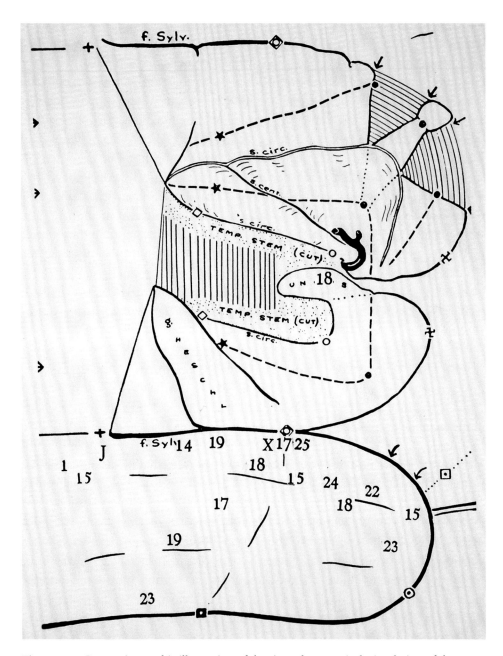

Figure 14.2. Composite graphic illustration of the sites where cortical stimulation of the temporal lobe in fifteen patients produced psychical hallucinations, to which Penfield later referred as experiential phenomena. Note that the responses cluster along the first temporal convolution but that they also occurred with stimulation of the uncus (no. 18). It would later be discovered that stimulation of the amygdala frequently produces such responses. Montreal Neurological Institute archives, Baldwin, "Functional Representation in the Temporal Lobe of Man."

Table 14.1
Manifestations of psychomotor seizures elicited by electrical stimulation of the temporal lobes

Stimulation of the lateral neocortex

Experiential Phenomena
Reactivation of a strip of the record of the stream of consciousness

Interpretive illusions (psychical illusions):
Alteration in the perception of the present:
    Auditory illusions of distance, loudness, and tempo
    Visual illusions of distance, dimension, erectness, and tempo
    Illusions of comparison – familiarity, strangeness, unreality
    Illusions of emotions – fear, loneliness, separation, sorrow, disgust

Stimulation of the amygdala

Automatisms and amnesia

Penfield considered that the function of the temporal lobes, exclusive of the area dedicated to language comprehension, was to activate the memory of past experiences when similar experiences were encountered, and join the past to the present through the bidirectional circuit between the temporal cortex and the brain stem.[17] Penfield was explicit in this regard, stating that the temporal lobes were the site of "a mechanism that unlocks the past and seems to scan it for the purpose of automatic *interpretation* [emphasis added] of the present."[18]

But why should the temporal cortex be so favoured?

THE INTERPRETIVE CORTEX

Let us suppose the mind to be white paper void of all characters, without any ideas; how comes it to be furnished? Whence has it all the materials of reason and knowledge? To this I answer, in one word, from experience –Locke[19]

Penfield initially referred to the temporal cortex as *uncommitted* because he believed that it was devoid of any function at birth. As the individual matured the uncommitted cortex of the dominant hemisphere became the seat of the interpretive aspect of language.[20] The remainder of the temporal cortices become the repository of life's experiences. They accumulated and stored them and recalled them as necessary to interpret new experiences as they were encountered.[21] Thus, Penfield came to the conclusion that "the temporal cortex plays an active role in the interpretation of each individuals present experience. [It] may be called *interpretive* as other areas of the cortex are called 'sensory' and still others 'motor.'"[22] The uncommitted cortex, like Locke's white paper, was a blank slate at birth upon which would be etched the experiences of a lifetime.[23] Its cells and circuits became the repository of human experience from birth to death. They were the banks of the stream of consciousness. The process by which the interpretative cortex acquired its functions, Penfield thought, was the conditioned reflex.

THE CONDITIONED REFLEX — WILL, SPEECH, AND PERCEPTION

Wilder Penfield and Ivan Pavlov are not often spoken of in the same breath. Nevertheless, they are inexorably linked through Pavlov's influence on Penfield's understanding of the physiology of the brain. The awe that Penfield felt for Pavlov is reflected in his reaction as he approached the Pavlov Institute of Physiology of the Academy of Sciences, Leningrad, while on a tour of the major scientific institutions of the Union of Soviet Socialist Republics in 1955:

> This institute is housed in a curiously curved building on the Neva River. From the front door a grand staircase of white marble leads upward to the second floor. As we climbed I could hear the faint echo of the barking dogs and I thought of how often Pavlov had himself climbed those stairs and savoured familiar smells and sights and sounds. A superstitious dualist, if one had been present, might have fancied that the spirit of Pavlov was walking with us through the laboratory.[24]

But Pavlov was more than a spectral presence to Penfield. Pavlov's work permeates Penfield's writings from the beginning of his career to the end of his life.

Penfield first invoked Pavlov and the conditioned reflex in a Harvey Lecture entitled "The Cerebral Cortex and Consciousness," given at Rockefeller University in 1936,[25] to explain the unusual responses produced by electrical stimulation in the case of the young girl the meadow. Penfield described how the process of conditioning resulted in the creation of an experiential experience in her case, its relationship to epileptic seizures, and its revival by the stimulating electrode, as well as the insight that it gave into the function of the temporal cortex:

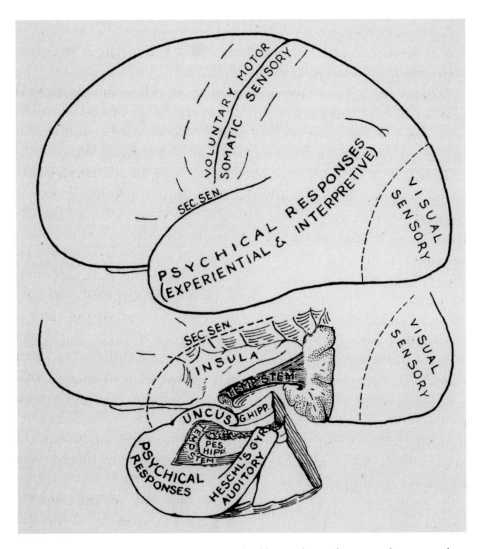

Figure 14.3. Penfield's drawing of the left cerebral hemisphere. The pre- and postcentral gyri are innately dedicated to motor and sensory functions, and the occipital cortex and Heschl's gyri are innately dedicated to vision and audition, respectively. The temporal lobe is represented as the interpretive cortex, which is conditioned by experience to be the storehouse of memories (experiential) and of perception (interpretive). Montreal Neurological Institute, McGill University.

That part of the cortex had been *conditioned* [emphasis added] by the original experience associated with fright. That is to say that the experience was recorded in a pattern of neuronal connections. The conditioning process was then reinforced by subsequent nightmares in which the same man appeared to frighten her. Later on, epileptiform seizures made their appearance … in the region where the above neurone pattern had been established. The epileptic discharge followed that pre-established pattern of neurone connections. The result was that in her aura the man approached again behind her and she was terrified. If the seizure went further one-sided convulsive movements appeared and spread to both sides ... Activation [by electrocortical stimulation] and conditioning of the cortex in one sense would seem to be identical processes. Thus activation may render accessible to the electrode the evidence of innate function present in all normal brains or it may reveal acquired experience peculiar to one individual.[26]

Penfield was clear: if stimulation of the temporal cortex involuntarily revives a memory, there is no reason to think that memories that are voluntarily recalled reside elsewhere in the brain – the temporal cortex is the storehouse of memory.

Penfield also linked the cortical pathways acquired by Pavlovian conditioning and the spread of epileptic seizures triggered by intra-operative electrocortical stimulation:

An habitual seizure, by virtue of frequent repetition, may eventually establish a complicated neurone pattern, so functionally organized that it may be stimulated electrically although no such complicated response could be obtained from stimulation of the normal brain. Induced seizures do not arise from distant stimulation. They begin by discharge in the neighbourhood of the stimulating electrode. This is followed by spread, which is not diffuse, but which is along a definite neurone system, which may be preformed or acquired. By "preformed" is meant a system of neuronal connections ordinarily recognized as physiologically functional in all normal brains. By "acquired" is meant a pattern of neuronal connections established by the conditioning influence of previous individual experience. In this sense *habitual seizures should be considered true conditioned reflexes in the cortex of any patient* [emphasis added.][27]

Conditioned reflexes were also the mechanism underlying voluntary motor tasks directed towards a goal. Penfield believed that there are inborn reflexes located in the brain stem and spinal cord. But like Pavlov, he also believed that there are acquired reflexes created by conditioning of the cerebral cortex.[28] Inborn reflexes are common to all humans and are responsible, for example, for homeostasis, simple stretch reflexes, and the more elaborate chains of reflexes responsible for maintaining upright posture. More skilful, voluntary motor tasks, such as voluntary movements of the head, the trunk, and the extremities, as well as movements of verbal articulation, were for Penfield "acquired mechanisms established in the primary (and probably also secondary and supplementary motor) somatic areas in the cerebral cortex ... as 'conditioned reflexes' as described by Ivan Pavlov."[29]

The same process of conditioning was responsible for the acquisition of higher cognitive functions, such as the acquisition of language, as Penfield bluntly stated:

"language learning may be looked upon as the process of setting up conditioned reflexes in certain parts of the uncommitted cortex of the dominant hemisphere."[30]

As for speech, so for perception. By *perception* Penfield meant the interpretation of the present in light of past experience, which was stored as experiential phenomena within the temporal cortex:

> For a short time, a man can recall all the details of his previous awareness. In minutes, some of it has faded ... in a week all of it seems to have disappeared ... But the detail is not really lost. During the subconscious interpretation of later contemporary experience, that detail is still available. This is a part of what we may call perception.[31]

This concept had also originated with Pavlov, who considered that the function of the conditioned reflex was to assure that an organism's response was conducive to survival in an ever-changing external environment.[32] Voluntary movement toward a goal, learning, speech, memory, and perception, all originated with Pavlovian conditioning of the human cortex in Penfield's physiology of mind.[33] But, Penfield was being surpassed by his reliance on Pavlov and eventually had to consider more substantive mechanisms to account for memory and learning, and address the concept of the engram.

The engram – the writing left behind in the brain

Penfield gave a lecture to the Royal Society of Medicine, London, in 1968, entitled "Engrams in the Human Brain."[34] The term *engram* was coined by Richard Semon, a late nineteenth-century German biologist, who used the term to refer to a memory trace created by a physical change in the substance of the brain in response to stimulation.[35] Semon's concept was purely theoretical, and it did not gain credibility until the work of Rafael Lorente de Nó, Donald Hebb, and Holger Hydén in the early and mid-twentieth century. Lorente de Nó, at the Rockefeller Institute for Medical Research, discovered that the cortex is the site of complex looped and reentrant circuits, and that repeated stimulation of these networks could activate one chain of neurons while simultaneously inhibiting others, thus creating a preferred pathway between different areas of the brain.[36] These pathways, Lorente de Nó also observed, are arranged as "self-re-exciting chains."[37] These chains of neurons were independent, Lorente de Nó found, of external sensory input and did not result in somatic motor output. It later occurred to Donald Hebb, then at McGill University, that "a group of neurons exciting and re-exciting each other" in the cortex and acting independently of the sensorimotor system could be "a possible basis of thought."[38] As Hebb later stated, "Lorente de Nó's work ... led me to write *The Organization of Behaviour*,"[39] in which he described his concept of the engram as a permanent, multisynaptic pathway formed in response to an individual's experience and reinforced by repeated stimulation.[40] The preferential transmission of an impulse across a synaptic cleft became known as the "Hebbian synapse," and it provided a theoretical explanation for the creation of memories. The concept of the engram was validated with the discovery of the molecular nature of synaptic transmission by Bernard Katz[41] and by Holger Hydén's demonstration that synaptic connections could be permanently modified by learning and memory.[42]

Penfield had been reticent to evoke the engram, stating, as late as 1960, "I have always avoided consciously using the word engram … because of the various types of thinking that have been carried out in regard to [it]."[43] He did, however, refer to the engram in his lecture to the Royal Society of Medicine, in which he defined his understanding of the term:

> the engram is the permanent impression left behind by psychical experience in the brain's cellular network. This "memory trace" makes all that came within the focus of a man's attention memorable in one way or another. It may modify or reinforce a skill. It, also, forms a part of the record of the stream of consciousness and may be summoned consciously or automatically for the purpose of recognition, interpretation, perception.[44]

However, despite the demonstration of its biochemical nature, Penfield's conception of the engram was still anchored to 1930s electrophysiology. For him, the engram was a product of electrical conduction through a neuronal circuit, not a molecular alteration of synaptic connections. Thus, Penfield turned to electrophysiology to define the engram: "The fact that the application of a gentle current, on certain portions of the temporal cortex, can switch on [a] recording, suggests that the engram is, in fact, a permanent and continuous thread of facilitation [which] lowers the threshold of resistance to the passage of nerve impulses."[5] Thus, the engram was simply a product of enhanced saltatory conduction within a neuronal circuit. The conditioned reflex remained for Penfield the mechanism responsible for the emergence of individual sensorimotor skills and cognitive functions.[46] His only concession to the engram was to assume that it could act in consort with the conditioned reflexes and to the sequential record of conscious experience.[47]

Nonetheless, whether electrical or biochemical or both, the conditioned reflex and the engram were a reflection of how Penfield understands the mind to work: "The mind is a communication system within the brain … although all parts of the cerebral cortex may make a contribution to its action when called upon, the essential part of the mechanism is subcortical."[48] Thus, the acquisition of memory, language, and perception, "the physiology of the mind,"[49] resided within a functional system based on the interaction of the cortex and the higher brain stem, to which Penfield referred as the centrencephalic integrating system.

The centrencephalic integrating system and the stream of consciousness – Where is the place of understanding[50]

Wilder Penfield first mentioned consciousness in 1932 in a description of the semiology of frontal lobe seizures, which, he observed, "are usually characterized by loss of consciousness."[51] This was in agreement, Penfield noted, with John Hughlings Jackson's concept of the hierarchical organization of the brain. For Jackson, the human brain consisted of three levels. The lowest level included the pons, the medulla oblongata, and the spinal cord. The motor and sensory convolutions of the frontal and parietal lobes constituted the middle level, and the frontal lobe anterior to the precentral gyrus and the occipital lobe constituted the highest level. Jackson held that consciousness resided within the highest level of organization, to which he referred as "the organ of the mind."[52] Penfield echoed Jackson, as he stated, the frontal lobes are "the indispensable accompaniment of conscious thought."[53]

Thus, when Penfield used the word "consciousness," he meant more than the state of wakefulness. In this he was explicit, if somewhat imprecise: "Consciousness," he wrote, "is an awareness, a thinking, a knowing, a focussing of attention, a planning of action, an interpretation of present experience, a perceiving."[54] And, referring to Alfred Fessard, the influential electrophysiologist, Penfield concluded that consciousness is the "integrated perception of the present."[55]

Penfield returned to the topic of consciousness in his Harvey lecture of 1936 subtitled, "The Cerebral Cortex and Consciousness."[56] Generalized seizures and loss of consciousness, he had observed, are often associated with loss of vasomotor function, such as blanching of the face; with visceral phenomena, such as urinary incontinence; and with vague epigastric sensations. These phenomena were accompanied by loss of muscular tone and falling to the ground. (The latter had given epilepsy its first appellation of *the falling sickness*.) These were not functions that resided in the frontal lobes and Penfield looked elsewhere for "the indispensable substratum of consciousness."[57] This should be, Penfield suggested, "near the representation of autonomic function in the hypothalamus, close to the third ventricle, in the region in which blanching of the face may be produced and visceral sense may be represented, and adjacent to the upper end of the nerve circuits in the midbrain which maintain standing."[58] Thus, Penfield narrowed his focus to the upper brain stem as the seat of consciousness. Penfield further reasoned that the highest level of neural activity could not reside within the cortical mantle because, although damage to the cortex could abolish motion and speech, it did not abolish the will to move or to speak, nor did extensive removal of the cortex lead to unconsciousness.[59] Damage to the brain stem, however, made consciousness impossible, and without consciousness, thoughts could not be generated, emotions could not be expressed, voluntary actions could not be undertaken.[60] Thus, for Penfield, the highest level of neural integration depended on the formation and maintenance of stable, bidirectional connections between the cortex and the upper brain stem.[61]

Penfield recognized the phylogenic expansion of the cerebral cortex, and especially of the frontal lobes, but he gave little weight to the process of encephalization in the evolution of consciousness, and stated,

> The human cerebral cortex has developed coincidentally with man's acquisition of new skills and new adjustments to his environment. A priori, there seems to be no reason that the neural mechanism essential to consciousness should migrate outward into the newly exfoliated hemisphere … [and concluded] … there is much evidence of a level of integration within the central nervous system that is higher than that to be found in the cerebral cortex, evidence of a regional localization of the neuronal mechanism involved in this integration … All regions of the brain may well be involved in normal conscious processes, but the indispensable substratum of consciousness lies outside the cerebral cortex, probably in the diencephalon.[62]

Thus, although Penfield considered that "all regions of the brain may well be involved in normal conscious processes, the indispensable substratum of consciousness" lay within the brain stem.[63] This is where he found "the place of understanding … the location of those neuronal circuits which are most intimately associated with the initiation of voluntary activity and with the sensory summation prerequisite to it."[64]

Penfield next spoke of the relationship of the brain, consciousness, and the mind in 1949, in a BBC radio transmission on the topic of "The Cerebral Cortex and the Mind of Man,"[65] during which he affirmed that the mind is a function of the brain.[66] He reiterated that "the higher brain-stem, together with that portion of the cortex which is being employed at the moment is the seat of consciousness," that it is the place "to which messages come and from which messages depart after appropriate decisions are reached, decisions that are based upon memories of previous experience and influenced by present desires."[67] But going a step further, he added that the interaction of cortex and brain stem, "this hypothetical mechanism of nerve cell connections … is the 'physiological basis of the mind.'"[68] Two years later, at the December 1951 meeting of the Association for Research in Nervous and Mental Disease, and after consulting with Stanley Cobb and Herbert Jasper, Penfield named this functional unit responsible for conscious awareness and the functions of the mind the *centrencephalic integrating system*,[69] which he defined anatomically as "the intralaminar system of the thalamus and the reticular system of the brain stem," and whose role was the integration of the function of the two cerebral hemispheres.[70]

Penfield's addressed the functions of the centrencephalic system at a "Symposium on Brain and Mind" hosted by the American Academy of Neurology in June 1951, when he spoke of "memory mechanisms."[71] The symposium included a number of distinguished speakers, including Horace Magoun, who spoke on the newly described reticular activating system; Herbert Jasper, who addressed the relationship of the cortex and brain stem; and Stanley Cobb, who spoke "On the Nature and Locus of Mind."[72] Karl Lashley was also in attendance, and he responded to Penfield's presentation by speaking "a word of warning against the present tendency to ascribe very complex functions to the thalamus and brain stem. These are regions of relatively few cells and poorly developed internuncial systems."[73] This gave Penfield the opportunity to clarify some misconceptions on the constituents and function of the centrencephalic system:

> I do not consider valid Dr Lashley's objection that the centrencephalic system is too small to do what we want it to do. He seems to think that we assume that the centrencephalic system is a sort of a room by itself that does all these things. The system does not function by itself. It functions together with all the other areas – cortex and other parts of the central nervous system. Thus, when it is functioning, all parts of the brain that are needed for that particular function come into action.[74]

Stanley Cobb, Penfield's lifelong friend, was also critical of one of the topics that Penfield had addressed in his presentation and unabashedly declared, "It is too much to believe that each memory has its separate neuron pathway."[75]

Cobb had the occasion to reflect at length upon Penfield's conception of the centrencephalic system in a review of Penfield's Sherrington Lecture, "The Excitable Cortex in Conscious Man," given at the University of Liverpool in 1958.[76] Cobb was circumspect in his criticism, but sharp nonetheless, and struck at the heart of Penfield's "physiology of the mind." Recognizing Penfield's reliance of the conditioned reflex as the foundation on which the centrencephalic system was built, Cobb was unequivocal: "The reflexology of the first quarter of this century … was too simple" to account for such a grandiose scheme.[77] Addressing Penfield's premise that the upper brain stem is the seat of consciousness because a small lesion within its substance can cause unconsciousness, while a lesion of the cortex cannot, Cobb countered that this was only to be expected since the neuronal circuits between the brain stem and cortex are more vulnerable in the latter, where they are more tightly packed, than in the cortex, where they are more widely spaced. And, as Cobb noted, "as these circuits spread out to many parts of both hemispheres they become less vulnerable to small lesions, but they are no less important to consciousness."[78] Thus, Cobb was of the opinion that "the complex and varying phenomena of consciousness and memory can only be explained by an hypothesis of many circuits, large and small, integrated at all levels of the neuraxis and including transcortical and transcallosal connection."[79]

Penfield was not swayed by Cobb's arguments. Theodore Erickson had studied the role of the corpus callosum in the spread of experimentally induced epileptic seizures, under Penfield's direction, for his master's thesis, which he published in 1939. Erickson observed that sectioning the corpus callosum arrested the spread of seizures from one hemisphere to the other, but it had no effect on consciousness.[80] This was confirmed one year later, when callosotomy was introduced to control epileptic seizures in man.[81] As Erickson had observed, sectioning the corpus callosum had no effect on the maintenance of human consciousness.

The stream of consciousness

> There can be no final organization, and no consciousness, *without centrencephalic organization* –Penfield, 1957

Penfield elaborated upon the functioning of the centrencephalic system during an address entitled "The Permanent Record of the Stream of Consciousness" that he gave at the International Congress of Psychology in Montreal, in June 1954.[82] Each sensation that reached the cortex, and the motor, cognitive, and emotional responses that it evoked, is transmitted to the upper brain stem, Penfield told his audience, where they are integrated into a complete experience. The newly created experiential event is then transmitted from the brain stem to the first temporal convolution, where it is stored within a specific volume of cortex. It returns to consciousness when a similar situation is encountered, so that an individual can perceive its significance based on past experience and react appropriately. The process as a whole constituted the stream of consciousness:

> It is evident that the brain of every man contains an unchanging ganglionic record of successive experience. The psychical responses which have been produced by electrical stimulation, during craniotomy and cortical exploration, demonstrate that this record embraces and retains the elements that once were incorporated in his stream of thought … Thousands of these conditioned ganglion cells may well be reached directly by the stimulation current and they have neuronal connections that pass through the grey matter that covers the temporal lobe and also inward to the central integrating circuits of the brainstem … Among the millions and millions of nerve cells that clothe certain parts of the temporal lobe on each

side, there runs a thread. It is the thread of time, the thread that has run through each succeeding wakeful hour of the individual's past life. Think of this thread, if you like, as a pathway through an unending sequence of nerve cells, nerve fibres and synapses. It is a pathway which can be followed again because of the continuing facilitation that has been created in the cell contacts. When, by chance, the neurosurgeon's electrode activates some portion of that thread, there is a response as though that thread were a wire recorder, or a strip of cinematographic film, on which are registered all those things of which the individual was once aware, the things he selected for his attention in that interval of time … As long as the electrode is held in place, the experience of a former day goes forward … When the electrode is withdrawn it stops as suddenly as it began. *We have found a way of activating the anatomical record of the stream of consciousness* [emphasis added].[83]

Penfield expanded on the function of the centrencephalic integrating system in addresses delivered at the First International Congress of Neurological Sciences[84] and at a symposium on the "Neurological Basis of Behaviour,"[85] held in Brussels and London, respectively, in 1957. The concept of the centrencephalic system, he told his Brussels audience, included more than the temporal lobes, and it did not apply solely to complex cognitive functions:

The brain is at once the target of bombardment from eye, ear, nose, skin and joint – and the origin of the travelling potentials sent out to the muscles to determine their movements during *voluntary action* [emphasis added]. But before planned voluntary action is possible, there must occur within the brain a complicated redirection of the entering potentials. The streams of sensory information must be arranged and organized. And to this organization must be added information from the individual's own past experience, pertinent data drawn from the memory storehouse of the brain. It is the organizing activity that comes between sensory input and voluntary motor output that constitutes the physical basis of mind.[86]

For the first time, Penfield invoked the *will* – to which he referred as "voluntary action," "volitional impulses," "planned initiative," "planned action," or "conscious planning" – as a function of the centrencephalic system: "The neural pathways that emerge from unidentified centrally placed ganglia carrying *volitional impulses* [emphasis added] to the precentral gyrus of each hemisphere do form a part of the centrencephalic system … From that target of grey matter the volitional stream of nerve impulses must emerge."[87] Further, "There must be a place toward which streams of sensory impulses converge. There must be a place from which streams of motor impulses emerge to move the hands in simultaneous *planned action* [emphasis added]. There must be neuronal circuits ... in which activity of both hemispheres is somehow summarized and fused – circuits the activation of which makes *conscious planning* [emphasis added] possible."[88] For Penfield that place was the centrencephalic integrating system, and the will to act arose from the higher brain stem:

> Many complicated neurone processes must take place before he can make up his mind just what the movement of his free hand is to be. He must call upon various areas of the cortex of each side for information. Those areas are all connected to the higher brain stem and it is from the higher brain stem that he seems to send out the neurone impulses that produce voluntary act.[89]

Milner and Penfield reported the effects of bilateral hippocampal lesions on memory,[90] in June 1955, a year after Penfield's address to the International Congress of Psychology on the stream of consciousness, and Penfield found that his model of the centrencephalic system was suddenly incomplete. Penfield now had to incorporate the function of the hippocampi into the centrencephalic theory of memory and experiential recall. In his new construct, the hippocampi acted as an intermediary between the temporal cortex and the brain stem. Thus, Penfield's "memory mechanism" – the act of scanning and recalling past experience – now had three components: the interpretive cortex, the hippocampi, and the upper brain stem. The upper brain stem kept its role of keeper of "the neuronal recording of the stream of consciousness,"[91] but the hippocampi took on a prominent role in the mechanism of conscious recall.[92] (See also figure 13.4.) Penfield was explicit in this regard, and whatever qualms he may have had in the past, he now entrusted his construct to the Hebbian engram:

> It may now be surmised that the hippocampi are involved with the interpretative cortex of both temporal lobes in the function of scanning and recall. It is the record of past consciousness that must be scanned. That record is a continuous pattern of neuron connections that have been permanently facilitated for the subsequent passage of neuronal currents. This continuous thread of facilitated passage is the experiential engram.[93]

PASCAL'S GAMBLE

Penfield died quietly at the Royal Victoria Hospital on 5 April 1976. One could easily conclude from his writings that he was a materialist, that he believed, as his closest friend Stanley Cobb did, that "the mind is what the brain does." But, as is so often the case, approaching death causes one to seek something everlasting, beyond "the scattered annals of our profession."[94] And so it was with Penfield, the centrencephalic

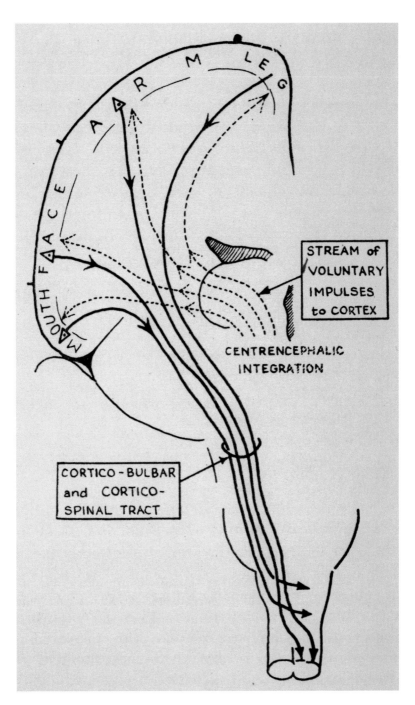

Figure 14.4 Penfield's drawing of the voluntary control of motion as a function if the centrencephalic integrating system. Montreal Neurological Institute, McGill University.

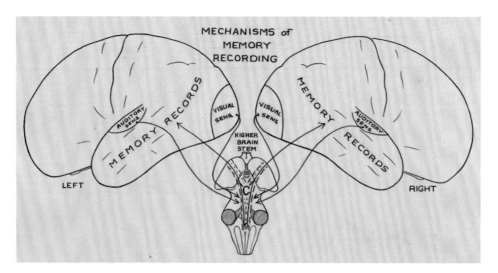

Figure 14.5. Drawing illustrating Penfield's conceptualization of the integration of memory into consciousness through the centrencephalic system, which he described before the discovery of the role of the hippocampus in short-term memory. Sounds and images that had reached the primary auditory and visual cortex were transmitted to the centrencephalic system in the upper brain stem, the seat of consciousness, indicated by the letter C. There, sounds and images were integrated with the thoughts and feelings with which they were accompanied when they were first perceived, creating a complete experience. The newly created experiential unit was then projected to the first temporal cortex where it was stored. Osler Library of the History of Medicine, McGill University.

system, and the mind. "Throughout my own scientific career," Penfield wrote shortly before his death,

> I, like other scientists, have struggled to prove that the brain accounts for the mind. But now, perhaps, the time has come when we may profitably consider the evidence as it stands, and ask the question: *Do brain-mechanisms account for the mind?* Can the mind be explained by what is now known about the brain? If not, which is the more reasonable of the two possible hypotheses: that man's being is based on one element, or two? … For my own part, after years of striving to explain the mind on the basis of brain-action alone, I have come to the conclusion that it is simpler if one adopts the hypothesis that our being does consist of two fundamental elements.[95]

This apparently clear statement is open to interpretation. Penfield was in awe of John Hughlings Jackson, and he would have been aware of his opinion on the brain–mind problem. Jackson held that there were three possible explanations for the relationship of the brain and the mind. First, that they are one and the same, as in the statement "the mind is what the brain does." Second, that they are distinct but interactive, as in the classical Cartesian view. Third, that they are distinct and independent one of the other, acting not in consort but in parallel. Jackson adhered to the latter view, to which he referred as "concomitance." Thus, when Penfield writes, "it is simpler if one adopts the hypothesis that our being does consist of two fundamental elements," he may be referring to Cartesian dualism or to Jacksonian concomitance.[96]

Herbert Jasper, Penfield's great collaborator, did not share Penfield's pessimism in uniting brain and mind, nor did he give much weight to his belated turn to dualism, and he later wrote a detailed note on this issue in his own biographical memoir:

> Penfield finally concluded, in his last publication, *The Mystery of the Mind*, that the brain–mind problem could not be solved since he had spent his entire life trying to do so without success. He allowed that conscious experience might be a separate form of reality. He suggested that I might be wasting my time seeking answers in electrophysiological or neurochemical functions of the brain, even though there were obviously close relationships.
>
> I am not prepared to agree with Penfield that there may be no solutions to the brain–mind problem although I do agree that we have not yet found that elusive link between the special brain mechanism involved in conscious awareness and mental activity. I do believe that there is some neuronal organization specialized for this purpose widely distributed throughout the brain and varying with behavioral activities each moment in the stream of consciousness, many centrencephalic mechanisms if you will, but they are too vague … in the present state of knowledge.
>
> However, the search is becoming more and more exciting and worth the effort in spite of its bewildering complexity.
>
> I have become convinced … that there are distributed systems of neurones in the brain stem, diencephalon, and cortex of particular importance in the control of states of consciousness and perceptual awareness.[97]

Jasper was also clear on Penfield's purpose in formulating the concept of the centrencephalic system, commenting,

> Penfield did not consider it to be limited to the reticular activating system of Moruzzi and Magoun, although probably included as part of it. It included two-way interconnections between all areas of cerebral cortex and an extensive network

of neurones in the diencephalon and brain stem. It was a *working hypothesis* [emphasis added], deliberately lacking in precise anatomical identity, to be worked out in the future.[98]

As it was.

A NEW PARADIGM

Penfield's focus on the interaction of the brain stem and cortex was very much at the forefront of mid-twentieth-century neurobiology. During this period, the concept of the reticular activating system was formulated, and its structure within the upper and lower brain stem was identified.[99] Herbert Jasper and his coworkers at the MNI studied the bidirectional interaction of the proximal reticular activating system and the cortex, while Horace Magoun and Giuseppe Moruzzi, at Northwestern University in Chicago, studied its function in the distal brain stem in priming the cortex into action. Jasper and his colleagues discovered that electrical stimulation of specific thalamic nuclei and intralaminar thalamic neurons activates specific layers of the cerebral cortex,[100] and Magoun and Moruzzi discovered that the activity of the lower brain stem maintains arousal and wakefulness.[101] These findings led Alexander Luria to conclude that

> the structures maintaining and regulating cortical tone do not lie in the cortex itself, but below it, in the subcortex [thalamus] and brain stem, [and] that these structures have a double relationship with the cortex, both influencing its tone and themselves experiencing its regulatory influence.[102]

These discoveries, according to Luria, brought about a new paradigm, that of the "vertical organization of all structures of the brain,"[103] and the recognition of the interaction of the cortex and brain stem in consciousness. This interaction became evident during the split-brain experiments performed by Michael Gazzaniga and Roger Sperry in the 1960s, when it was observed that consciousness is fully preserved in patients whose hemispheres have been disconnected by sectioning of the corpus callosum. Penfield had been aware of this since at least 1966 when Sperry gave the thirty-second Hughlings Jackson Lecture at the Montreal Neurological Institute, entitled "Mental Unity Following Surgical Disconnection of the Cerebral Hemispheres."[104]

Conscious awareness is preserved in callosotomized patients, according to Gazzaniga, "because the connections between the cortex and thalamus in each hemisphere remain intact."[105] Current electrophysiological experimentations have

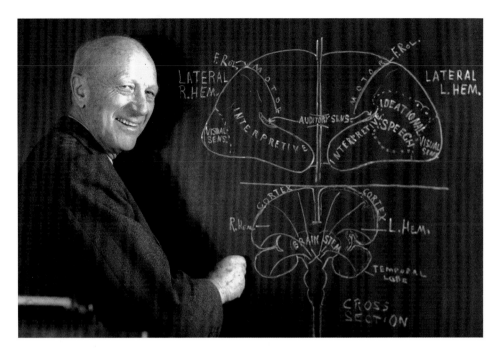

Figure 14.6. Penfield at the blackboard, illustrating the centrencephalic integrating system. Montreal Neurological Institute, McGill University.

confirmed Jasper's findings of three decades previously, that "the thalamus represents a hub from which any site in the cortex can communicate with any other such site or sites"[106] and have "emphasized the importance of the thalamo–cortical system of the brain in generating conscious awareness,"[107] which Penfield had recognized in 1936. The last word, then, should be Penfield's:

> Those who would come upon the truth should elaborate their incomplete hypotheses, keeping always clear in mind what is proven fact and what is fancy. You never know which, if any, of your theories will be verified in your lifetime. But chance does favour the "prepared mind" and the man who formulates hypotheses and waits.[108]

2010 – Looking Back

M.P. was eighty-two years old when she returned to the MNI in 2014 for her final postoperative assessment.[1]

When she was first admitted to the MNI in 1954, Brenda Milner had found that her verbal fluency was restricted and her test scores for verbal memory were low. Her nonverbal memory was intact. Thus, the patient's psychometric test results were compatible with an epileptogenic focus in the left, dominant temporal lobe. The clinical pattern of her seizures – automatism and amnesia – the radiological findings of left hemisphere atrophy, a left temporal EEG focus, and the neuropsychological confirmation of left temporal lobe cognitive deficiencies were concordant. She was confidently brought to the operating room but intraoperative cortical stimulation did not produce an epileptic attack or even the warning of an attack, and this had worried Penfield. Nonetheless, what was by then his standard resection of the lateral cortex and extensive resection of the hippocampus was performed.

The patient had two postoperative seizures, one in the first year after surgery and the other six years later in the last trimester of her first pregnancy. She remained seizure-free thereafter for the next fifty years, the last twenty-five years off all medication. M.P. completed her studies in visual arts and enjoyed a successful career as a painter, despite the loss of half of her visual field as a result of the extensive resection that Penfield had performed. She married and had two children. She divorced in 1980.

The patient returned to the MNI in 2010 as part of a project to assess the long-term cognitive effects of temporal lobe surgery. It was found that her deficits in verbal fluency and the memory for verbal material had worsened with time, but she had not been aware of either deficit. She tested at the same level as her peers in all other cognitive tasks. No comparison could be made, of course, with individuals with medially refractory epilepsy who had not undergone surgery and had suffered a lifetime of epileptic attacks. Gabriel Leonard, a neuropsychologist at the MNI, had previously demonstrated, however, that patients whose seizures were controlled by surgery did better on a variety of cognitive tests than patients whose seizures had persisted postoperatively.[2] Specifically, patients whose surgery had been successful in alleviating seizures scored significantly higher on general intelligence tests than patients whose seizures had persisted after surgery. This was also the case for tests for delayed verbal memory and verbal fluency. Safe to say, then, that whatever verbal deficits were teased out by neurocognitive tasks did not interfere with M.P.'s education, raising a family, having a successful career, and enjoying life well into her eighties. None of this would have been possible with uncontrolled seizures.

The extent of hippocampal resection became a concern when it was found that it was related to the loss of verbal or of nonverbal memory. Philip Corsi's thesis, which had brought this relationship to the fore, was published by McGill University in 1972, two years after Penfield had retired from surgery. Subsequently, hippocampal resections were more parsimonious and limited to the *pes hippocampi* or to that part of its anterior aspect from which epileptic activity was recorded or from which stimulation produced a seizure. Nonetheless, there were patients in whom a limited resection of the hippocampus was ineffectual in controlling their seizures. Further resection of the hippocampus in those patients converted an unsuccessful operation into a successful one in the majority of cases.[3]

Results of Surgery

SURGERY OF EPILEPSY

Theodore Rasmussen published the outcome of surgery in patients operated upon at the MNI between 1928 and 1971.[1] Rasmussen separated the results of surgery into five categories depending on the pre- and postoperative frequency of a patient's seizures. Class I consisted of patients who were seizure free since discharge from hospital.[2] Class II patients became seizure free after some postoperative attacks. Class III patients had been seizure free for three to twenty years and subsequently had had rare or occasional attacks. Class IV patients were not seizure free, but had a 98–99% reduction in seizure frequency. Class V included patients who had a moderate or less reduction in seizure frequency. Some had only 5–10% as many attacks as preoperatively, many had a 40–60% reduction in the frequency of their seizures, and a few had little or no reduction. Rasmussen also observed that reoperation to resect an area of persistence epilpetogenesis converted a failed operation into a successful one in slightly more than half of the cases.[3]

TEMPORAL LOBE EPILEPSY

Wilder Penfield began operating on patients with temporal lobe epilepsy in 1928, but, despite this early start, temporal resections accounted for only one-tenth of his epilepsy cases through the 1930s. The proportion of temporal cases rose to one-quarter by the mid-1940s, and temporal resections accounted for half of the epilepsy cases after the discovery of incisural sclerosis. The proportion of temporal lobe cases reached two-thirds over the following decades.[4]

Theodore Rasmussen reviewed the results of surgery in patients with temporal lobe epilepsy operated upon from 1928 to 1972, a span that covers Penfield's surgical career. Rasmussen's study included 653 patients who had been followed up for at least two years after surgery. The longest follow up was thirty-eight years and 80% of patients had been followed from the time of their operation to the end of their life.

Table A.1
Results of surgery for epilepsy, 1928–71

Outcome	No. of cases	%
Class I	237	21
Class II	179	15
Class III	122	11
Class IV	198	17
Class V	409	36

Modified from Rasmussen, "Cortical Resection in the Treatment of Focal Epilepsy.

Table A.2
Results of reoperation, 1928–71

Outcome	No. of cases	%
Class I	13	11
Class II	16	14
Class III	13	11
Class IV	18	16
Class V	55	36

Modified from Rasmussen, "Cortical Resection in the Treatment of Focal Epilepsy."

Table A.3
Results of surgery for temporal lobe epilepsy, 1928–72

Outcome	No. of cases	%
Class I	158	24
Class II	99	15
Class III	69	11
Class IV	140	21
Class V	187	29

Modified from Rasmussen, "Surgical Treatment of Patients with Complex Partial Seizures."

Table A.4

Resuts of surgery for temporal lobe epilepsy, 1928–72 (%)

Outcome	Etiology			
	Birth injury	Inflammatory	Postnatal trauma	Unknown
Class I	31	30	16	19
Class II	18	16	6	14
Class III	10	10	16	10
Class IV	18	14	28	18
Class V	22	30	35	39

Modified from Rasmussen, "Surgical Treatment of Patients with Complex Partial Seizures."

Rasmussen found that 24% of patients fell into Class I, 15% were in Class II, 11% were in Class III, and 21% were in Class IV. Thus, a total of 71% of patients had a complete or nearly complete reduction in seizure frequency as a result of surgery. This left a group of 29% patients whose outcome was less than satisfactory. Some of the patients in this group experienced a 90–95% reduction in the frequency of their attacks, and many had a 40–60% reduction.[5]

Rasmussen went further in his analysis and considered outcome according to the type of lesion that had been at the origin of the temporal seizures. Seventy-seven percent of patients who had sustained birth trauma had a complete or nearly complete reduction in seizure frequency. A similar outcome was attained in 70% of patients whose epilepsy had been caused by an inflammatory process. Sixty-six percent of patients who had sustained postnatal trauma, and 61% patients in whom the ethology was unknown were also seizure free or saw a marked reduction in seizure frequency.

Notes

INTRODUCTION

1 W. Penfield, "The Radical Treatment of Traumatic Epilepsy and Its Rationale," *Canadian Medical Association Journal* 23 (1930): 189–97; O. Foerster and W. Penfield, "The Structural Basis of Traumatic Epilepsy and Results of Radical Operation," *Brain* 53 (1930): 99–119.
2 Penfield, "The Radical Treatment of Traumatic Epilepsy and Its Rationale," 197.

A NOTE ON ANATOMY

1 P.C. Ritterbush, *The Art of Organic Forms* (Washington, DC: Smithsonian Institution Press, 1968), 70.

CHAPTER ONE

1 M.P.'s consultant was Robert G. Armour, a well-regarded neurologist at the University of Toronto. Penfield was asked to take on Margaret's case by Kenneth G. McKenzie, the first neurosurgeon at the same institution.
2 Penfield used a thyratron stimulator that delivered a short pulse at a relatively high 10 to 30 volts until 1945. He used a Rahm stimulator, which produced a voltage of one-half to 3v or more, after that date; O.H.A. Schmitt and F.O. Schmitt, "A Universal Precision Stimulator," *Science* 76 (1932): 328–30; W.E. Rham and J.E. Scarf, "Electrical Excitation of the Cerebral Cortex," *Archives of Neurology and Psychiatry* 50 (1943): 183–9; W. Penfield and W. Rasmussen, *The Cerebral Cortex of Man* (New York: Macmillan, 1950), 6–7.

CHAPTER TWO

1 Victoria ascended to the throne in 1837. Construction of the Royal Victoria Hospital was begun in 1887, and it opened in 1893. The hospital relocated to its current site in 2015.
2 N. Terry, *The Royal Vic: The Story of Montreal's Royal Victoria Hospital, 1894–1994* (Montreal & Kingston: McGill-Queen's University Press, 1994). The Royal Victoria Hospital was relocated to the west of the city in 2015, where it is at the heart of a huge hospital complex.
3 R. Leblanc, "The Royal Victoria Hospital," in *The Wounded Brain Healed: The Golden Age of the Montreal Neurological Institute, 1934–1984*, W. Feindel and R. Leblanc (Montreal & Kingston: McGill-Queen's University Press, 2016), 41–5.
4 Now Wroclaw, Poland.
5 E. Archibald, "Surgical Affections and Wounds of the Head," in *American Practice of Surgery: A Complete System of the Science and Art of Surgery, by Representative Surgeons*

of the United States and Canada, vol. 5, eds. J.D. Bryant and A.H. Buck (New York: William Wood and Co., 1908), 3–378.

6 M. Entin, *Edward Archibald: Surgeon of the Royal Vic* (Montreal & Kingston: McGill-Queen's University Press, 2004), 2.

7 W. Penfield, *No Man Alone: A Neurosurgeon's Life* (Boston, Toronto: Little, Brown and Company, 1977), 9.

8 Ibid., 5.

9 Ibid., 3.

10 Ibid., 4.

11 Ibid., 6.

12 Ibid., 18.

13 Ibid., 33.

14 I.W. Brown, Jr, "The Amazing Adventures of Wilburt C. Davison, Wilder G. Penfield, and Emile F. Holman while Rhodes Scholars in Medicine at Oxford during World War I, 1913–1917," *Annals of Surgery* 211 (1990): 224–34.

15 Penfield, *No Man Alone*, 33.

16 Ibid., 37.

17 Ibid.

18 J.F. Fulton, *Harvey Cushing: A Biography* (Springfield: Thomas, 1946), 197–200.

19 Penfield, *No Man Alone*, 42.

20 W. Penfield, "Alterations of the Golgi Apparatus in Nerve Cells," *Brain* 43 (1920): 290–305.

21 H.C. Bazett and W. Penfield, "A Study of the Sherrington Decerebrate Animal in the Chronic as Well as the Acute Condition," *Brain* 45 (1922): 185–264.

22 Penfield, *No Man Alone*, 42.

23 W. Penfield, "Obituary: Sir Percy Sargent, 1873–1933," *Archives of Neurology and Psychiatry* 30 (1933): 413–14.

24 Penfield, *No Man Alone*, 87–8.

25 W. Penfield, "Osteogenetic Dural Endothelioma: The True Nature of Hemicraniosis," *Journal of Neurology and Psychopathology* 4 (1923): 27–34.

26 Archibald, "Surgical Affections and Wounds of the Head," 3–378.

27 H. Cushing, "Surgery of the Head," in *Surgery: Its Principles and Practice*, vol. 3, ed. W.W. Keen (Philadelphia: W.B. Saunders, 1908), 17–276.

28 F. Krause, *Chirurgie des Gehirns und Rückenmarks nach eigenen Erfahrungen*, vols. 1, 2 (Berlin: Urban und Schwarzenburg, 1908 and 1911); F. Krause, *Surgery of the Brain and Spinal Cord: Based on Personal Experiences*, vols. 1–3 (New York: Rebman Co, 1909–12).

29 Krause, *Surgery of the Brain and Spinal Cord*, vol. 2, 320–53; R. Leblanc, "The Contributions of Fedor Krause," in *A History of Neurosurgery*, ed. S.H. Greenblatt (Park Ridge, IL: The American Association of Neurological Surgeons, 1997), 468–71.

30 C.F. Costea, D.M. Turliuc, A. Sava, G.F. Dumitrescu, A.I. Cucu, E. Patraşcanu, D. Trandafir, and Ş. Turliuc, "Fedor Krause (1857–1937): The Father of German Neurosurgery," *Romanian Neurosurgery* 30 (2016): 241–7.

31 Krause, *Surgery of the Brain and Spinal Cord*, 288.

32 Ibid., 322–3.

33 Ibid.

34 Ibid., 390.

35 Penfield, *No Man Alone*, 60.

36 Ibid.

37 Ibid., 71–2.

38 M.C. Preul and W. Feindel, "Origins of Wilder Penfield's Surgical Technique: The Role of the 'Cushing Ritual' and Influences from the European Experience," *Journal of Neurosurgery* 75 (1991): 812–20; M.C. Preul and W. Feindel, "The Art Is Long and the Life Short: The Letters of Wilder Penfield and Harvey Cushing," *Journal of Neurosurgery* 95 (2001): 148–61.

39 Penfield, *No Man Alone*, 63–5.

40 W. Penfield, "Meningocerebral Adhesions: A Histological Study of the Results of Cerebral Incision and Cranioplasty," *Surgery, Gynecology and Obstetrics* 39 (1924): 803–10.

41 Penfield, *No Man Alone*, 94.

42 W. Penfield, "Oligodendroglia and Its Relationship to Classical Neuroglia," *Brain* 47 (1924): 440.

43 Ibid., 430–52.

44 Ibid., 452.

45 P. del Rio Hortega and W. Penfield, "Cerebral Cicatrix: The Reaction of Neuroglia and Microglia to Brain Wounds," *Bulletin of Johns Hopkins Hospital* 41 (1927): 278–303.

46 W. Penfield and R.C. Buckley, "Punctures of the Brain: The Factors Concerned in Gliosis and Cicatricial Contraction," *Transactions of the American Neurological Association* 1927: 34–46. W. Penfield and R.C. Buckley, "Punctures of the Brain: The Factors Concerned in Gliosis and in Cicatricial Contraction," *Archives of Neurology and Psychiatry* 20 (1928): 1–13.

47 W. Penfield, "The Mechanism of Cicatricial Contraction of the Brain," *Brain* 50 (1927): 499–517.

48 Ibid., 516.

CHAPTER THREE

1   W. Penfield, "The Mechanism of Cicatricial Contraction of the Brain," *Brain* 50 (1927): 499–517.

2   Ibid., 501. Emphasis in original.

3   Ibid., 500.

4   Ibid., 504.

5   Ibid., 511.

6   W. Penfield and W. Cone, "Acute Swelling of Oligodendroglia: A Specific Type of Neuroglia Change," *Transactions of the American Neurological Association* 1925: 182–204.

7   W. Penfield, "Dr. William Vernon Cone 1897–1959," *Canadian Medical Association Journal* 81 (1959): 55–6.

8   M.C. Preul, J. Stratford, G. Bertrand, and W. Feindel, "Neurosurgeon as Innovator: William V. Cone (1897–1959)," *Journal of Neurosurgery* 79 (1993): 621.

9   Ibid., 619–31.

10 Ibid., 621.

11 W. Feindel and E. Maloney, "Wilder Penfield: His Journey to Montreal," in *The Wounded Brain Healed: The Golden Age of the Montreal Neurological Institute, 1934–1984*, W. Feindel and R. Leblanc (Montreal & Kingston: McGill-Queen's University Press, 2016), 14–19.

12 R. Leblanc, "Otfrid Foerster and the Surgical Treatment of Epilepsy," in *The Wounded Brain Healed: The Golden Age of the Montreal Neurological Institute, 1934–1984*, W. Feindel and R. Leblanc (Montreal & Kingston: McGill-Queen's University Press, 2016), 29–39.

13 O. Foerster and W. Penfield, "The Structural Basis of Traumatic Epilepsy and Results of Radical Operation," *Brain* 53 (1930): 99–119. Emphasis added.

14 R. Leblanc, "Otfried Foerster," 31–9.

15 Foerster and Penfield, "The Structural Basis of Traumatic Epilepsy and Results of Radical Operation," 102.

16 Ibid., 117–18.

17 O. Foerster and W. Penfield, "Der Narbenzug am und in Gherin bei Traumatischer Elilepsie in seiner Bedeutung fur das Zustandekommen der Angalle und fur die Therapeurische Bekampfung derselbe," *Zeitschfift fur die Gesamte Neurologie und Psychiatrie* 125 (1930): 475–572; Penfield published an abridged version of this paper: Foerster and Penfield, "The Structural Basis of Traumatic Epilepsy and Results of Radical Operation," *Brain* 53 (1930): 99–119.

18 Ibid., 118. Emphasis added.

19 Ibid.

20 W. Penfield, "The Radical Treatment of Traumatic Epilepsy and Its Rationale," *Canadian Medical Association Journal* 23 (1930): 189–97.

21 Ibid., 196. Emphasis in original.

22 W. Penfield, "Epilepsy and Surgical Therapy," *Archives of Neurology and Psychiatry* 36 (1936): 450.

23 W. Penfield and A.A. Ward, "Calcifying Epileptogenic Lesion," *Archives of Neurology and Psychiatry* 60 (1948): 20–36.

24 A. Torkildsen, "The Gross Anatomy of the Lateral Ventricles," *Journal of Anatomy* 68 (1934): 480–91.

25 A.E. Childe and W. Penfield, "Anatomic and Pneumographic Studies of the Temporal Horn with a Further Note on Pneumographic Analysis of the Cerebral Ventricles," *Archives of Neurology and Psychiatry* 37 (1937): 1021–34.

26 MNI archives, case I.H.

27 A. Torkildsen and W. Penfield, "Ventriculographic Interpretation," *Archives of Neurology and Psychiatry* 30 (1933): 1011–21.

28 This was achieved initially using an electrode that delivered a pulse of galvanic current to the cortex, while stimulation to identify a putative epileptogenic focus by provoking an aura or a seizure was performed with a Faradic coil. As technology advanced, a thyratron stimulator was used in both cases.

29 C. Vogt and O. Vogt, "Die Vergleichend-Architektonische und die Vergleichend-Reiz-physiologische Felderung der Grosshirnrinde unter Besonderer Berucksichtigung der Menschlichen," *Naturwissenschaften* 14 (1926): 1190–4.

30 R. Leblanc, "Mr Hodge," in in *The Wounded Brain Healed: The Golden Age of the Montreal Neurological Institute, 1934–1984*, W. Feindel and R. Leblanc (Montreal & Kingston: McGill-Queen's University Press, 2016) 356–8.

31 I. Klatzo, *Cécile and Oskar Vogt: The Visionaries of Modern Neuroscience* (Wein, New York: Springer-Verlag, 2002), 21.

CHAPTER FOUR

The quote is taken from K.R. Popper, *Conjectures and Refutations: The Growth of Scientific Knowledge* (New York: Harper, 1962).

1 W. Penfield, "The Evidence for a Cerebral Vascular Mechanism in Epilepsy," *Annals of Internal Medicine* 7 (1933): 303–4.

2 Ibid., 118. Emphasis added.

3 J.R. Reynolds, *Epilepsy: Its Symptoms, Treatment and Relation to Other Chronic Convulsive Diseases* (London: John Churchill, 1861), 25–6; M.G. Echeverria, *On Epilepsy* (New York: William Wood & Company, 1870).

4 C. Bernard, "Influence du Grand Sympathique sur la Sensibilité et sur la Calorifica-
   tion," *Comptes Rendus et Mémoires de la Société de Biologie* 3, 1851 (1852): 163–4; C. Ber-
   nard, "Sur les Effets de la Section de la Portion Encéphalique du Grand Sympathique,"
   Comptes Rendus et Mémoires de la Société de Biologie 4, 1852 (1853): 168–70; C. Bernard,
   Leçons sur la Physiologie et la Pathologie du Système Nerveux, vol. 2 (Paris: J.B. Baillière et
   Fils, 1858), 491–5; C. Bernard, "Recherches Expérimentales sur les Nerfs Vasculaires et
   Calorifiques du Grand Sympathique," *Comptes Rendus Hebdomadaire de l'Académie des
   Sciences* 55 (1862): 228–36, 305–12.

5 J. Choróbski, "Part 1. A Vasodilator Nervous Pathway to the Cerebral Vessels from the
   Central Nervous System. Part 2. On the Occurrence of Afferent Nerve Fibers in the
   Internal Carotid Plexus" (master's thesis, McGill University, 1932), http://digitool.
   Library.McGill.CA:80/R/-?func=dbin-jump-full&object_id=135010&silo_library=
   GEN01; Choróbski and W. Penfield, "Cerebral Vasodilator Nerves and their Pathway
   from the Medulla Oblongata with Observations on the Pial and Intracerebral Vascular
   Plexus," *Archives of Neurology and Psychiatry* 28 (1932): 1257–89.

6 A. Kussmaul and A. Tenner, "On the Nature and Origin of Epileptiform Convolutions
   Caused by Profuse Bleeding, and Also Those of True Epilepsy," trans. E. Bonner, *The
   New Sydenham Society* 5 (1859): 22; italics in original.

7 S. Van der Kolk, "On the Minute Structure and Functions of the Spinal Cord and
   Medulla Oblongata and the Proximate Cause and Rational Treatment of Epilepsy,"
   trans. W.D. Moore, *The New Sydenham Society* 4 (1859): 211.

8 G. Fritsch and E. Hitzig, "Ueber die Elektrische Erregbarkeit des Grosshirns," *Archiv fur
   Anatomie und Physiologie* 37 (1870): 316; Translated and reprinted in T. Crump and L.
   Shari, "Electric eExcitability of the Cerebrum," *Epilepsy and Behavior* 15 (2009): 317; D.
   Ferrier, "Pathological Illustrations of Brain Function," *West Riding Lunatic Asylum Med-
   ical Reports* 4 (1874): 30–62; M. Eadie, "Cortical Epileptogenesis and David Ferrier,"
   Journal of the History of the Neurosciences 27 (2018): 107–16.

9 J.H. Jackson, "A Study of Convulsions," *St Andrews Medical Graduates' Association
   Transactions* 3 (1870): 162–204; J.H. Jackson, "On the Anatomical, Physiological, and
   Pathological Investigation of Epilepsies," *West Riding Lunatic Asylum Medical Reports* 3
   (1873): 317n, 318, 321–2.

10 J.H. Jackson, "A Study of Convulsions," 202.

11 R. Leblanc, "Wilder Penfield and the Vascular Hypothesis of Focal Epilepsy," *Journal of
   Neurosurgery* (in press).

12 P. Sargent, "Some Observations on Epilepsy," *Brain* 24 (1921): 312–28, emphasis added.

13 Ibid., 313.

14 Ibid., 314.

15 Ibid., 323–5.

16 Ibid., 326.

17 Ibid., 328.

18 W. Spielmeyer, "The Anatomic Substratum of the Convulsive State," *Archives of Neurology and Psychiatry* 23 (1930): 869–75.

19 Ibid., 873.

20 Penfield, "The Evidence for a Cerebral Vascular Mechanism in Epilepsy," 303–10.

21 W. Penfield, "Intracerebral Vascular Nerves," *Archives of Neurology and Psychiatry* 27
   (1932): 44.

22 Penfield, "The Evidence for a Cerebral Vascular Mechanism in Epilepsy," 308.

23 W. Penfield, "The Circulation of the Epileptic Brain," *Proceedings of the Association for
   Research in Nervous and Mental Disease* 28 (1937): 605–37.

24 Penfield, "The Evidence for a Cerebral Vascular Mechanism in Epilepsy," 309.
25 Ibid.
26 Ibid., 305.
27 Ibid., 304–5.
28 Ibid., 310.
29 W. Penfield, "Epilepsy and Surgical Therapy," *Archives of Neurology and Psychiatry* 36 (1936): 449–84.
30 Penfield revealed the patient's name in his autobiography, *No Man Alone: A Neurosurgeon's Life* (Boston, Toronto: Little, Brown and Company, 1977).
31 Ibid., 180–1.
32 R. Leblanc, "Madeleine Louise Ottmann," in *The Wounded Brain Healed: The Golden Age of the Montreal Neurological Institute, 1934–1984*, W. Feindel and R. Leblanc (Montreal & Kingston: McGill-Queen's University Press, 2016), 45–8.
33 Penfield, "Epilepsy and Surgical Therapy."
34 Penfield, *No Man Alone*, 238–43.
35 W. Penfield, "Intracerebral Vascular Nerves," *Transactions of the American Neurological Association* 57 (1931): 426–40.
36 Choróbski and Penfield, "Cerebral Vasodilator Nerves," 1282.
37 E.L. Gage, "The Effect of Vasomotor Nerve Section on Experimental Epilepsy" (master's thesis, McGill University, 1931), http://digitool.Library.McGill.CA:80/R/-?func=dbin-jump-full&object_id=136480&silo_library=GEN01.
38 W. Penfield, "Intracerebral Vascular Nerves" (1931), 440; Penfield, "Intracerebral Vascular Nerves" (1932), 30–44.
39 J. Choróbski, "Part 1, A Vasodilator Nervous Pathway to the Cerebral Vessels from the Central Nervous System. Part 2. On the Occurrence of Afferent Nerve Fibers in the Internal Carotid Plexus" (master's thesis, McGill University, 1932), http://digitool.library.mcgill.ca/R/?func=dbin-jump-full&object_id=135010.
40 Ibid.
41 S.H. Forbes, "The Cerebral Circulation. 1. Observation and Measurement of Pial Vessels," *Archives of Neurology and Psychiatry* 19 (1928): 751–61.
42 S. Cobb and J.E. Finesinger, "The Vagal Pathway of the Vasodilator Impulses," *Archives of Neurology and Psychiatry* 28 (1932): 1234–56; Choróbski and Penfield, "Cerebral Vasodilator Nerves," 1257–89.
43 Anonymous, "In Memoriam: René Leriche (1879–1955): Honorary Fellow of the College; Membre de l'Institut de France," *Annals of the Royal College of Surgeons of England* 18 (1956): 132–3.
44 R. Leriche, "De la Résection du Carrefour Aortico-Iliaque avec Double Sympathectomie Lombaire pour Thrombose Artéritique de l'Aorte: le Syndrome de l'Oblitération Termino-Aortique par Artérite," *La Presse Medicale* 48 (1940): 601–7.
45 Despite this facade, Leriche collaborated with the Germans during the occupation of France.
46 W. Penfield, "Surgical Aspects of the Sympathetic Nervous System in the Work of René Leriche," *Bulletin of the Johns Hopkins Hospital* 37 (1925): 369–75.
47 W. Penfield, "Epilepsy and Surgical Therapy," *Archives of Neurology and Psychiatry* 36 (1936): 462–3. (Read before the International Neurologic Congress, London, 30 July 1935.)
48 W. Alexander, *The Treatment of Epilepsy* (Edinburgh: Y.J. Pentland, 1889).
49 Penfield, *No Man Alone*, 23.
50 Ibid., 336, note 42.

51 Penfield, "Epilepsy and Surgical Therapy," 461–3.

52 F.A. Echlin, "Cerebral Ischemia and Its Relation to Epilepsy" (master's thesis, McGill University, 1939), http://digitool.Library.McGill.CA:80/R/-?func=dbin-jump-full &object_id=131669&silo_library=GEN01.

53 Ibid.

54 H.W. Florey, "Microscopical Observations on the Circulation of the Blood in the Cerebral Cortex," *Brain* 48 (1925): 43–64; Florey was awarded the Nobel Prize in 1945 for his role in the synthesis of penicillin.

55 A. Ecker and P.A. Riemenschneider, "Arteriographic Demonstration of Spasm of the Intracranial Arteries with Special Reference to Saccular Arterial Aneurysms," *Journal of Neurosurgery* 8 (1951): 660–7.

56 W. Penfield and T.C. Erickson *Epilepsy and Cerebral Localization* (Springfield and Baltimore: Charles C. Thomas, 1941).

57 T.C. Erickson, "The Nature and Spread of the Epileptic Discharge" (PhD dissertation, McGill University, 1939), http://digitool.Library.McGill.CA:80/R/-?func=dbin-jump-full&object_id=130214&silo_library=GEN01.

58 I.P. Pavlov, *Conditioned Reflexes: An Investigation of the Physiological Activity of the Cerebral Cortex*, trans. G. Anrep (London: Oxford University Press, 1926).

59 I.P. Pavlov, Lecture XIX in *Conditioned Reflexes: An Investigation of the Physiological Activity of the Cerebral Cortex*, trans. G. Anrep (London: Oxford University Press, 1926).

60 Ibid., 321–2.

61 F.A. Gibbs, "A Thermoelectric Blood Flow Recorder in the Form of a Needle," *Proceedings of the Society for Experimental Biology and Medicine* 31 (1933): 141–6.

62 Erickson, "The Nature and Spread of the Epileptic Discharge," 45.

63 Ibid., 55.

64 W.H. Bridgers, "A Study of Epileptogenic Lesions of the Brain" (master's thesis, McGill University, 1941), 81, http://digitool.Library.McGill.CA:80/R/-?func=dbin-jump-full &object_id=129629&silo_library=GEN01.

65 "Now it is far from obvious, from a logical point of view, that we are justified in inferring universal statements from singular ones, no matter how numerous; for any conclusion drawn in this way may always turn out to be false: no matter how many instances of white swans we may have observed, this does not justify the conclusion that *all* swans are white." K. Popper, *The Logic of Scientific Discovery* (New York: Harper & Row, 1968), 27.

66 W. Penfield, "The Circulation of the Epileptic Brain," *Proceedings of the Association for Research in Nervous and Mental Disease* 28 (1937): 605–37.

67 F.A. Gibbs, "A Thermoelectric Blood Flow Recorder in the Form of a Needle," *Experimental Biology and Medicine* 31 (1933): 141.

68 F.A. Gibbs, "Cerebral Blood Flow Preceding and Accompanying Experimental Convulsions," *Archives of Neurology and Psychiatry* 30 (1933): 1003–10.

69 F.A. Gibbs, W.G. Lennox, and E.L. Gibbs, "Cerebral Blood Flow Preceding and Accompanying Epileptic Seizures in Man," *Archives of Neurology and Psychiatry* 32 (1934): 257–72.

70 H.H. Jasper, "The Early Development of Neuroscience in Canada," *Canadian Journal of Neurological Sciences* 12 (1985): 221–9.

71 N.C. Norcross, "Studies in Cerebral Circulation" (master's thesis, McGill University, 1936), http://digitool.Library.McGill.CA:80/R/-?func=dbin-jump-full&object_id=134035&silo_library=GEN01; N.C. Norcross, "Intracerebral Blood Flow: Experimental Study," *Archives of Neurology and Psychiatry* 40 (1938): 291–9.

72 Jasper, "The Early Development of Neuroscience in Canada," 221–9.

73 K. von Santha and A. Cipriani, "Focal Alterations in Subcortical Circulation Resulting from Stimulation of the Cerebral Cortex," *Association for Research in Nervous and Mental Disease* 18 (1937): 346–62.

74 W. Penfield, K. von Santha, and A. Cipriani, "Cerebral Blood Flow During Induced Epileptiform Seizures in Animals and Man," *Journal of Neurophysiology* 2 (1939): 257–67.

75 Ibid.

76 Ibid., 265. Emphasis added.

77 K.R. Popper, *The Logic of Scientific Discovery* (London and New York: Harper Torchbooks, 1968).

78 W. Penfield, "Remarks in Incomplete Hypotheses for the Control of Cerebral Circulation," *Journal of Neurosurgery* 35 (1971): 127.

79 Pavlov, *Conditioned Reflexes*, 327.

80 Penfield, "Epilepsy and Surgical Therapy," 449–84.

81 Ibid., 476.

CHAPTER FIVE

1 R. Leblanc, "Herbert Jasper and the Electrical Activity of the Brain," in *The Wounded Brain Healed: The Golden Age of the Montreal Neurological Institute, 1934–1984*, W. Feindel and R. Leblanc (Montreal & Kingston: McGill-Queen's University Press, 2016), 123–8.

2 H.H. Jasper and L. Carmichael, "Electrical Potentials from the Intact Human Brain," *Science* 81 (1935): 51–3.

3 H.H. Jasper, "Memoirs Autobiography of Seventy Years Adventures in Neuroscience Research and with Neuroscientists," William Feindel Fond, McGill University.

4 O. Foerster and H. Altenburger, "Elektrobiologische Vorgänge an der Menschlichen Hirnrinde," *Dtsch Z Nervenheilkd* 135 (1935): 277–88.

5 Case J.T. MNI archives.

6 W. Penfield and T.C. Erickson, *Epilepsy and Cortical Localization* (Baltimore: Charles C. Thomas, 1941): 451–2.

7 MNI neuropathology reports, S-138-39, 26 June 1939. MNH archives.

8 Penfield and Erickson, *Epilepsy and Cortical Localization*.

9 V. Salanova, F. Andermann, T. Rasmussen, A. Olivier A, and L.F. Quesney, "Parietal Lobe Epilepsy: Clinical Manifestations and Outcome in 82 Patients Treated Surgically between 1929 and 1988," *Brain* 118 (1995): 607–27.

10 W. Penfield and L. Gage, "Cerebral Localization of Epileptic Manifestations," *Archives of Neurology and Psychiatry* 30 (1933): 721–2.

11 W. Penfield and E. Boldrey, "Cortical Spread of Epileptic Discharge and the Conditioning Effect of Habitual Seizures," *American Journal of Psychiatry* 96 (1939): 280–1.

12 Penfield's reliance on the conditioned reflex to explain the acquisition of higher order cognitive functions is discussed in chapter 14.

13 V. Salanova, F. Andermann, T. Rasmussen, A. Olivier A, and L.F. Quesney, "Occipital Lobe Epilepsy: Electroclinical Manifestations, Electrocorticography, Cortical Stimulation and Outcome in 42 Patients Treated between 1930 and 1991: Surgery of Occipital Lobe Epilepsy," *Brain* 115 (1992): 1655–80.

14 W. Penfield and L. Gage, "Cerebral Localization of Epileptic Manifestations," *Proceedings of the Association for Research in Nervous and Mental Disease* 13 (1934): 593–613; Penfield and Gage, "Cerebral Localization of Epileptic Manifestations," 709–27.

15 J.H. Jackson, "Epileptiform Seizures – Aura from the Thumb – Attacks of Coloured Vision," *Medical Times and Gazette* 1 (1863): 588.

16 Ibid.

17 J.H. Jackson, "On Temporary Mental Disorders after Epileptic Paroxysms," *West Riding Lunatic Asylum Medical Reports* 5 (1875): 123.

18 Penfield and Gage, "Cerebral Localization of Epileptic Manifestations," 709–27; W. Penfield and J.P. Evans, "Functional Defects Produced by Cerebral Lobectomies," *Association for Research in Nervous and Mental Disease* 1934: 352–77; W. Penfield, J.P. Evans, and J.A. MacMillan, "Visual Pathways in Man with Particular Reference to Macular Representation," *Archives of Neurology and Psychiatry* 33 (1935): 816–34.

19 Case C.F., MNI archives.

20 Penfield, Evans, and MacMillan, "Visual Pathways in Man," 816, 832–4.

CHAPTER SIX

1 W. Penfield, "Osteogenic Dural Endothelioma: The True Nature of Hemicraniosis," *Journal of Neurology and Psychopathology* 4 (1923): 27–34.

2 Ibid., 31.

3 W. Penfield, "A Paper on Classification of Brain Tumours and Its Practical Application," *British Medical Journal* 1 (1931): 340–1.

4 W. Penfield, "The Encapsulated Tumors of the Nervous System: Meningeal Fibroblastomata, Perineural Fibroblastomata, and Neurofibroblastomata of von Recklinghausen," *Surgery, Gynecology and Obstetrics* 45 (1927): 178–88.

5 W. Penfield, "Oligodendroglia and Its Relation to Classical Neuroglia," *Brain* 47 (1924): 430–52.

6 W. Penfield and A.W. Young, "The Nature of von Recklinghausen's Disease and the Tumours Associated with It," *Transactions of the American Neurological Association* 1929: 319–43.

7 Anonymous, "Captain F.A.C. Scrimger, V.C., M.D.," *Canadian Medical Association Journal* 6 (1916): 334–6; W.B. Howell, "Colonel F.A.C. Scrimger, V.C.," *Canadian Medical Association Journal* 38 (1938): 279–81.

8 The Schwannoma is named for Theodor Schwann who discovered the Schwann cell, which invests nerves with a layer of insulating myelin. The oligodendrocyte performs the same task in the brain.

9 Penfield, "The Encapsulated Tumors of the Nervous System," 188; See also Penfield and Young, "The Nature of von Recklinghausen's Disease," 331.

10 Penfield, "The Encapsulated Tumors of the Nervous System," 178–88.

11 Penfield and Young, "The Nature of von Recklinghausen's Disease," 320–44.

12 Ibid.

13 Penfield, "A Paper on Classification of Brain Tumours," 337.

14 Ibid., 340–1; W. Penfield, "The Classification of Gliomas and Neuroglia Cell Types," *Archives of Neurology and Psychiatry* 26 (1931): 745–53.

15 W. Penfield, ed., *Cytology and Cellular Pathology of the Nervous System* (New York: Paul B. Hoeber, 1932).

16 W. Penfield, "Tumours of the Sheaths of the Nervous System," in *Cytology and Cellular Pathology of the Nervous System*, vol. 3, 953–90; W. Penfield, "Neuroglia: Normal and Pathological," in *Cytology and Cellular Pathology of the Nervous System*, vol. 2, 423–79.

17 W. Penfield, "Neuroglia: Normal and Pathological."

18 W. Penfield, "A Paper on Classification of Brain Tumors and Its Practical Application," *British Medical Journal* 1 (1931): 339.

19 W. Penfield, *No Man Alone: A Neurosurgeon's Life* (Boston, Toronto: Little, Brown and Company, 1977), 214–16.

20 Penfield, "A Paper on Classification of Brain Tumours," 339.

21 P. Bailey and P. Bucy, "Oligodendrogliomas of the Brain," *Journal of Pathology* 34 (1929): 735–51.

22 Ibid., 102.

23 Penfield, "A Paper on Classification of Brain Tumours."

24 Ibid., 339.

25 W. Penfield and J. Evans, "Functional Defects Produced by Cerebral Lobectomies," *Association for Research in Nervous and Mental Disease* 13 (1933): 352–77.

26 W. Penfield and J. Evans, "The Frontal Lobe in Man: A Clinical Study of Maximum Removals," *Brain* 58 (1935): 115–33.

27 Ibid., 131.

28 W. Penfield and D. MacEachern, "Intracranial Tumours" in *Oxford Medicine*, ed. H.F. Christian (New York: Oxford University Press), 137–216.

29 C. Vogt and O. Vogt, "Die Vergleichend-Architektonische und die Vergleichend-Reiz-physiologische Federung der Großhirnrinde unter Besonderer Berücksichtigung der Menschlichen," *Naturwissenschaften* 14 (1926): 1190–4.

30 E.B. Boldrey, "The Architectonic Subdivision of the Mammalian Cerebral Cortex Including a Report of Electrical Stimulation of One Hundred and Five Human Cerebral Cortices" (MSc thesis, McGill University, 1936), http://digitool.Library.McGill. CA:80/R/-?func=dbin-jump-full&object_id=133257&silo_library=GEN01.

31 Harriet Blackstock Thompson trained in medical illustration with Max Brodel at Johns Hopkins University. Brodel, a master artisan, had been Harvey Cushing's illustrator. Blackstock came to McGill and the Royal Victoria Hospital's medical illustration department in 1924, which she eventually led. After seven years in that position, she returned to Johns Hopkins to work with Brodel's successor, Racine Crosby; See L.R. Thomson, "Medical Illustration: Our Early Years. Reminiscing in Letters: Harriet Blackstock Thomson to Ranice Crosby," *Journal of Biocommunication* 8 (1981): 13–15; M. Mackay, "Elizabeth Blackstock (1911–2009) Artist, Mentor and Friend," BMCAA *Alumni News* 22 (2009): 8; Anonymous, "Harriet Blackstock Thompson," DFSI *Database of Scientific Illustrators 1450–1950*, http://www.uni-stuttgart.de/hi/gnt/dsi2/index.php?table_name=dsi&function=details&where_field=id&where_value=1258, accessed 6 August 2016.

32 MNH archives, case D.H.

33 Erickson was one of the most distinguished of MNI fellows and made significant contributions to neurobiology, both with Penfield and Clinton Woolsey; See R. Leblanc, "Theodore Charles Erickson," in Feindel and Leblanc, *The Wounded Brain Healed*, 163–5. Tarlov was later professor and chair of neurosurgery of New York Medical College.

34 W. Penfield, T.C. Erickson, and I. Tarlov, "Relations of Intracranial Tumors and Symptomatic Epilepsy," *Archives of Neurology and Psychiatry* 44 (1940): 315.

CHAPTER SEVEN

1 R. Leblanc, "Deceptive Monstrosity," in *The Wounded Brain Healed: The Golden Age of the Montreal Neurological Institute, 1934–1984*, W. Feindel and R. Leblanc (Montreal & Kingston: McGill-Queen's University Press, 2016), 211–12.

2 R. Leblanc, "Nature Unveiling Herself before Science," in *The Wounded Brain Healed:*

The Golden Age of the Montreal Neurological Institute, 1934–1984, W. Feindel and R. Leblanc (Montreal & Kingston: McGill-Queen's University Press, 2016), 441–58.

3 For authoritative reviews see: J.E. Scarff, "Primary Cortical Centers for Movements of the Upper and Lower Limbs in Man," *Archives of Neurology and Psychiatry* 44 (1940): 243–99; E.A. Walker, "The Development of the Concept of Cerebral Localization in the Nineteenth Century," *Bulletin of the History of Medicine* 31(1957): 99–121; C.G. Gross, "The Discovery of Motor Cortex and Its Background," *Journal of the History of the Neurosciences* 16 (2007): 320–31.

4 The laminar structure of the occipital cortex had been descried in the preceding century by Félix Vicq d'Azyr (1748–1794) and Francesco Gennari (1750–1797).

5 R. Leblanc, *Fearful Asymmetry Bouillaud, Dax, Broca, and the Localization of Language. Paris 1825–1879* (Montreal & Kingston: McGill-Queen's University Press, 2017).

6 H.A. Whitaker and S.C. Etlinger, "Theodor Meynert's Contributions to Classical 19th Century Aphasia Studies," *Brain and Language* 45 (1993): 560–71.

7 C. Wernicke, "The Aphasia Symptom Complex: A Psychological Study on an Anatomic Basis" (1874), in *Wernicke's Works on Aphasia: A Sourcebook and Review,* ed. G.H. Eggert (Mouton Publishers, 1977), 91–145.

8 J. Dejerine, "Sur un Cas de Cécité Verbale avec Agraphie, Suivi d'Dutopsie," *Comptes Rendus Hebdomadaires des Séances et Mémoires de la Société de Biologie*, series 9, 3 (1891): 197–201; J. Dejerine, "Contribution à l'Étude Anatomo-Pathologique et Clinique des Différentes Variétés de Cécité Verbale," *Comptes Rendus Hebdomadaires des Séances et Mémoires de la Société de diologie Paris*, series 9, 4 (1892): 61–90.

9 J.M. Charcot and A. Pitres, *Les Centres Moteurs Corticaux chez l'Homme* (Paris: Rueff, 1895).

10 R. Leblanc, *Fearful Asymmetry.*

11 G.T. Fritsch and E. Hitzig, "On the Electrical Excitability of the Cerebrum," in *Some Papers on the Cerebral Cortex*, trans. G. von Bonin (Springfield, IL: Charles C. Thomas, 1960).

12 D. Ferrier, "Experimental Researches in Cerebral Physiology and Pathology," *West Riding Lunatic Asylum Medical Reports* 3 (1873): 30–96.

13 F. Krause, *Surgery of the Brain and Spinal Cord: Based on Personal Experiences*, vols. 1–3 (New York: Rebman Co, 1909–12).

14 H. Cushing, "A Note Upon the Faradic Stimulation of the Postcentral Gyrus in Conscious Patients," *Brain* 32 (1909): 44–53.

15 V. Horsley, "The Function of the So-Called Motor Area of the Brain (Linacre Lecture)," *British Medical Journal* 11 (1909): 125–32.

16 O. Foerster and W. Penfield, "The Structural Basis of Traumatic Epilepsy and Results of Radical Operation," *Brain* 53 (1930): 99–119.

17 W. Feindel, R. Leblanc, and J.-G. Villemure, "History of the Surgical Treatment of Epilepsy," in *A History of Neurosurgery in Its Scientific and Professional Contexts*, eds. S.H. Greenblatt, T.F. Dagi, and M.H. Epstein (Park Ridge, IL: The American Association of Neurological Surgeons, 1997), 465–88; W. Feindel, R. Leblanc, and A.N. de Almeida, "Epilepsy Surgery: Historical highlights 1909–2009," *Epilepsia* (Suppl 3) 50 (2009): 131–51.

18 P. Wolf, "History of Epilepsy Surgery in Europe," in *Epilepsy Surgery*, ed. H. Lüders (New York: Raven Press, 1992), 9–17.

19 R. Leblanc, "Fedor Krause and Epilepsy Surgery," in Feindel, Leblanc and de Almeida, "Epilepsy Surgery," 133–5.

20 F. Krause and H. Schurn, "Die Spezielle Chirurgie der Gehirn Krankheiten," *Die Epileptischen Erkrankungen* 2bd. (Stuttgart: Enke, 1931, 1932).

21 H. Cushing, "A Note upon the Faradic Stimulation of the Postcentral Gyrus in Conscious Patients," *Brain: A Journal of Neurology* 32 (1909): 44–53.

22 R. Leblanc, "Cushing, Penfield, and Cortical Stimulation," *Journal of Neurosurgery* 130, no. 1 (January 2019): 76–83.

23 Foerster and Penfield, "The Structural Basis of Traumatic Epilepsy," 99–119.

24 W. Penfield, "The Radical Treatment of Traumatic Epilepsy and Its Rationale," *Canadian Medical Association Journal* 23 (1930): 189–97.

25 W. Penfield and E.B. Boldrey, "Somatic Motor and Sensory Representation in the Cerebral Cortex of Man as Studied by Electrical Stimulation," *Brain* 60 (1937): 389–443.

26 C. Gere, "'Nature's Experiment': Epilepsy, Brain Localization, and the Emergence of the Cerebral Subject," in *Neurocultures: Glimpses into an Expanding Universe*, eds. F. Ortega and F. Vidal (Frankfurt am Main: Peter Lang, 2011), 235–48.

27 R. Elder, "Speaking Secrets: Epilepsy, Neurosurgery, and Patient Testimony in the Age of the Explorable Brain, 1934–1960," *Bulletin of the History of Medicine* 89 (2015): 761–98.

28 W. Penfield and T. Erickson, *Epilepsy and Cortical Localization* (Baltimore: Charles C. Thomas, 1941), 48.

29 E.B. Boldrey, "Architectonic Subdivision of the Mammalian Cerebral Cortex Including a Report of the Electrical Stimulation on One Hundred and Five Human Cerebral Cortices" (master's thesis, McGill University, 1936), http://digitool.Library.McGill.CA: 80/R/-?func=dbin-jump-full&object_id=133257&silo_library=GEN01.

30 Penfield and Boldrey, "Somatic Motor and Sensory Representation in the Cerebral Cortex of Man as Studied by Electrical Stimulation," 389–443.

31 Hortense Douglas Cantlie drew the original homunculus as it appeared in 1937, as well as its more familiar incarnation published in Penfield and Rasmussen's *Cerebral Cortex of Man*.

32 Penfield and Boldrey, "Somatic Motor and Sensory Representation in the Cerebral Cortex of Man," 439.

33 F.M.R. Walshe to W. Penfield, 6 August 1946, file C/G20; W. Penfield to F.M.R. Walshe, 20 August 1946, file C/G20. Wilder Penfield Fond, Osler Library of the History of Medicine, McGill University.

34 W. Penfield to F.M.R. Walshe, 20 August 1946, file C/G20; Penfield's correspondence with Walshe can also be found in R. Leblanc, "Deceptive Monstrosity."

35 W. Penfield and T. Rasmussen, *The Cerebral Cortex of Man: A Clinical Study of Localization of Function* (New York: MacMillan, 1950), 13.

36 Ibid.

37 T. Rasmussen and W. Penfield, "Movement of the Head and Eye from Stimulation of the Human Frontal Cortex," *Proceedings of the Association for Research in Nervous and Mental Disease* 27 (1948): 346–61; W. Penfield and T. Rasmussen, "Vocalization and Arrest of Speech," *Archives of Neurology and Psychiatry* 61 (1949): 21–7; W. Penfield, "A Secondary Somatic Sensory Area in the Cerebral Cortex of Man," *Transactions of the American Neurological Association* 74 (1949): 184–6.

38 W. Penfield and T. Rasmussen, "Further Studies of the Sensory and Motor Cortex in Man," *Federation Proceedings* 6 (1947): 452–60.

39 Hortense Douglas Cantlie studied drawing at the Montreal Art Association and anatomical illustration with Max Brodel at Johns Hopkins Medical School. She was employed as medical illustrator at the Montreal General Hospital, but, recognizing her talent, Penfield called upon her to illustrate the 1937 and 1950 homunculi. She also cre-

ated a charming bronze representation of the homunculus entitled "Children of the Brain/Brain Babies," which adorns the MNI; Anonymous, "Cantlie, Hortense Pauline Douglas, 1901–1979," McGill University Archives, https://pams.library.mcgill.ca/index.php/cantlie-hortense-pauline-douglas-1901-1979; R. Leblanc, "The McConnell Wing," in *The Wounded Brain Healed: The Golden Age of the Montreal Neurological Institute, 1934–1984*, W. Feindel and R. Leblanc (Montreal & Kingston: McGill-Queen's University Press, 2016), 257–9.

40 Pathological examination of the biopsy specimens taken during surgery confirmed the presence of a diffuse astrocytoma, which put an end to the patient's life thirteen years after diagnosis.

41 W. Penfield and H. Jasper, *Epilepsy and the Functional Anatomy of the Human Brain* (Boston: Little, Brown and Company, 1954), 69.

42 E.D. Adrian, "Double Representation of the Feet in the Sensory Cortex of the Cat," *Journal of Physiology* 98 Suppl. (1940): 16–8.

43 Ibid., 16–17.

44 E.D. Adrian, "Sensory Areas of the Brain," *Lancet* 242 (1943): 33–5.

45 W. Penfield, "Ferrier Lecture: Some Observations on the Cerebral Cortex of Man," *Proceedings of the Royal Society B* 134 (1947): 336–7.

46 Penfield and Rasmussen, "Further Studies of the Sensory and Motor Cortex in Man," 459.

47 Penfield, "A Secondary Somatic Sensory Area in the Cerebral Cortex of Man," 184.

48 Penfield and Jasper, *Epilepsy and the Functional Anatomy of the Human Brain*, 77–88.

CHAPTER EIGHT

1 Cited in W. Penfield and K. Welch, "The Supplementary Motor Area of the Cerebral Cortex," *Archives of Neurology and Psychiatry* 66 (1951): 291.

2 E.P. Sparrow and S. Finger, "Edward Albert Schäfer (Sharpey-Schafer) and His Contributions to Neuroscience: Commemorating of the 150th Anniversary of His Birth," *Journal of the History of the Neurosciences* 10 (2001): 41–57.

3 V. Horsley and E.A. Schäfer, "Experimental Research in Cerebral Physiology I: On the Function of the Marginal Convolution," *Proceedings of the Royal Society of London* 36 (1883): 437–42.

4 V. Horsley and E.A. Schäfer, "A Record of Experiments upon the Functions of the Cerebral Cortex," *Philosophical Transactions of the Royal Society of London. B* 179 (1888): 1–45.

5 Horsley and Schäfer, "Experimental Research in Cerebral Physiology I," 438–9.

6 Cited by Penfield and Welch, "The Supplementary Motor Area," 294.

7 O. Foerster, "Motor Cortex in Man in the Light of Hughlings Jackson's Doctrines," *Brain* 59 (1936): 135–59.

8 Anonymous, "Second International Neurological Congress," *Archives of Neurology and Psychiatry* 33 (1935): 447–9.

9 C. Vogt and O. Vogt, "Die Vergleichend-Architektonische und die Vergleichend-Reizphysiologische Felderung der Großhirnrinde unter Besonderer Berucksichtigungder Menschlichen," *Naturwissenschaften* 14 (1926): 1190–4.

10 Foerster, "Motor Cortex in Man in the Light of Hughlings Jackson's Doctrines," 148–9.

11 Ibid., 156–7.

12 Ibid., 149.

13 R. Brickner, "A Human Cortical Area Producing Repetitive Phenomena when Stimulated," *Journal of Neurophysiology* 3 (1940): 128–30.

14 The anterior cingulate gyrus.

15 Brickner, "A Human Cortical Area Producing Repetitive Phenomena When Stimulated."

16 Ibid., 128.

17 Penfield and Welch, "The Supplementary Motor Area of the Cerebral Cortex of Man," 289.

18 W. Penfield and K. Welch, "The Supplementary Motor Area in the Cerebral Cortex of Man," *Transactions of the American Neurological Association* 74 (1949): 179–84.

19 Ibid., 183.

20 W. Penfield, "A Secondary Somatic Sensory Area in the Cerebral Cortex of Man," *Transactions of the American Neurological Association* 74 (1949): 184–6.

21 Penfield and Welch acknowledge Foerster and Brickner in their address.

22 E.B. Boldrey, "The Architectonic Subdivision of the Mammalian Cerebral Cortex Including a Report of Electrical Stimulation of One Hundred and Five Human Cerebral Cortices" (master's thesis, McGill University, 1936), http://digitool.Library.McGill.CA:80/R/-?func=dbin-jump-full&object_id=133257&silo_library=GEN01.

23 W. Penfield and E.B. Boldrey, "Somatic Motor and Sensory Representation in the Cerebral Cortex of Man as Studied by Electrical Stimulation," *Brain* 60 (1937): 389–443.

24 W. Penfield and T. Rasmussen, "Vocalization and Arrest of Speech," *Archives of Neurology and Psychiatry* 61 (1949): 21–7.

25 Penfield and Welch, "The Supplementary Motor Area" (1949), 180.

26 Ibid., 181.

27 Ibid.

28 W. Penfield, "Observations on Cerebral Localization of Function," *Comptes Rendus, IV Congres Neurologique International* 3 (1949): 425–34; W. Penfield, "The Clinical Classification of the Epilepsies with Notes on Surgical Therapy," *Comptes Rendus, IV Congres Neurologique International* 3 (1949): 435–49.

29 Penfield, "Observations on Cerebral Localization of Function," 427.

30 W. Penfield, "The Supplementary Motor Area in the Cerebral Cortex of Man," *Archiv fur Psychiatrie und Zeitschrift Neurologie*, 185 (1950): 670–4.

31 Penfield, "The Supplementary Motor Area in the Cerebral Cortex of Man," 673. Emphasis in original.

32 Bertrand was later neurosurgeon-in-chief at the MNI.

33 G. Bertrand, "Studies on Cortical Localization in the Monkey 'the Supplementary Motor Area'" (master's thesis, McGill University, 1953), http://digitool.Library.McGill.CA:80/R/-?func=dbin-jump-full&object_id=108668&silo_library=GEN01.

34 Ibid., 69, 76.

35 Ibid., 79.

36 Penfield and Welch, "The Supplementary Motor Area" (1951), 289–317.

37 Ibid., 299.

38 Ibid., 312–13.

39 A Corvette was a Second World War antisubmarine escort vessel.

CHAPTER NINE

1 R. Descartes, "Lettre au Marquis de Newcastle du 23 Novembre 1646," *Œuvres* (Paris: La Pléiade, Éditions Gallimard, 1953): 1254–6.

2 W. Penfield and T. Rasmussen, "Vocalization and Arrest of Speech," *Archives of Neurology and Psychiatry* 61 (1949): 21.

3 Ibid., 21–7.

4 W. Penfield, "The Cerebral Cortex of Man. 1: The Cerebral Cortex and Consciousness," *Archives of Neurology and Psychiatry* 40 (1938): 423.

5 Ibid., 421–6.

6 Penfield and Rasmussen, "Vocalization and Arrest of Speech," 21–7.

7 Ibid., 27.

8 J.-B. Bouillaud, "Discussion sur la Faculté du Langage Articulé," *Bulletin de l'Académie Impériale de Médecine* 30 (1865): 584.

9 G.T. Fritsch and E. Hitzig (1870), "On the Electrical Excitability of the Cerebrum," in *Some Papers on the Cerebral Cortex*, trans. G. von Bonin (Springfield, IL: Charles C. Thomas, 1960).

10 Leblanc, *Fearful Asymmetry: Bouillaud, Dax, Broca, and the Localization of Language, Paris 1825–1879* (Montreal & Kingston: McGill-Queen's University Press, 2017), 65.

11 F. Krause, *Surgery of the Brain and Spinal Cord: Based on Personal Experiences,* vols. 1–3 (New York: Rebman Co, 1909–12).

12 H. Cushing, "A Note upon the Faradic Stimulation of the Postcentral Gyrus in Conscious Patients," *Brain* 32 (1909): 44–53.

13 V. Horsley, "The Function of the So-Called Motor Area of the Brain (Linacre Lecture)," *British Medical Journal* 11 (1909): 125–32.

14 O. Foerster and W. Penfield, "The Structural Basis of Traumatic Epilepsy and Results of Radical Operation," *Brain* 53 (1930): 99–119.

15 R. Leblanc, "Preston Robb," in *The Wounded Brain Healed: The Golden Age of the Montreal Neurological Institute, 1934–1984*, W. Feindel and R. Leblanc (Montreal & Kingston: McGill-Queen's University Press, 2016), 193–5.

16 P. Robb, "A Study of the Effects of Cortical Excision on Speech in Patients with Previous Cerebral Injuries" (master's thesis, McGill University, 1946) http://digitool.Library.McGill.CA:80/R/-?func=dbin-jump-full&object_id=125827&silo_library=GEN01; P. Robb, "Effects of Cortical Excision and Stimulation of the Frontal Lobe on Speech," *Association for Research in Nervous and Mental Disease* 27 (1947): 587–609.

17 L. Roberts, "A Study of Certain Alterations in Speech during Stimulation of Specific Cortical Regions" (master's thesis, McGill University, 1949), 20, http://digitool.Library.McGill.CA:80/R/-?func=dbin-jump-full&object_id=124462&silo_library=GEN01.

18 See chapter 10, case T.E.

19 Robb, "Effects of Cortical Excision and Stimulation of the Frontal," 603.

20 Robb, "A Study of the Effects of Cortical Excision on Speech," 93–6.

21 Ibid., 56–7.

22 Ibid., 94.

23 Ibid., 96.

24 Ibid., 61.

25 Robb, "Effects of Cortical Excision and Stimulation of the Frontal Lobe," 587–609.

26 Ibid., 606.

27 Roberts, "A Study of Certain Alterations in Speech," 23–9.

28 Ibid., 28–9.

29 Ibid.

30 L. Roberts, "Alterations in Speech Produced by Cerebral Stimulation and Excision" (PhD dissertation, McGill University, 1952), http://digitool.Library.McGill.CA:80/R/-?func=dbin-jump-full&object_id=123892&silo_library=GEN01.

31 Ibid., 1.

32 G. Gradenigo, "Sulla Leptomeningite Circonscritta e Sulla Paralisi dell'Abducenta di Origine Otitica," *Giornale dell'Accademia di Medicina di Torino* 10 (1904): 59–84, 361.

33 W. Penfield and L. Roberts, *Speech and Brain Mechanisms* (Princeton, NJ: Princeton University Press, 1959).

34 Ibid., 136.

35 Ibid., 72.

36 J. Dejerine and A. Dejerine-Klumpke, *Anatomie des Centres Nerveux* (Paris: Rueff, 1895), 247–8.

37 Leblanc, *Fearful Asymmetry*, 196.

38 J.-B. Bouillaud, "Discussion sur la Faculté du Langage Articulé," *Bulletin de l'Académie Impériale de Médecine* 30 (1865): 583.

39 P. Eling, "Broca and the Relation between Handedness and Cerebral Speech Dominance," *Brain and Language* 22 (1984): 158–9.

40 Robb, "A Study of the Effects of Cortical Excision on Speech," 62.

41 Roberts, "Alterations in Speech," 185.

42 P. Broca, "Sur le Siège de la Faculté du Langage Articulé," *Bulletins de la Société d'anthropologie de Paris* 6 (1865): 377–94.

43 C. Branch, B. Milner, and T. Rasmussen, "Intracarotid Sodium Amytal for the Lateralization of Cerebral Speech Dominance: Observations in 123 Patients," *Journal of Neurosurgery* 21 (1964): 399–405.

44 T. Rasmussen and B. Milner, "The Role of Early Left-Brain Injury in Determining Lateralization of Cerebral Speech Functions," *Annals of the New York Academy of Sciences* 299 (1977): 355–69.

45 J.B. Parchappe, "Sur la Faculté du Langage Articulé," *Bulletin de l'Académie Impériale de Médecine* 30 (1865): 679–703.

46 Penfield and Roberts, *Speech and Brain Mechanisms*, 191.

47 Ibid., 188.

48 William Feindel, personal communication.

49 André Olivier, personal communication.

50 Penfield and Roberts, *Speech and Brain Mechanisms*, 203.

51 Leblanc, *Fearful Asymmetry*, 196–7.

52 H.L. Roberts, "Functional Plasticity in Cortical Speech Areas and Integration of Speech," *Archives of Neurology and Psychiatry* 79 (1956): 275–83.

53 Leblanc, *Fearful Asymmetry*.

54 F. Leuret and P. Gratiolet, *Anatomie Comparé du Système Nerveux Considéré Dans Ses Rapports avec l'Intelligence,* vol. 2 (Paris: J.B. Baillière et Fils, 1839–57), 241–2, 263; P. Gratiolet, *Mémoire Sur Les Plis Cérébraux de l'Homme et des Primates* (Paris: Arthus Bertrand, 1854).

55 R. Leblanc, *Fearful Asymmetry*, 149–61.

56 E.B. Marsh, A.E. Hillis, "Recovery from Aphasia Following Brain Injury: The Role of Reorganization," *Progress in Brain Research* 157 (2006): 143–56.

PART TWO, SECTION TWO

1 W. Penfield and H. Flanigin, "Surgical Therapy of Temporal Lobe Seizures," *Archives of Neurology and Psychiatry* 64 (1950): 491–500.

CHAPTER TEN

1 MNI archives, case R.M. William Feindel published a short note on this case. See W.

Feindel, "Development of Surgical Therapy of Epilepsy at the Montreal Neurological Institute," *Canadian Journal of Neurological Sciences* 18 (1991): 549.

2 W. Penfield and T.C. Erickson, *Epilepsy and Cerebral Localization* (Springfield and Baltimore: Charles C. Thomas, 1941).

3 W. Penfield and H. Steelman, "The Treatment of Focal Epilepsy by Cortical Excision," *Annals of Surgery* 126 (1947): 743.

4 Ibid.

5 Emphasis added. Penfield and Erickson, *Epilepsy and Cerebral Localization*, 301.

6 R. Leblanc, "Home Front," in *The Wounded Brain Healed: The Golden Age of the Montreal Neurological Institute, 1934–1984*, W. Feindel and R. Leblanc (Montreal & Kingston: McGill-Queen's University Press, 2016), 157–77.

7 A local anesthetic.

8 T. Rasmussen and B. Milner, "The Role of Early Left-Brain Injury in Determining Lateralization of Cerebral Speech Functions," *Annals of the New York Academy of Sciences* 299 (1977): 355–69.

9 Penfield and Steelman, "The Treatment of Focal Epilepsy by Cortical Excision," 740–61.

10 W. Penfield, "The Epilepsies: With a Note on Radical Therapy," *New England Journal of Medicine* 221 (1939): 209–18; S.P. Humphreys, "Study of the Vascular and Cytological Changes in the Cerebral Cicatrix" (master's thesis, McGill University, 1939), http://digitool.Library.McGill.CA:80/R/-?func=dbin-jump-ull&object_id=130199&silo_library=GEN01; R. Leblanc, "Microgyria," in *The Wounded Brain Healed: The Golden Age of the Montreal Neurological Institute, 1934–1984*, W. Feindel and R. Leblanc (Montreal & Kingston: McGill-Queen's University Press, 2016), 130–4.

11 Ibid., 760.

12 Ibid.

13 W. Penfield and H. Steelman, "The Treatment of Focal Epilepsy," 747.

14 Ibid., 760.

15 Ibid., 750.

CHAPTER ELEVEN

1 E.L. Gibbs, F.A. Gibbs, and B. Fuster, "Psychomotor Epilepsy," *Archives of Neurology and Psychiatry* 60 (1948): 332.

2 J.H. Jackson, "On a Particular Variety of Epilepsy ('Intellectual Aura'), One Case with Symptoms of Organic Brain Disease," *Brain* 11 (1888): 179–207.

3 Ibid., 179.

4 The term petit mal was used at the time to indicate a nonconvulsive seizure.

5 Jackson, "On a Particular Variety of Epilepsy," 206–7.

6 Ibid., 179.

7 J.H. Jackson and W.S. Colman, "Case of Epilepsy with Tasting Movements and 'Dreamy State' – Very Small Patch of Softening in the Left Uncinate Gyrus," *Brain* 21 (1898): 580–90.

8 Ibid., 588–9.

9 D.C. Taylor and S.M. Marsh, "Hughlings Jackson De. Z: The Paradigm of Temporal Lobe Epilepsy Revealed," *Journal of Neurology, Neurosurgery, and Psychiatry* 43 (1980): 758–67.

10 E.L. Gibbs, F.A. Gibbs, and B. Fuster, "Psychomotor Epilepsy," 331–9.

11 Ibid.

12 F.K.D. Naham and K.H. Pribram, "Heinrich Klüver," in *Biographical Memoirs,* vol. 73 (Washington, DC: National Academy Press, 1998), 289–306.

13 H. Klüver, "Mescal Visions and Eidetic Vision," *American Journal of Psychology* 37 (1926):

502–15; H. Klüver, *Mescal: The Divine Plant and Its Psychological Effects* (Oxford: Kegan Paul, 1928).

14 H. Klüver and P.C. Bucy, "'Psychic Blindness' and Other Symptoms Following Bilateral Temporal Lobectomy in Rhesus Monkeys," *American Journal of Physiology* 119 (1937): 352–3.

15 H. Klüver and P.C. Bucy, "An Analysis of Certain Effects of Bilateral Temporal Lobectomy in the Rhesus Monkey, with Special Reference to 'Psychic Blindness,'" *Journal of Psychology* 5 (1938): 33–54; H. Klüver and P.C. Bucy, "Preliminary Analysis of Functions of the Temporal Lobes in Monkeys," *Archives of Neurology and Psychiatry* 42 (1939): 979–1000; H. Klüver and P.C. Bucy, "Anatomic Changes Secondary to Temporal Lobectomy," 44 (1940): 1142–6; H. Klüver and P.C. Bucy, "An Anatomical Investigation of the Temporal Lobe in the Monkey (Macaca mulatta)," *Journal of Comparative Neurology* 103 (1955): 151–251.

16 Klüver and Bucy, "An Anatomical Investigation of the Temporal Lobe," 151–251.

17 Ibid.

18 P.F. Bladin, "Murray Alexander Falconer and the Guy's-Maudsley Hospital Seizure Surgery Program," *Journal of Clinical Neuroscience* 11 (2004): 577–83.

19 W. Penfield and H. Flanigin, "Surgical Therapy of Temporal Lobe Seizures," *Archives of Neurology and Psychiatry* 64 (1950): 491–500.

20 H. Jasper and J. Kershman, "Electroencephalic Classification of the Epilepsies," *Archives of Neurology and Psychiatry* 45 (1941): 932.

21 W. Penfield and H. Steelman, "The Treatment of Focal Epilepsy by Cortical Excision," *Annals of Surgery* 126 (1947): 760.

22 H.H. Jasper, B. Pertuiset, and H. Flanigin, "EEG and Cortical Electrogram in Patients with Temporal Lobe Seizures," *Archives of Neurology and Psychiatry* 65 (1951): 272–90.

23 Ibid., 278.

24 Ibid., 497.

25 The part of the skull in which the temporal lobe resides.

26 Jasper, Pertuiset, and Flanigin, "EEG and Cortical Electrogram in Patients with Temporal Lobe Seizures," 278.

CHAPTER TWELVE

1 Comment by William Mixter on W. Penfield and M. Baldwin, "Temporal Lobe Seizures and the Technic of Subtotal Temporal Lobectomy," *Annals of Surgery* 136 (1952): 634.

2 Penfield and Baldwin, "Temporal Lobe Seizures," 625–34.

3 K.M. Earle, M. Baldwin, and W. Penfield, "Incisural Sclerosis and Temporal Lobe Seizures Produced by Hippocampal Herniation at Birth," *Archives of Neurology and Psychiatry* 69 (1953): 27–42.

4 W. Feindel, W. Penfield, and H.H. Jasper, "Localization of Epileptic Discharge in Temporal Lobe Automatism," *Transactions of the American Neurological Association* 77 (1952): 14–17.

5 J.H. Jackson and P. Stewart, "Epileptic Attacks with a Warning of Crude Sensation of Smell and with Intellectual Aura (Dreamy State) in a Patient Who Had Symptoms Pointing to Gross Organic Disease of the Right Temporo-Sphenoidal Lobe," *Brain* 22 (1899): 534–49.

6 Ibid., 538–9.

7 Penfield and Baldwin, "Temporal Lobe Seizures," 625–34.

8 M. Baldwin, "Functional Representation in the Temporal Lobe of Man (A Study

of Response to Electrical Stimulation)" (master's thesis, McGill University, 1952), http://digitool.Library.McGill.CA:80/R/-?func=dbin-jump-full&object_id=107456 &silo_library=GEN01.

9 Penfield and Baldwin, "Temporal Lobe Seizures and the Technic of Subtotal Temporal Lobectomy."

10 Feindel, Penfield, and Jasper, "Localization of Epileptic Discharge," 14–17.

11 W. Feindel and W. Penfield, "Localization of Discharge in Temporal Lobe Automatism," *Archives of Neurology and Psychiatry* 72 (1954): 605–30.

12 J.H. Jackson and W.S. Colman, "Case of Epilepsy with Tasting Movements and 'Dreamy State' – Very Small Patch of Softening in the Left Uncinate Gyrus," *Brain* 21 (1898): 580–90.

13 Feindel and Penfield, "Localization of Discharge in Temporal Lobe Automatism," 605–30.

14 W.E. Le Clark, "The Thalamic Connections of the Temporal Lobe of the Brain in the Monkey," *Journal of Anatomy* 70 (1936): 447–64.

15 A. Brodal, "The Hippocampus and the Sense of Smell: A Review," *Brain* 70 (1947): 179–222; A. Brodal, "The Amygdaloid Nucleus in the Rat," *Journal of Comparative Neurology* 87 (1947): 1–16.

16 W. Feindel, P. Gloor, and W. Penfield, "Diffuse Electrocorticographic Effects Produced by Stimulation of the Amygdaloid Region in Human Subjects and Cats," *Proceedings of the IXX International Physiology Congress* 343 (1953); W. Feindel and P. Gloor, "Comparison of Electrographic Effects of Stimulation of the Amygdala and Brain Stem Reticular Formation in Cats," *Electroencephalography and Clinical Neurophysiology* 6 (1954): 389–402.

17 P. Gloor, "The Pattern of Conduction of Amygdaloid Seizure Discharge: An Experimental Study in the Cat," *Archives of Neurology and Psychiatry* 77 (1957): 246–58.

18 H.H. Jasper and J. Kershman, "Electroencephalographic Classification of the Epilepsies," *Archives of Neurology and Psychiatry* 45 (1941): 932.

19 Ibid., 940.

20 P. Chaslin, "Note Sur l'Anatomie Pathologique de l'Epilepsie Essentielle: La Sclerose Nevroglique," *Comptes Rendus Hebdomadaires des Seances et Memoires de la Societe de Biologie* 1 (1889): 169–71.

21 W. Spielmeyer, "The Anatomic Substratum of the Convulsive State," *Archives of Neurology and Psychiatry* 23 (1930): 869–75.

22 K.M. Earle, M. Baldwin, and W. Penfield, "Temporal Lobe Seizures: The Anatomy and Pathology of the Probable Cause," *Journal of Neuropathology and Experimental Neurology* 12 (1953): 98–9.

23 Earle, Baldwin, and Penfield, "Incisural Sclerosis," 28.

24 Earle, Baldwin, and Penfield, "Temporal Lobe Seizures," 98–9.

25 Earle, Baldwin, and Penfield, "Incisural Sclerosis," 28.

26 Earle, Baldwin, and Penfield, "Temporal Lobe Seizures," 99.

27 Ibid.

28 Earle, Baldwin, and Penfield, "Incisural Sclerosis," 27–42.

29 Ibid., 39–40.

30 Ibid., 29.

31 Comment by William Mixter on Penfield and Baldwin, "Temporal Lobe Seizures," 634.

32 Penfield and Baldwin, "Temporal Lobe Seizures," 625–34.

33 H. Silfvenius, P. Gloor, and T. Rasmussen, "Evaluation of Insular Ablation in Surgical

Treatment of Temporal Lobe Epilepsy," *Epilepsia* 5 (1964): 307–20; W. Penfield, R.A. Lende, and T. Rasmussen, "Manipulation Hemiplegia: An Untoward Complication in the Surgery of Focal Epilepsy," *Journal of Neurosurgery* 18 (1961): 760–76.

34 W. Feindel and T. Rasmussen, "Temporal Lobectomy with Amygdalectomy and Minimal Hippocampal Resection: Review of 100 Cases," *Canadian Journal of Neurological Sciences* 18 (1991): 603–5.

35 T. Rasmussen and W. Feindel, "Temporal Lobectomy: Review of 100 Cases with Major Hippocampectomy," *Canadian Journal of Neurological Sciences* 18 (1991): 601–2.

PART TWO, SECTION THREE

1 W. Penfield, "The Cerebral Cortex of Man. 1: The Cerebral Cortex and Consciousness," *Archives of Neurology and Psychiatry* 40 (1938).

CHAPTER THIRTEEN

1 F.J. Gall, *Organologie ou Exposition des Instincts, des Penchans, des Senti-mens et des Talens, ou des Qualites Morales et des Facultes Intellectuelles Fondamentales de l'Homme et des Animaux et du Siege de Leurs Organes*, vol. 5 (Paris: Boucher, 1823), 12–13.

2 R. Leblanc, *Fearful Asymmetry: Bouillaud, Dax, Broca, and the Localization of Language. Paris 1825–1879* (Montreal & Kingston: McGill-Queen's University Press, 2017).

3 P. Broca, "Atrophie Cerebrale. Remarques sur le Siege, le Diagnostique et la Nature de l'Aphemie. Discussion a Propos de la Communication de M. Parrot," *Bulletins de la Societe Anatomique de Paris* 2, no. 8 (1863): 397–8.

4 Much of P.B.'s chart has been lost. The archival documents that exist are augmented here by the fragments of P.B.'s case published over the years. See W. Penfield and H. Jasper, *Epilepsy and the Functional Anatomy of the Human Brain* (Boston: Little, Brown and Company, 1954), 508–9; B. Milner and W. Penfield, "Effects of Hippocampal Lesions on Recent Memory," *Transactions of the American Neurological Association* 1955: 42–8; W. Penfield and B. Milner, "Memory Deficit Produced by Bilateral Lesions in the Hippocampal Zone," *Archives of Neurology and Psychiatry* 79 (1958): 474–97; Scoville and Milner, "Loss of Recent Memory after Bilateral Hippocampal Lesions," *Journal of Neurology, Neurosurgery and Psychiatry* 20 (1957): 11–21; W. Penfield and G. Mathieson, "Memory Autopsy Findings and Comments on the Role of Hippocampus in Experiential Recall," *Annals of Neurology* 31 (1974): 145–54; Most useful, however, were conversations with Brenda Milner about Penfield's two cases and patient H.M.

5 Penfield and Milner, "Memory Deficit Produced by Bilateral Lesions in the Hippocampal Zone," 483.

6 Penfield and Mathieson, "Memory Autopsy Findings and Comments on the Role of Hippocampus in Experiential Recall," 147.

7 B. Milner, "Intellectual Effects of Temporal-lobe Damage" (PhD dissertation, McGill University, 1952), http://digitool.Library.McGill.CA:80/R/-?func=dbin-jump-full &object_id=123923&silo_library=GEN01.

8 Penfield and Mathieson, "Memory Autopsy Findings and Comments on the Role of Hippocampus in Experiential Recall," 147.

9 Penfield and Milner, "Memory Deficit Produced by Bilateral Lesions in the Hippocampal Zone," 484.

10 Penfield and Mathieson, "Memory Autopsy Findings and Comments on the Role of Hippocampus in Experiential Recall," 147.

11 Ibid., 142.

12 Ibid., 147.

13 P.B. was operated upon Thursday, 9 October 1952, and J.O. had been operated upon Wednesday, 3 October 1951.

14 Penfield and Jasper, *Epilepsy and the Functional Anatomy of the Human Brain*, 509.

15 Milner and Penfield, "The Effect of Hippocampal Lesions on Recent Memory," 41–8.

16 Penfield and Mathieson, "Memory Autopsy Findings and Comments on the Role of Hippocampus in Experiential Recall," 148.

17 Penfield and Milner, "Memory Deficit Produced by Bilateral Lesions in the Hippocampal Zone," 477.

18 Ibid., 478.

19 Ibid., 479.

20 Ibid., 480. Emphasis added.

21 Milner and Penfield, "The Effect of Hippocampal Lesions on Recent Memory." It was Penfield's practice to invite his fellows to give the first presentation of a combined paper. The full-length paper was published in 1958 as Penfield and Milner, "Memory Deficit Produced by Bilateral Lesions in the Hippocampal Zone."

22 Milner and Penfield, "The Effect of Hippocampal Lesions on Recent Memory," 43.

23 Ibid., 42; Penfield and Milner, "Memory Deficit Produced by Bilateral Lesions in the Hippocampal Zone," 491.

24 Milner and Penfield, "The Effect of Hippocampal Lesions on Recent Memory," 42–3.

25 K.M. Earle, M. Baldwin, and W. Penfield, "Temporal Lobe Seizures: The Anatomy and Pathology of the Probable Cause," *Journal of Neuropathology and Experimental Neurology* 12 (1953): 98–9.

26 W. Penfield, "Engrams in the Human Brain: Mechanisms of Memory," *Proceedings of the Royal Society of Medicine* 61 (1968): 837n.

27 Penfield and Mathieson, "Memory Autopsy Findings and Comments on the Role of Hippocampus in Experiential Recall," 145–54.

28 P. Glees and H.B. Griffith, "Bilateral Destruction of the Hippocampus (Cornus Ammonis) in a Case of Dementia," *Monatsschrift für Psychiatrie und Neurologie* 123 (1952): 193–204.

29 G. Gopinath, "Paul Glees – An Obituary," http://www.iisc.ernet.in/currsci/nov25/articles32.htm.

30 Glees and Griffith, "Bilateral Destruction of the Hippocampus (Cornus Ammonis) in a Case of Dementia," 193–204.

31 Brenda Milner, personal communication, March 2014.

32 Scoville and Milner, "Loss of Recent Memory after Bilateral Hippocampal Lesions," 11.

33 H.M. was recently revealed to be Henry Molaison; S. Corkin, *Permanent Present Tense: The Unforgettable Life of the Amnesic Patient, H.M.* (New York: Basic Books, 2014).

34 W.B. Scoville, "The Limbic Lobe in Man," *Journal of Neurosurgery* 11 (1954): 64–6.

35 One patient was Henry Molaison. The other was a schizophrenic patient whose test results, Milner thought, could be assailed by critics in view of his or her underlying condition. (Brenda Milner, personal communication, March 2014.)

36 Milner and Penfield, "The Effect of Hippocampal Lesions on Recent Memory," 43.

37 Scoville and Milner, "Loss of Recent Memory after Bilateral Hippocampal Lesions."

38 Penfield and Milner, "Memory Deficit Produced by Bilateral Lesions in the Hippocampal Zone."

39 Brenda Milner, personal communication, March 2014.

40 B. Milner, S. Corkin, and H.L. Teuber, "Further Analysis of the Hippocampal Amnesic Syndrome: 14-Year Follow-up Study of H.M," *Neuropsychologia* 6 (1968): 215–34. See also Corkin, *Permanent Present Tense*.

41 B. Milner, "Disorders of Memory after Brain Lesions in Man," *Neuropsychologia* 6 (1968): 177.

42 Penfield and Mathieson, "Memory Autopsy Findings and Comments on the Role of Hippocampus in Experiential Recall," 148–9.

43 Ibid., 145–54.

44 Ibid., 150.

45 W. Penfield, "The Interpretive Cortex," *Science* 129 (1959): 1719–25.

46 Ibid., 1722.

47 Penfield, "The Interpretive Cortex."

48 B. Milner, "Memory Mechanisms," *Canadian Medical Association Journal* 116 (1977): 1376.

49 Ibid., 1374–6.

50 Ibid., 1376.

51 Corkin, *Permanent Present Tense.*

52 S. Corkin, D.G. Amaral, R.G. González, K.A. Johnson, and B.T. Hyman, "H.M.'s Medial Temporal Lobe Lesion: Findings from Magnetic Resonance Imaging," *Journal of Neuroscience* 17 (1997): 3964–79.

53 D.H. Salat, A.J. van der Kouwe, D.S. Tuch, B.T. Quinn, B. Fischl, A.M. Dale, and S. Corkin, "Neuroimaging H.M.: A 10-Year Follow-up Examination," Hippocampus 16 (2006): 936–45.

54 J.C. Augustinack, A.J. van der Kouwe, D.H. Salat, T. Benner, A.A. Stevens, J. Annese, B. Fischl, M.P. Frosch, and S. Corkin, "H.M.'s Contributions to Neuroscience: A Review and Autopsy Studies," *Hippocampus* 24 (2014): 1267–86.

55 J. Annese, N.M. Schenker-Ahmed, H. Bartsch, P. Maechler, C. Sheh, N. Thomas, J. Kayan, A. Ghatan, N. Bresler, M.P. Frosch, R. Klaming, and S. Corkin, "Postmortem Examination of Patient H.M.'s Brain Based on Histological Sectioning and Digital 3D Reconstruction," *Nature Communication* 5 (2014): 3122.

56 Corkin, *Permanent Present Tense,* 276.

57 Ibid.; L. Dittrich, *Patient H.M.: A Story of Memory, Madness, and Family Secrets* (Random House: 2016).

58 L.R. Squire, "The Legacy of Patient H.M. for Neuroscience," *Neuron* 61 (2009): 6–9.

59 C. Branch, B. Milner, and T. Rasmussen, "Intracarotid Sodium Amytal for the Lateralization of Cerebral Speech Dominance: Observations in 123 Patients," *Journal of Neurosurgery* 21 (1964): 399–405.

60 B. Milner, "Clues to the Cerebral Organization of Memory, in P.A. Buser and A. Rougeul-Buser," *Cerebral Correlates of Consciousness* INSERM Symposium No. 6 (Amsterdam: Elsevier/North-Holland Biomedical Press, 1978), 149.

61 B. Milner, C. Branch, and T. Rasmussen, "Study of Short Term Memory after Intracarotid Sodium Amytal Procedure," *Transactions of the American Neurological Association* 87 (1962): 224–6.

62 B. Milner, "Brain Mechanisms Suggested by Studies of Temporal Lobes," in *Brain Mechanisms Underlying Speech and Language*, ed. F.L. Darley (New York. Grune and Stratton, 1967), 122–32.

63 B. Milner, "Psychological Defects Produced by Temporal Lobe Excision," *Research Publication of the Association for Research in Nervous and Metal Disease* 36 (1958): 44–57.

64 Ibid., 55.

65 Milner, "Brain Mechanisms Suggested by Studies of Temporal Lobes," 125.

66 Ibid., 128.

67 P.M. Corsi, "The Effects of Contralateral Noise upon the Perception and Immediate Recall of Monaurally-Presented Verbal Material" (master's thesis, McGill University, 1967),

http://digitool.Library.McGill.CA:80/R/-?func=dbin-jump-full&object_id=43892&silo_library=GEN01.

68 MNI Annual Report 1966–1967, 51.

69 MNI Annual Report, 1967–1968, 52.

70 MNI Annual Report, 1968–1969, 55.

71 P.M. Corsi, "Human Memory and the Medial Temporal Region of the Brain" (PhD dissertation, McGill University, 1972), http://digitool.Library.McGill.CA:80/R/-?func=dbin-jump-full&object_id=70754&silo_library=GEN01.

72 Ibid., 29, 36.

73 Ibid., 50.

CHAPTER FOURTEEN

1 L. Tolstoy, *Anna Karenina*, trans. C. Garnett. Part I, chapter 7, 1901.

2 W. Penfield, "The Cerebral Cortex and Consciousness," *The Harvey Lectures* 36 (1937): 35–69.

3 Penfield followed J.V. for twenty-one years. She was not cured by the first resection, and required two other operations to achieve a satisfactory result; W. Penfield, "A Surgeon's Chance Encounters with Mechanisms Related to Consciousness," *The Royal College of Surgeons, Edinburgh* 5 (1960): 173–190.

4 The "dreamy state" is a term coined by John Hughlings Jackson to describe the elaborate mental symptoms of varying complexity that came to be recognized as a hallmark of temporal lobe – or psychomotor– epilepsy. These include what Jackson referred to as "reminiscences," exemplified *by déjà vu* and *déjà entendu* phenomena, distortions of perception of the size and distance of objects – the Alice in Wonderland syndrome, feelings of depersonalization and out of body sensations, and automatisms, the performance of complex everyday tasks of which the patient is unaware and for which he has no memory. See: J.H. Jackson, "Notes on Cases of Diseases of the Nervous System," *Medical Times and Gazette* 2 (1876): 702; J.H. Jackson, "On a Particular Variety of Epilepsy ('Intellectual Aura'), One Case with Symptoms of Organic Brain Disease," *Brain* 11, no. 2 (1988): 179–207; Jackson and Colman, "Case of Epilepsy With Tasting Movements and 'Dreamy State' – Very Small Patch of Softening in the Left Uncinate Gyrus," *Brain* 21, no. 4 (1898): 580–90.

5 R. Leblanc, "Home Front," in *The Wounded Brain Healed: The Golden Age of the Montreal Neurological Institute, 1934–1984*, W. Feindel and R. Leblanc (Montreal & Kingston: McGill-Queen's University Press, 2016), 157–77.

6 W. Penfield, "Psychical Seizures," *British Medical Journal* 2 (1946): 639–41; See also, W. Penfield and H.H. Jasper, "Highest Level Seizures," *Epilepsy: Proceedings of the Association Held Jointly with the International League Against Epilepsy December 13 and 14, 1946, New York* (Baltimore: Williams and Willkins, 1947): 252–71.

7 Penfield used Jackson's definition of psychical "to denote the more complicated mental phenomena made possible by final neuronal integration within the brain." See W. Penfield, "The Permanent Record of the Stream of Consciousness," Proceedings of the 14th International Congress of Psychology, Montreal, 9 June 1954, *Acta Psychologia* 11 (1955): 48n.

8 Penfield, "Psychical Seizures," 640.

9 W. Penfield, "Ferrier Lecture: Some Observations on the Cerebral Cortex of Man," *Proceedings of the Royal Society B* 143 (1947): 344.

10 W. Penfield, "Observations on the Anatomy of Memory," *Folia Psychiatrica, Neurologica et Neurichirurgica Neerlandica* 53 (1950): 349–51.

11 M. Baldwin, "Functional Representation in the Temporal Lobe of Man (A Study of Response to Electrical Stimulation)" (master's thesis, McGill University, 1952), http://digitool.Library.McGill.CA:80/R/-?func=dbin-jump-full&object_id=107456 &silo_library=GEN01.

12 Ibid., 1.

13 Penfield, "The Permanent Record of the Stream of Consciousness," 59. Penfield referred to these complex responses under a variety of names – psychical phenomena, psychical hallucinations, experiential hallucinations – before settling on experiential phenomena.

14 Penfield, "The Permanent Record of the Stream of Consciousness," 47–69.

15 W. Penfield, "'The Mechanism of Memory': The Gordon Wilson Lecture 12 October 1950," *Transactions of the American Clinical and Climatological Association* 62 (1950): 169.

16 Penfield, "The Permanent Record of the Stream of Consciousness," 68.

17 W. Penfield, "Some Mechanisms of Consciousness Discovered during Electrical Stimulation of the Brain," *Proceedings of the National Academy of Sciences* 44 (1958): 51–66.

18 Ibid., 65.

19 J. Locke (1689), *An Essay Concerning Human Understanding*, book II, chapter 2, s2 in *The Works of John Locke in Nine Volumes*, 12th ed., vol. 1 (London: Rivington, 1824), http://oll.libertyfund.org/titles/761#Locke_0128-01_207.

20 W. Penfield, "Speech, Perception and the Uncommitted Cortex," in *Brain and Conscious Experience: Study Week September 28 to October 4, 1964, of the Pontificia Academia Scientiarum*, ed. J.C. Eccles (Berlin and Heidelberg: Springer, 1965), 217–37; W. Penfield, "Conditioning the Uncommitted Cortex for Language Learning," *Brain* 88 (1965): 787–98.

21 W. Penfield, "The Role of the Temporal Cortex in Recall of Past Experience and Interpretation of the Present," in *Ciba Foundation Symposium on the Neurological Basis of Behaviour*, eds. E.W. Wolstenholme and C. O'Connor (London: J. & A. Churchill, 1958): 149–74.

22 W. Penfield, "The Interpretive Cortex," *Science* 129 (1959): 1719–25.

23 Penfield, "The Permanent Record of the Stream of Consciousness," 47–69; W. Penfield, "The Twenty-Ninth Maudsley Lecture: The Role of the Temporal Cortex in Certain Psychical Phenomena," *Journal of Mental Science* 101 (1955): 451–65.

24 W. Penfield, "The Cerebral Cortex and Consciousness," 35–69.

25 W. Penfield, "The Cerebral Cortex of Man. 1: The Cerebral Cortex and Consciousness," *Archives of Neurology and Psychiatry* 40 (1938): 417–42.

26 W. Penfield and E. Boldrey, "Cortical Spread of Epileptic Discharge and the Conditioning Effect of Habitual Seizures," *American Journal of Psychiatry* 96 (1939): 255–81. (Emphasis added.)

27 Ibid.

28 W. Penfield, "Consciousness, Memory and Man's Conditioned Reflexes," in *On the Biology of Learning*, ed. K.H. Pribram (New York, Chicago, San Francisco, Atlanta: Harcourt, Brace & World, 1969), 130.

29 Ibid., 136

30 Ibid., 149

31 Ibid., 165

32 I.P. Pavlov, *Conditioned Reflexes: An Investigation of the Physiological Activity of the Cerebral Cortex*, trans. G. Anrep (London: Oxford University Press, 1926).

33 Penfield, "Consciousness, Memory and Man's Conditioned Reflexes," 130.

34 W. Penfield, "Engrams in the Human Brain: Mechanisms of Memory," *Proceedings of the Royal Society of Medicine* 61 (1968): 831.

35 R. Semon, "Engraphic Action of Stimuli on the Individual," *The Mneme* (London: George Allen & Unwin, 1921), 24.

36 R. Lorente de Nó, "Analysis of the Activity of the Chains of Internuncial Neurons," *Journal of Neurophysiology* 1 (1938): 207–44.

37 Ibid., 232.

38 D.O. Hebb, "D.O. Hebb," in *A History of Psychology in Autobiography*, vol. 7, ed. G. Lindzey (San Francisco: W.H. Freeman 1980), 295; D.O. Hebb, "Devising an Improbable Theory," in *Essay on Mind* (New York and London: Psychology Press, 1980), 85.

39 D.O. Hebb, "D.O. Hebb," 292.

40 D.O. Hebb, *The Organization of Behaviour* (Mahwah and New Jersey: Lawrence Erlbaum Associates, 2002), 62.

41 P. Fatt and B. Katz, "Spontaneous Subthreshold Activity at Motor Nerve Endings," *Journal of Physiology* 117 (1952): 109–128.

42 H. Hyden and E. Egyhazi, "Nuclear RNA Changes in Nerve Cells during Learning Experiments in Rats," *Proceedings of the National Academy of Sciences* 48 (1962): 1366–73.

43 P. Perot and W. Penfield, "Hallucinations of Past Experiences and Experiential Responses to Stimulation of Temporal Cortex," *Transactions of the American Neurological Association* 1960, 84.

44 Penfield, "Engrams in the Human Brain. Mechanisms of Memory," 840.

45 Ibid., 839.

46 Ibid., 838, 840.

47 W. Penfield, "The Mind and the Highest Brain-Mechanism," *The American Scholar* 43 (1974): 241.

48 W. Penfield, "The Electrode, the Brain and Mind," *Zeitschrift fur Neurologie* 201 (1972): 297–309.

49 Penfield, "The Mechanism of Memory," 165–9.

50 W. Penfield, "The Cerebral Cortex of Man. 1: The Cerebral Cortex and Consciousness," *Archives of Neurology and Psychiatry* 40 (1938): 417–42.

51 W. Penfield and L. Gage, "Cerebral Localization of Epileptic Manifestations," *Archives of Neurology and Psychiatry* 30 (1933): 727.

52 J.H. Jackson, "A Contribution to the Comparative Study of Convulsions," *Brain* 9 (1886): 1–23; G.K. York III and D.A. Steinberg, "Hughlings Jackson's Neurological Ideas," *Brain* 134 (2011): 3106–13.

53 Penfield and Gage, "Cerebral Localization of Epileptic Manifestations," 715.

54 W. Penfield and L. Roberts, *Speech and Brain Mechanisms* (Princeton, NJ: Princeton University Press, 1959): 38–9.

55 Penfield and Roberts, *Speech and Brain Mechanisms*, 39.

56 Penfield, "The Cerebral Cortex of Man. 1: The Cerebral Cortex and Consciousness," 417–42.

57 Ibid., 437.

58 Ibid., 436.

59 W. Penfield and J. Evans, "The Frontal Lobe in Man: A Clinical Study of Maximum Removals," *Brain* 58 (1935): 115–33; Penfield, "The Cerebral Cortex of Man. 1: The Cerebral Cortex and Consciousness," 440; Penfield, "Consciousness, Memory and Man's Conditioned Reflexes," 136.

60 Penfield, "The Cerebral Cortex of Man. 1: The Cerebral Cortex and Consciousness," 441–2.

61 Ibid., 440; W. Penfield, "Memory Mechanism," *Archives of Neurology and Psychiatry* 67 (1952a): 178–91 (delivered as the presidential address at the Seventy-Sixth Annual

Meeting of the American Neurological Association, Atlantic City, NJ, 18 June 1951), 185. W. Penfield, "Epileptic Automatism and the Centrencephalic Integrating System," *Association for Research in Nervous and Mental Disorder* 30 (1952): 513.

62 Penfield, "The Cerebral Cortex of Man. 1: The Cerebral Cortex and Consciousness," 441–2.

63 Ibid.

64 Ibid.

65 W. Penfield, "Evidence of Brain Operations," *The Listener*, 23 June 1949 (London: British Broadcasting Corporation). Later published as W. Penfield, "The Cerebral Cortex and the Mind of Man," in *The Physical Basis of Mind: A Series of Broadcast Talks*, ed. P. Laslett (Oxford: Basil Blackwell, 1950), 56–64.

66 Penfield, "The Cerebral Cortex and the Mind of Man," 57–8.

67 Ibid., 58.

68 Ibid., 63–4

69 Penfield, "Epileptic Automatism and the Centrencephalic Integrating System," 514.

70 Ibid., 513–14.

71 Penfield, "Epileptic Automatism and the Centrencephalic Integrating System," 178–98.

72 H.W. Magoun, "An Ascending Reticular Activating System in the Brain Stem," *Archives of Neurology and Psychiatry* 67 (1952): 145–54; H. Jasper and C. Ajmone-Marsan, "Corticofugal Projections to the Brain Stem," *Archives of Neurology and Psychiatry* 67 (1952): 155–71. S. Cobb, "On the Nature and Locus of Mind," *Archives of Neurology and Psychiatry* 67 (1952): 172–7.

73 K. Lashley, comment in Penfield, "Memory Mechanism," 196.

74 Penfield, "Memory Mechanism," 198.

75 S. Cobb, "On the Nature and Locus of Mind," *Archives of Neurology and Psychiatry* 67 (1952): 176.

76 W. Penfield, *The Excitable Cortex in Conscious Man: The Fifth Sherrington Lecture* (Liverpool: Liverpool University Press, 1958); S. Cobb, "The Excitable Cortex of Conscious Man," *Clinical Neurophysiology* 11 (1959): 621–3.

77 Cobb, "The Excitable Cortex of Conscious Man," 623.

78 Ibid., 621–3.

79 Ibid., 623.

80 T.C. Erickson, "The Nature and Spread of the Epileptic Discharge" (PhD dissertation, McGill University, 1939), http://digitool.Library.McGill.CA:80/R/-?func=dbin-jump-full&object_id=130214&silo_library=GEN01.

81 W.P. Van Wagenen and R.Y. Herren, "Surgical Division of Commissural Pathways in the Corpus Callosum: Relation to Spread of an Epileptic Attack," *Archives of Neurology and Psychiatry* 44 (1940): 740–59.

82 Penfield, "The Permanent Record of the Stream of Consciousness," 47–69.

83 Ibid., 67–8.

84 W. Penfield, "Consciousness and Centrencephalic Organization," in *Proceedings of the First International Congress of Neurological Sciences*, eds. L. Van Bogaert and J. Rademecker (London: Pergamon Press, 1957), 7–18

85 Penfield, "Some Mechanisms of Consciousness Discovered," 149–74.

86 Penfield, "Consciousness and Centrencephalic Organization," 8.

87 Ibid., 11, 13.

88 Penfield and Roberts, *Speech and Brain Mechanisms*, 20.

89 Osler Library of the History of Medicine, Penfield fond W/U 109.

90 Milner and Penfield, "Effects of Hippocampal Lesions on Recent Memory," 42–8.

91 Penfield and Mathieson, "Memory: Autopsy Findings and Comments on the Role of Hippocampus in Experiential Recall," 152.

92 Ibid., 152.

93 Ibid., 154.

94 R. Polonsky, *Molotov's Magic Lantern: A Journey in Russian History* (New York: Farrar, Strauss and Giroux, 2010), 18.

95 W. Penfield, *The Mystery of the Mind* (New Jersey, Princeton University Press, 1978), xiii.

96 J.H. Jackson, "Remarks on Evolution and Dissolution of the Nervous System," *Journal of Mental Science* 23 (1887): 25–48.

97 H.H. Jasper, "Memoirs Autobiography of Seventy Years Adventures in Neuroscience Research and with Neuroscientists," MNI Archives, McGill University.

98 Ibid.

99 J. Olszewski, "The Cytoarchitecture of the Human Reticular Formation," in *Brain Mechanism and Consciousness*, ed. J.L. Delafresnaye (Springfield: Charles C. Thomas, 1954), 54–80.

100 H. Jasper, "Diffuse Projection Systems: The Integrative Action of the Thalamic Reticular System," *Electroencephalography and Clinical Neurophysiology* 1 (1949): 405–20; H.H. Jasper and C. Ajmone-Marsan, "Thalamo-Cortical Integrating Mechanisms," *Proceedings of the Association for Research in Nervous and Mental Disease* 30 (1950): 493–512; H. Jasper, C. Ajmone-Marsan, and J. Stoll, "Corticofugal Projections to the Brain Stem," *Archives of Neurology and Psychiatry* 67 (1952): 155–71; H.H. Jasper, "Functional Properties of the Thalamic Reticular System," in *Brain Mechanism and Consciousness*, ed. J.L. Delafresnaye (Oxford: Blackwell, 1954), 374–401.

101 G. Moruzzi and H.W. Magoun, "Brain Stem Reticular Formation and Activation of the EEG," *Electroencephalography Clinical Neurophysiology* 1 (1949): 455–73; H.W. Magoun, "An Ascending Reticular Activating System in the Brain Stem," *Archives of Neurology and Psychiatry* 67 (1952): 145–54.

102 A.R. Luria, *The Working Brain* (New York: Basic Books, 1973), 45.

103 L.M. Ward, "The Thalamic Dynamic Core Theory of Conscious Experience," *Consciousness and Cognition* 20 (2011): 464–86.

104 R. Leblanc, "Academia," in *The Wounded Brain Healed: The Golden Age of the Montreal Neurological Institute, 1934–1984*, W. Feindel and R. Leblanc (Montreal & Kingston: McGill-Queen's University Press, 2016), 139, 241–2, 264, 336–7, 366, 407. Sperry's lecture was published as R.W. Sperry, "Mental Unity Following Surgical Disconnection of the Cerebral Hemispheres," *Harvey Lectures* 62 (1966–1967): 293–323.

105 N.L. Marinsek, M.S. Gazaniga, and M.B. Miller, "Split-Brain, Split-Mind," in *The Neurology of Consciousness*, eds. S. Laureys, O. Gosseries, and G. Tononi (San Diego, CA: Academic Press, 2016), 271–9.

106 R. Llinas, U. Ribary, D. Contreras, and C. Pedroarena, "The Neuronal Basis for Consciousness," *Philosophical Transactions: Biological Sciences* 353 (1998): 1841.

107 Ward, "The Thalamic Dynamic Core Theory of Conscious Experience," 464; See also R. Linás and U. Ribary, "Consciousness and the Brain: The Thalamocortical Dialogue in Health and Disease." *Annals of the New York Academy of Sciences* 929 (2002): 166–75; J.S. Crone, A. Soddu, Y. Holler, A. Vanhaudenhuyse, M. Schurz, et al., "Altered Network Properties of the Fronto-Parietal Network and the Thalamus in Impaired Consciousness" *Neuroimage: Clinical* 4 (2014): 204–48.

108 W. Penfield, "Remarks on Incomplete Hypotheses for the Control of Cerebral Circulation," *Journal of Neurosurgery* 35 (1971): 217.

POSTSCRIPT

1 S.J. Banks, W. Feindel, B. Milner, and M. Jones-Gotman, "Cognitive Function Fifty-Six Years after Surgical Treatment of Temporal Lobe Epilepsy: A Case Study," *Epilepsy and Behavioral Case Reports* 2 (2014): 31–6.

2 G. Leonard, "Temporal Lobe Surgery for Epilepsy: Neuropsychological Variables Related to Surgical Outcome," *Canadian Journal of Neurological Sciences* 18 (1991): 503–97.

3 I.M. Germano, N. Poulin, and A. Olivier, "Reoperation for Recurrent Temporal Lobe Epilepsy," *Journal of Neurosurgery* 81 (1994): 31–6.

APPENDIX

1 T. Rasmussen, "Cortical Resection in the Treatment of Focal Epilepsy," *Advances in Neurology* 8 (1975): 139–54.

2 Patients in this class might have had sensory auras without motor manifestation, interruption of though process, or loss of contact.

3 T. Rasmussen, "Surgical Treatment of Patients with Complex partial Seizures," *Advances in Neurology* 11 (1975): 415–42.

4 Ibid., 415.

5 Ibid., 430–1.

Index